Short Essays, MCQs and OSCEs

MR(

Short Essays, MCQs and OSCEs for MRCOG Part 2

A comprehensive guide

Justin C. Konje MBA, MD, MRCOG
Senior Lecturer and Honorary Consultant Obstetrician and Gynaecologist
Leicester Royal Infirmary
University of Leicester, UK

A member of the Hodder Headline Group
LONDON

First published in Great Britain in 2003 by
Arnold, a member of the Hodder Headline Group,
338 Euston Road, London NW1 3BH

http://www.arnoldpublishers.com

Distributed in the United States of America by
Oxford University Press Inc.,
198 Madison Avenue, New York, NY10016
Oxford is a registered trademark of Oxford University Press

Whilst the advice and information in this book are believed to be true and
accurate at the date of going to press, neither the author nor the publisher
can accept any legal responsibility or liability for any errors or omissions
that may be made. In particular (but without limiting the generality of the
preceding disclaimer) every effort has been made to check drug dosages;
however it is still possible that errors have been missed. Furthermore,
dosage schedules are constantly being revised and new side-effects
recognized. For these reasons the reader is strongly urged to consult the
drug companies' printed instructions before administering any of the drugs
recommended in this book.

British Library Cataloguing in Publication Data
A catalogue record for this book is available from the British Library

Library of Congress Cataloging-in-Publication Data
A catalog record for this book is available from the Library of Congress

ISBN 0 340 80928 0

1 2 3 4 5 6 7 8 9 10

Commissioning Editor: Joanna Koster
Project Editor: Anke Ueberberg
Production Controller: Bryan Eccleshall
Cover Design: Terry Griffiths

Typeset in 10 on 12 pt Minion by Phoenix Photosetting, Chatham, Kent
Printed and bound in Malta by Gutenberg Press

What do you think about this book? Or any other Arnold title?
Please send your comments to feedback.arnold@hodder.co.uk

Contents

Preface   vii

Section One: **How to approach the Part 2 examination**   1
           Chapter 1   The structure of the MRCOG Part 2 examination   3
           Chapter 2   How to answer short essays   5
           Chapter 3   How to fail the examination   9

Section Two: **Short essay questions: obstetrics**   11
           Chapter 1   Prenatal diagnosis and congenital malformations   13
           Chapter 2   Hypertensive disorders in pregnancy   27
           Chapter 3   Medical disorders in pregnancy   39
           Chapter 4   Infections in pregnancy   51
           Chapter 5   Isoimmunization   63
           Chapter 6   Abnormal fetal growth   73
           Chapter 7   Epidemiology, social obstetrics, drugs in pregnancy   81
           Chapter 8   Abnormal presentation   89
           Chapter 9   Premature labour/premature rupture of fetal
                        membranes   95
           Chapter 10   Anaesthetic disorders in pregnancy   105
           Chapter 11   Intrauterine and intrapartum stillbirth   113
           Chapter 12   Labour, including induction – normal/abnormal   123
           Chapter 13   Intrapartum care and complications of labour   135
           Chapter 14   Operative obstetrics   147
           Chapter 15   Postpartum complications   157
           Chapter 16   Neonatology   167

Section Three: **Short essay questions: gynaecology**   177
           Chapter 1   Adolescent gynaecology   179
           Chapter 2   Menstrual disorders   191
           Chapter 3   Gynaecology, endocrinology   203
           Chapter 4   Termination of pregnancy and early pregnancy
                        complications   213
           Chapter 5   Benign uterine lesions and endometriosis   225
           Chapter 6   Benign ovarian lesions   239

CONTENTS

Chapter 7   Vulval and vaginal disorders   247
Chapter 8   Infertility   255
Chapter 9   Family planning   269
Chapter 10   Pelvic infections, pelvic pain, chronic vaginal discharge   279
Chapter 11   Menopause   289
Chapter 12   Genital prolapse and urinary incontinence   299
Chapter 13   Cervical malignancy   313
Chapter 14   Uterine malignancy   329
Chapter 15   Ovarian malignancy   339
Chapter 16   Gestational trophoblastic disease   349
Chapter 17   Operative gynaecology   357
Chapter 18   Ethics, medico-legal   369

Section Four: **Practice papers for revision**   **381**
Chapter 1   Introduction   383
Chapter 2   Multiple-choice questions (MCQs)   385

Section Five: **The structured oral examination (OSCE)**   **407**
Chapter 1   Introduction   409
Chapter 2   Sample OSCE questions   411
Chapter 3   Marking schemes   419
Chapter 4   Recommended reading   449

Index   450

Preface

The MRCOG Part 2 examination has evolved over the past decade. The impetus for the various changes has come from a desire to make the examination reflect its aims. The overall objective of the examination is to assess clinical competencies, most of which are pitched at experienced SHO specialist registrar level. The problems created by 'Calmanization' of training have meant that some candidates sitting the examination would inevitably have had little or no experience at specialist registrar level. The attitudes of such candidates towards the examination are, therefore, not surprisingly immature. It is hoped that, with the changes being introduced from 2002, a greater number of candidates will have had that much-valued experience.

The examination itself now consists of short essays, multiple-choice questions (MCQs) and an oral examination otherwise known as the objective structured clinical examination (OSCE). Although the introduction of this type of examination has eliminated the previous problems of candidates regurgitating chapters from textbooks, especially *Progress in Obstetrics and Gynaecology*, many candidates have experienced and continue to experience difficulties with the examination. This is not because of lack of knowledge but owing to a poor approach to the short essays. Experience from various revision courses, and from the examination itself, suggests that given the correct points required for each question, candidates still find difficulties in presenting the facts in a way that will convince examiners.

This book aims to provide candidates with a different approach to preparing for the examination, especially the short essays. It is based on the experience gained from running one of the most successful revision courses at Leicester and also from examining. The aim is not to provide a prescriptive format for answering questions, but to guide candidates in the right direction and, more importantly, to show them how to avoid the path to failure. The book is divided into five sections: the first focuses on how to approch the examination; the second concentrates on short essay questions in obstetrics; the third section, short essay questions in gynaecology; the fourth section looks at practice papers for revision; and the fifth section considers the oral examination itself.

Individual chapters in Sections One and Two consist of several questions. Each question is followed by common mistakes made by candidates, the important points required for a good answer and, lastly, a sample of a good essay. Some of the sample answers may be much longer than would be expected from candidates within the time allocated for each question. This is deliberate to ensure that as much as possible is covered. Candidates must appreciate that the answers are by no means definitive. Indeed, some points may not be discussed. Their absence does not imply that they are irrelevant.

Section Three contains 300 multiple-choice questions (MCQs) in the format of the examination. They are included to encourage the candidates to practise.

Section Four introduces the objective structured clinical examination (OSCE). The principles of the examination are similar to those of the DRCOG OSCE, but the stations are longer and more details are required. Candidates should practise answering the questions during their preparation for the examination. More sample questions for practice may be found in the author's book listed in Recommended reading.

I know that most candidates preparing for the MRCOG Part 2 examination are terrified, but good clinicians should have no difficulties in passing – provided their approach to the short essays is the correct one. I hope that this book will provide all the ingredients you need for the examination and I wish you the very best of luck.

Justin C. Konje

This book is dedicated to my grandmother Mambotoh Tabe, who died in August 1969

Section One

How to approach the Part 2 examination

1

The structure of the MRCOG Part 2 examination

The examination consists of two parts:

1. The written examination – the multiple-choice question (MCQ) paper and the two short essay papers.
2. The oral examination.

The multiple-choice question (MCQ) paper consists of 300 true or false questions. There is no negative marking. Although there may be several 'twigs' to a statement, each statement should be read independently. There are two short essay papers – one consisting of five obstetric questions and the other of five gynaecology questions. Each question carries 20 marks. Before each examination, candidates are sent instructions. These include the pass mark for the various parts of the examination. As of the time of going to press, the pass mark for the written examination is 183 out of 300. The MCQ paper is marked out of 100 and the short essays out of 200. It is very likely that this mark will vary with each examination. Only candidates who attain the pass mark will proceed to the oral part of the examination.

The oral or objective structured clinical examination (OSCE) consists of 12 stations each lasting 15 minutes. Two of these stations are preparatory stations. Details of this part of the examination are provided under the appropriate section in this book.

2

How to answer short essays

There are many textbooks on MCQs in obstetrics and gynaecology. All candidates sitting the MRCOG Part 2 examination will have had the experience of this type of examination from Part 1. The short essays are different and require a completely new approach. The questions are clinical and require logic and structure. Most questions require a matured and well-reasoned approach; a personal rather than a generic one. Although the questions may appear straightforward, candidates fail to provide the correct answers because of their lack of under-standing of the key issues within them. It is expected that these questions will be approached from a clinical perspective rather from a theoretical basis. The MCQs test theory, whereas the short essays and the oral or objective structured clinical examination (OSCE) assess clinical competencies. Here, some guidance is provided on how to approach the short essays. Always remember that the question is asking what *you* would do rather than what your consultant, another colleague or the textbook would do. If in doubt, imagine that you are faced with a patient in the clinic, on the wards or in theatre and you have to explain to your consultant how and why you would manage that patient in a particular way. Below are some guiding principles for the short essays.

Important questions to ask before starting any question

- What does the examiner want (what is the question asking)?
- What does the question not ask?
- Have you read and understood the question?
- What do I have to write to convince the examiner that I am clinically competent?
- What exactly do I need to write and how do I need to argue my point?
- Do I need an introduction and a conclusion? – this is often unnecessary.

Answering the questions

- Do you have a plan?
- What are the relevant issues and have you written them down?
- What is the logical approach to the question?
- Do you have to make many sentences to get your point across?
- Is it in essay form or bullet points, lines, notes, short phrases, etc.?
- How easy is it to read your handwriting?

Understanding the wording in the question (commonly used instructions)

- *Evaluate*
- *Critically appraise*
- *Consider the options*
- *Justify*
- *Summarize*
- *Compare*
- *What steps will you take?*
- *Debate*
- *Outline*
- *Consider the options*

Read the question and underline the key words or phrases first.

Evaluate

- Place a value on – literally what price will you place on something?
- No need to place a price on what you put down
- Need to have some order or preferencing in your answer

Critically appraise

- Two words – *critical* and *appraise*
- *Critical* – fault-finding, discerning, decisive, skilled in judgement
- *Appraise* – estimate value of
- *Critically appraise* – combine fault-finding and estimation of value

Justify

- Prove right, vindicate – you must give reasons for your answer

Debate

- Argue – advantages and disadvantages (similar to *critically appraise*, except more structured)

Suggested approach to the short essay papers

- First, read through the whole paper very quickly
- Go through each question and underline the key words

- Jot down a rough plan for each question – starting with the difficult ones
- Wipe you hands before you start writing if they are sweaty
- Start with the easy questions – builds confidence
- Do not finish with the difficult question (may not have enough time)
- Time yourself – and be disciplined
- Read though your answers if possible

You do not need to fill the two pages to pass the examination. In fact, most candidates score most of their marks from the first two paragraphs of their answer. It is better to have a concise and well-structured answer than a lengthy, meaningless one. If you present your work neatly, examiners will find it easier to read and assess. If you create extra lines on the answer sheet, write across the paper and fail to paragraph your essay, you run the risk of losing marks. Remember that persistent factual errors and incorrect and dangerous statements are penalized by deduction of marks (you could lose up to four marks out of 20 for this). Candidates are in the habit of quoting figures to impress examiners. It is dangerous to quote incorrect figures. You are advised not to quote figures unless you are very sure of them. You may lose marks for incorrect figures.

You must aim to complete all 10 questions. If you concentrate on seven, eight or nine and hope to make up for the one (s) you do not know, you are very unlikely to pass. It is better to spend your time equally on each question, as this strategy will offer you a better chance of passing. Each question should take 24 minutes. My advice is for candidates to spend the first 10 minutes of the examination writing a plan for the five essays (of each paper) and the last 10–15 minutes reading through each answer to correct spelling mistakes. Some of these mistakes may alter the content of your answer.

3

How to fail the examination

Irrespective of how much advice candidates receive, some will continue to make mistakes. In order to facilitate this task for these candidates, some pointers are provided here on how to fail the examination:

- Failing to write your candidate number on each page of the answer booklet
- Continuing to write when told to stop (remember that when you are caught, it will mean automatic disqualification)
- Failing to write in essay form – listing, use of bullet points
- Ignoring the instructions (for example, not justifying, appraising, evaluating, etc.)
- Use of unfamiliar abbreviations
- Making dangerous and persistent factual errors
- Answering your own questions rather than those on the paper
- Discussing what a consultant, a textbook or a journal author would do rather than what you will do

Section Two
Short essay questions: obstetrics

1

Prenatal diagnosis and congenital malformations

1. Critically appraise the methods of prenatal screening in the first trimester.

2. Mrs BT attended for a detailed ultrasound scan and the baby was found to have an exomphalus. Justify your management of the patient.

3. Critically appraise the management of a 16-year-old girl whose baby has been found to have a congenital cardiac abnormality.

4. Critically appraise the role of ultrasound scan in the diagnosis of trisomy 21.

5. Debate the statement that amniocentesis is soon to supersede chorionic villus sampling in prenatal diagnosis.

6. How will you counsel a couple whose baby was found at 15 weeks' gestation to have a diaphragmatic hernia?

1. Critically appraise the methods of prenatal screening in the first trimester.

Common mistakes

- Listing all the malformations which may be diagnosed in the first trimester
- Restricting yourself to chromosomal abnormalities
- Failing to mention biochemical screening
- Excluding history as a screening method

A good answer will include some or all of these points

- Starts with identifying the high-risk group – problem is most cases have no history
- Ultrasound scan: nuchal translucency (NT) – identify those at risk of chromosome and cardiac and other structural anomalies; problems of NT; advantages of NT; other soft markers – cystic hygromas; structural anomalies – transvaginal scans – central nervous system (CNS), renal, anterior abdominal wall; understand the limitations imposed by the normal anatomical development of organs, especially the anterior abdominal wall
- Biochemistry: human chorionic gonadotrophin (HCG), alpha-fetoprotein (AFP) – still rising therefore unreliable; inhibin; PAPP1; fetal blood in maternal circulation

Sample answer

Prenatal diagnosis is an important part of contemporary perinatal medicine. There are currently different approaches to screening, most of which are in the second trimester. Recently, however, an increasing number of screening methods have becoming available in the first trimester. These include family and obstetric history, radiological and biochemical screening.

A positive history in the family or previous pregnancies may identify the at-risk population for prenatal diagnosis. Other factors from the personal history include exposure to drugs, infections, systemic diseases and teratogens, such as radiation. This screening is often identified during the booking history. Ideally, at-risk groups should be identified before pregnancy and counselled on how to minimize risk factors that are teratogenic. Unfortunately, some of the subtle pointers to these at-risk groups are often missed, either because of an inadequate history or a failure to recognize their significance. Diseases considered significant in this regard include diabetes mellitus, connective tissue diseases and epilepsy. Some systemic diseases may also increase the risk of abnormalities. A combination of this method of identifying the at-risk population with biochemical analytes significantly improves the accuracy of the screening test.

Biochemical screening is becoming a recognized tool in the first trimester. The analytes measured in maternal serum include inhibin, PAPP1, βhCG and αFP. Because these analytes rise at a very fast rate in the first trimester they require very accurate dating of the pregnancy for interpretation. An ideal screening with these analytes must, therefore, be combined with a dating ultrasound scan in the first trimester, otherwise margins of error will be too wide for accurate interpretation.

Nuchal translucency (NT) is the most commonly applied screening test in the first trimester. This is performed between 11 and 13 weeks' gestation. It is a marker for chromosomal abnormalities and cardiac malformations. The accuracy of this screening depends on training. A large study in the south-east of England demonstrated that most radiographers can be trained to provide a reliable service. When combined with biochemistry, approximately 80 per cent of chromosomally abnormal fetuses are identified.

Very recently, nasal bone hypoplasia at 11–13 weeks' gestation has been shown to be a soft marker for chromosomal abnormalities. Preliminary results suggest that this is a feasible screening tool, but it needs refining before widespread application in clinical practice. Fetal cells or DNA in the maternal circulation are currently being investigated as a screening tool in the first trimester. Although there are several published studies of the successful application of this non-invasive screening/diagnostic aid, it remains primarily a research tool.

Although screening in the first trimester is fast becoming an important part of perinatal care, the rationale for its widespread application remains controversial. There are those, for example, who argue that most pregnancies with major chromosomal or structural abnormalities will be aborted spontaneously before the early second trimester. Screening and identifying these pregnancies therefore pressurizes prospective parents into options to terminate pregnancies that would otherwise have ended spontaneously. Such psychological stress, it is argued, may be avoided by restricting screening to the second trimester.

Ultrasound scan in the first trimester is an important screening tool. It allows the dating of the pregnancy, which is crucial for interpretation of biochemical screening tests, identifies multiple pregnancies and chorionicity, and is able not only to diagnosis structural abnormalities but also to to identify soft markers for chromosomal abnormalities. Structural abnormalities that may be identified in the first trimester vary from those of the central nervous system (CNS) and skeletal to the gastrointestinal tract. The use of transvaginal ultrasound scanning and machines with a better resolution, and a greater understanding of the structural embryology of the fetus, have significantly improved the accuracy of the early identification of some of these anomalies. However, because several organs may be too small at these early gestations, difficulties may be encountered clearly defining some important abnormalities.

2. Mrs BT attended for a detailed ultrasound scan and the baby was found to have an exomphalus. Justify your management of the patient.

Common mistakes

- Discussing how to diagnose exomphalus
- Involving surgeons to make the diagnosis
- Assuming the baby has a chromosomal abnormality
- Discussing termination of pregnancy as the only option

A good answer will contain some or all of these points

- Explain the findings to the patient
- Offer further ultrasound screening for anomalies
- Discuss the implications for the diagnosis – exclude the differentials
- Options – amniocentesis, chorionic villus sampling (CVS), continuation if normal or abnormal
- Extent of lesions – presence of other viscera in hernia sac
- Involve paediatric surgeons
- Inovolve geneticits for syndromic diagnosis
- Involve neonatologist
- Follow-up management – looking for prognostic features

Sample answer

The diagnosis of any congenital structural abnormality is devastating to any couple. The approach to such cases must therefore be sensitive, supportive and honest. The management of this patient should involve experts who will provide the correct information in the right way and offer further investigations and counselling if necessary.

The first step is to explain the diagnosis to the patient. In the first instance, the patient may refuse to accept the diagnosis and a skilled counsellor may be necessary. Alarming the patient of the risk of severe abnormality may be counterproductive as some patients will automatically opt for a termination of pregnancy. It is important to approach it sensibly, emphasizing that the diagnosis of such a problem does not necessarily mean that the baby will be severely handicapped. Exomphalus is associated with a chromosomal abnormality in about 40 per cent of cases. In the other 60 per cent, there is no karyotypic abnormality but the baby may be syndromic.

Whether or not the baby has a chromosomal abnormality, there may be associated structural abnormalities (e.g. cardiac). The patient should be offered a further, detailed ultrasound scan at a tertiary level. The presence of such abnormalities, though, may not be diagnostic of a chromosomal abnormality but when combined with the exomphalus may fit into a syndrome the prognosis of which may be easy to assign (if known syndrome).

In view of the high risk of chromosomal abnormalities with exomphalus, invasive testing for fetal karyotype should be offered in the form of amniocentesis or chorionic villus sampling (CVS). The choice for either will depend on the patient. However, it may be advisable for her to opt for an amniocentesis as the risk of mosaicism is not as high as that with CVS. She must understand how long it takes for the results to be available. With modern fluorescent *in situ* hybridzation (FISH) techniques, results may be available within two to three days. This technique is, however, not yet available in all units.

If the chromosomes are normal, the prognostic factors need to be assessed and the patient counselled appropriately. If the hernia is large, and the liver and other viscera are outside the abdominal cavity, the prognosis is poor. In these circumstances, a termination may be offered. A paediatric surgeon and a neonatologist should be involved in the patient's care. The paediatric surgeon will explain the management after delivery, whereas the neonatologist will explain the neonatal care of the fetus. An important part of the management is to follow up the pregnancy with serial ultrasound scans to assess the exomphalus and prognostic factors such as polyhydramnios. Where the defect is small and only small parts of the abdominal viscera are in the hernia sac, the prognosis is good. It may be advisable to introduce the patient and her husband/partner to families that have had affected children and or to associations that provide support for such parents. The timing and method of delivery will depend on the presence of complications. In the absence of complications, there is no reason why the pregnancy should not be allowed to proceed to term. Delivery should be as gentle as possible to avoid rupturing the hernia sac.

3. Critically appraise the management of a 16-year-old girl whose baby has been found to have a congenital cardiac abnormality.

Common mistakes

- Terminate pregnancy
- Offer neonatal surgery
- Perform chromosome investigations
- Involve social workers

A good answer will include some or all of these points

- Explain the diagnosis to the patient
- She is young – any effects on her understanding?
- Involve paediatric cardiologist
- Counselling about the diagnosis
- Further investigations – karyotyping – normal or abnormal? Normal does not exclude other problems
- Management – neonatal period
- Other undiagnosed abnormalities not diagnosed
- Problems of diagnosis

Sample answer

The first step in the management of this patient is to explain the findings and its implications to her. She is very young and it may therefore be difficult for her to come to terms with the diagnosis and explanations offered. It is therefore preferable to assess her ability to assimilate the information before proceeding to in-depth counselling. It may be necessary to involve her parents or partner at a later date if no one is available at the time of the diagnosis.

The counselling will depend on the clinician or ultrasonographer who has made the diagnosis. It is likely that this was made by a radiographer or at the secondary level ultrasound scan. In these circumstances, counselling must be undertaken with extreme caution as, unless a fetal echocardiography has been undertaken, counselling may be misleading as to the outlook and the subsequent management options after delivery. It is important that the diagnosis and the severity of the abnormality is confirmed by a fetal cardiologist. Subsequent counselling must be offered by the cardiologist and the obstetrician. Other structural abnormalities need to be excluded by further ultrasound scanning.

Major structural cardiac abnormalities may be associated with chromosome abnormalities. Such abnormalities include deletion of the short arm of chromosome 22. The type of cardiac abnormality is therefore important. If it is a minor abnormality there will be no need to exclude this abnormality. If it is a major abnormality, karyotyping must be discussed and

19

offered if acceptable. Irrespective of the findings, the counselling should emphasize that cardiac scanning is difficult and, although major abnormalities may be identified, subtle ones may not be excluded confidently. To this end, therefore, subsequent monitoring and repeat detail cardiac scans need to be performed during the pregnancy. These will increase the chances of identifying other abnormalities as the fetal heart gets bigger.

Malformations of the heart may co-exist with other structural abnormalities. The antenatal exclusion of these structural or chromosomal abnormalities does not, unfortunately, completely guarantee their co-existence. Counselling must therefore emphasize that definitive answers will only be provided after delivery. In some cases, these may not even be too obvious until after the neonatal period. The neonatal care of the baby and possible complications need to be discussed. Ample opportunity should be provided for repeated counselling to reinforce the information offered. The timing and place of delivery need to be discussed antenatally. It is advisable for the baby to be delivered in a unit where there is a neonatal cardiologist and *in utero* transfer is better than *ex utero* transfer. The recurrence risk will depend on the type of malformation and its association with chromosomal abnormalities. The definitive counselling will however only be offered after delivery and must involve a neonatologist.

4. Critically appraise the role of ultrasound scan in the diagnosis of trisomy 21.

Common mistakes

- Discussion of prenatal diagnosis of trisomy 21
- Ultrasound features of Down syndrome
- Amniocentesis
- Chorionic villus sampling (CVS)
- Biochemical analytes for screening for trisomy 21
- Therefore no point discussing all the soft markers for Down syndrome; amniocentesis versus CVS; biochemical analytes and Down syndrome; advantages of first trimester versus second trimester scanning; accuracy of soft markers versus biochemical versus invasive procedures

A good answer should include some or all of these points

- Recognize that ultrasound is not a diagnostic tool for Down syndrome
- Its role is mainly as an adjunct in: screening; diagnostic procedures
- Screening: dating of pregnancy – important as 40 per cent of women do not remember their last menstrual period (LMP) and therefore interpretation of nuchal translucency (NT) and biochemical screening will be inaccurate; soft markers – first trimester, second trimester
- Adjunct to diagnostic procedures: amniocentesis and CVS done under ultrasound guidance
- Disadvantages: operator dependent; machine quality important; not reliable in picking up cases of Down's syndrome; markers may generate unnecessary parental anxiety (false negative results)
- Conclusion: key role in prenatal diagnosis of Down's syndrome but only in conjuction with invasive procedures of amniocentesis and CVS

Sample answer

Trisomy 21 is the most common chromosomal abnormality in the UK, with an incidence of one in 600 live births. Diagnosis is based on chromosome analysis and is not radiological, therefore ultrasound is not a diagnostic method for this abnormality. Its role in the diagnosis is, however, mainly as an adjunct to screening and in the performance of the invasive diagnostic procedures.

Although maternal age and family history are important risk factors for screening for Down's syndrome, biochemistry has become a common screening method. This depends on an accurately dated pregnancy. Since about 40 per cent of women are uncertain of their last menstrual period (LMP), to be able to interpret the biochemical screening correctly, the pregnancy must be dated accurately. In the first trimester, ultrasound scan will date the pregnancy to within four days and to within seven to 10 days in the second trimester. In the first trimester, ultrasound is also used to measure the nuchal translucency (NT), which is now a well-recognized marker for both chromosomal and structural or compression thoracic and cardiac abnormalities. Increasingly, sonoembryology is allowing early identification of soft markers for karyotypic abnormalities. In the second trimester ultrasound scan is useful in the identification of soft markers for trisomy 21. It is also an adjunct for diagnostic purposes as the procedures of amniocentesis, chorionic villus sampling (CVS) and fetal blood sampling are all performed under ultrasound guidance.

Although ultrasound is important, there are disadvantages of using this tool in the antenatal diagnosis of trisomy 21. It is operator-dependent and, therefore, soft markers may be missed. On the other hand, the quality of the machine is extremely important. With better machines, soft markers and other structural abnormalities of uncertain significance may become more evident and thus cause more uncertainty and anxiety to prospective parents. Ultrasound is not reliable in the diagnosis of Down syndrome and some of the soft markers may be transient. The absence of these markers does not therefore imply the absence of trisomy 21. In fact, about 50 per cent of cases of trisomy 21 have no associated soft markers.

Ultrasound scan plays a key role in the prenatal diagnosis of trisomy 21, but only as a screening tool or when used to guide the operator in various invasive diagnostic procedures. Unfortunately, it generates significant anxiety in prospective parents when it identifies soft markers, especially as most of these fetuses are chromosomally normal.

5. Debate the statement that amniocentesis is soon to supersede chorionic villus sampling in prenatal diagnosis.

Common errors

- Describing the procedure of chorionic villus sampling (CVS)
- Describing the complications of amniocentesis
- Complications of both procedures
- Early amniocentesis/CVS: limb defects?; aneuploidy?; amniocentesis between nine and 11 weeks and at 11–12 weeks?; polymerase chain reaction (PCR) for prenatal diagnosis

A good answer will include some of the following

- CVS: timing; skilled operator; results; mosaicism; complications
- Amniocentesis: timing; results – role of fluorescent *in situ* hybridization (FISH) (limitations to specific probes), expensive; lower complication rate
- Termination of pregnancy – STOP or medical
- Unlikely to be superseded but will remain as an alternative under specific indications

Sample answer

Amniocentesis and chorionic villus sampling (CVS) are the two most common methods of prenatal karyotyping. Amniocentesis was the first of these procedures introduced into obstetrics. When CVS was introduced it was generally believed that this procedure may supersede amniocentesis. However, both procedures continue to be offered to women throughout the world. Each has advantages and disadvantages. The concept that one will supersede the other is fuelled by these differences.

CVS offers prenatal diagnosis between nine and 11 weeks' gestation. Although it was initially offered as early as eight weeks' gestation, reports of association with terminal limb defects discouraged many perinatologist from offering it before nine weeks' gestation. The advantages of CVS include early and quicker diagnosis – usually within 48 hours (from direct preparations) thereby allowing surgical terminations. In addition, these terminations may be performed without the patient feeling fetal movements or other signs of pregnancy becoming too obvious. The procedure is only available in a few centres where the expertise exists and enough procedures are undertaken to ensure that standards are maintained. The complications of the procedure include miscarriages which may occur in about one to two per cent of all cases. Placental mosaicism occurs in about one per cent of CVS. Although the results may be available within 48 hours, this may fail. For quality assurance cultures are necessary to confirm results. These tend to take about 10 days. The need for a skilled operator and facilities to process these samples mean that this option is not readily available to all patients in some hospitals.

Amniocentesis, on the other hand is, recommended to be performed from 14 completed weeks of gestation upwards. The procedure is easy to perform and most units offer it. The main disadvantage is the time it takes for results to be available. In most units, this takes between 14 and 21 days, and in some, it may even take up to four weeks. By the time the results are known, it is often too late for a surgical termination and most units will therefore offer medical terminations. Some patients find this very distressing. With the advent of fluorescent *in situ* hybridization (FISH) this may no longer be applicable. This technique can produce results from amniocentesis within 48 hours. The main disadvantage is its restriction to specific chromosomes for which there are probes. Although it will identify most of the major chromosomal abnormalities and the sex chromosome disorders, the subtle or uncommon chromosomal abnormalities are unlikely to be diagnosed. The complications of amniocentesis are less frequent that those of CVS with a miscarriage risk of 0.5–1.0 per cent. The risk of mosaicism is also lower. Unlike CVS, this procedure can be performed by trained specialist registrars and in most units in the UK.

The two procedures may be interchangeable in some situations, but in some cases they serve different purposes. The concept of one superseding the other is therefore very unlikely. These two procedures complement each other and are offered for specific indications. It is therefore likely that they will remain available to couples.

6. How will you counsel a couple whose baby was found at 15 weeks' gestation to have a diaphragmatic hernia?

Common mistakes

- Offer termination of pregnancy
- Refer patient to a feto-maternal specialist
- Diagnose chromosomal abnormalities
- Discuss amniocentesis and chorionic villus sampling (CVS)
- Complications of the prenatal diagnostic test

A good answer will include some or all of these points

- Explain the diagnosis
- Outline difficulties to predict prognosis antenatally
- Early diagnosis may indicate poorer prognosis
- Need for scan to exclude other abnormalities
- Isolated – need for karyotype
- Exclude cardiac malformations
- Involvement of geneticist, neonatologist and paediatric surgeon
- Monitor for factors for adverse outcome: level in the chest; polyhydramnios; associated congenital malformations; need for long term follow-up

Sample answer

The diagnosis of a fetal abnormality is distressing to both the prospective parents and the clinician. Management requires skill in communication, sensitivity in discussing the options and empathy in the way the patient is treated. The first step in the management of this couple is to explain the diagnosis to them. It is important to be sure that the diagnosis is certain and, to this effect, a further ultrasound scan by a perinatologist (tertiary level ultrasound scan) must be offered to the couple if one has not already been performed. During this ultrasound scan examination, not only must the diagnosis be confirmed but other structural abnormalities should be excluded.

The diagnosis of diaphragmatic hernia poses several questions – one of which is prognosis. The abnormality may be associated with other structural abnormalities, especially of the cardiovascular system. Fetal echocardiography should therefore be performed. Where the abnormality is isolated, the prospective parents must be informed that the prognosis for the condition is difficult to predict. There are currently no predictive tests to gauge prognosis. However, monitoring during pregnancy may identify polyhydramnios, which is a poor prognostic factor. In addition, because the diagnosis has been made so early, this is likely to be associated with a large defect in the diaphragm and therefore a poor prognosis. Another factor, which may predict prognosis is the inclusion of other abdominal viscera such as the liver and bowel in the thorax.

Although diaphragmatic hernias are not necessarily associated with a significantly higher incidence of chromosomal abnormalities, these need to be excluded as their co-existence is associated with a poor prognosis. On the basis of this, therefore, prenatal karotyping by amniocentesis or chorionic villus sampling (CVS) should be discussed and offered. If the karyotype is normal then subsequent management of the pregnancy must be multidisciplinary – involving a paediatrician, paediatric surgeon and a geneticist. The paediatrician will counsel the couple about neonatal management, whereas the paediatric surgeon will discuss the surgical correction of the defect. The geneticist will introduce the concept of syndromic babies. Although there may be no other structural abnormality on ultrasound scan, or no chromosomal abnormality, there may be subtle abnormalities which, combined with the hernia, would be indicative of a syndrome. This possibility must be discussed and a priori recognition of some of these subtle abnormalities may make their identification after delivery easier.

The place and timing of delivery need to be discussed with the couple and the team managing them. If the pregnancy is allowed to continue, the baby must be delivered in a unit with neonatal intensive care facilities and those for paediatric surgery. The best option is to deliver the baby by Caesarean section. This allows immediate intubation and ventilation rather than awaiting the onset of spontaneous breathing, which allows air into the stomach which may prevent the expansion of the lungs. The outcome for this baby must remain guarded until after delivery and surgery. In about 50 per cent of isolated cases, the outcome is good. In the others this will depend on various factors, some of which may be identified antenatally but most of which may not be obvious until delivery. Whatever the decision, there is a need to follow up the couple and the pregnancy long term to provide appropriate support and information about future pregnancies.

2
Hypertensive disorders in pregnancy

1. Justify your management of a primigravida presenting with hypertension and proteinuria at 35 weeks' gestation.

2. A 32-year-old primigravida with pre-eclampsia at 39 weeks' gestation has just had a fit in labour. Justify your management of this patient.

3. What steps will you take to improve the outcome of pregnancy in a 27-year-old known hypertensive, in her first pregnancy, booking for antenatal care at 10 weeks' gestation?

4. A 26-year-old is admitted at 30 weeks' gestation with pre-eclampsia. Justify your subsequent management.

5. Mrs BOC is 36 years old, in her first pregnancy, at 38 weeks' gestation. She attended the antenatal clinic and was found to have a blood pressure of 160/120 mmHg and two plusses of protein. She has had a headache associated with nausea and vomiting over the past two days. Critically appraise your management.

1. Justify your management of a primigravida presenting with hypertension and proteinuria at 35 weeks' gestation.

Common mistakes

- Discussing the diagnosis of pre-eclampsia
- Listing the complications of pre-eclampsia
- Manage in the community
- Refer to hypertensive team
- Deliver by Caesarian section
- Monitor fetus

A good answer will include some or all of these points

- Diagnosis – pre-eclampsia
- Need to assess severity of disease
  - Physical examination for signs of severity – reflexes
  - Full blood count (FBC) – platelets
  - Urea and electrolytes (U&E) – creatinine and urea
  - Clotting screen – fibrinogen and fibrinogen degradation products (FDPs)
  - Liver function test (LFT) – alanine transferase (AST)/alkaline phosphatase (ALP)
- Monitor fetus – ultrasound scan for growth and Doppler scans/CTGs
- 24-hour ambulatory blood pressure monitoring (ABPM)
- Admit and monitor – four-hourly blood pressure, urinalysis, regular biochemistry and haematology tests
- Blood pressure – high – treat
- Deliver – when and how, Caesarian section, induce, etc.
- Manage as outpatient or inpatient – inpatient management on outpatient basis?
- Complications of the disease on the baby and the mother

Sample answer

Hypertensive disorders of pregnancy are the second most common cause of maternal mortality and an important cause of premature (iatrogenic) birth in the UK. This patient presents with features of pre-eclampsia – a common complication of pregnancy. Management should aim to minimize the complications of this disease on the mother and the fetus.

Specific management of this patient will be determined by the severity of the disease, which depends on associated symptoms and signs, and the results of various investigations. These symptoms include headaches, visual disturbances, right upper abdominal pain and altered sensorium. Their presence, though of significance, does not necessarily equate to severity. Signs of severe disease, such as hyper-reflexia, ankle clonus and right hypochondrial tenderness, need to be excluded.

For most patients, severe disease will be associated with abnormal biochemical and haematological indices. Investigations to ascertain or exclude these derangements will include a full blood count (FBC) for platelet levels (thrombocytopenia), urea and electrolytes (U&E) (high urea and creatinine), high serum uric acid, low fibrinogen and high fibrinogen degradation products (PDPs), and high alanine transaminases and alkaline phosphatases. The degree of derangement in these indices will provide guidance to the severity of the disease. Quantification of urinary protein over a 24-hour period will indicate the severity of proteinuria. Before this, however, semi-quantitative estimation should be undertaken by urinary dipstick. Three or more plusses of proteinuria indicate significant proteinuria.

Although some of these investigations may be performed on an outpatient basis, this patient should be admitted for initial assessment. However, she may be allowed home after the initial assessment, for close monitoring, but this decision can only be made after collating all the information identified above.

Her initial inpatient monitoring should include a strict fluid input/output chart, four-hourly blood pressure measurements and observation for early signs of imminent eclampsia, such as nausea and vomiting, severe headaches, epigastric pain and visual disturbances. Pre-eclampsia is associated with intrauterine growth restriction (IUGR); an ultrasound scan for fetal growth and liquor volume should therefore be performed. This may not be necessary if, clinically, there is no suspicion of IUGR. However, since the accuracy of clinical diagnosis of IUGR is poor it would be advisable. In addition, umbilical artery Doppler velocimetry could be performed as part of the ultrasound scan.

Assuming the disease is mild (blood pressure remains below 150/95 mmHg) and the biochemical and haematological indices are normal, or only slightly deranged, there may be a case for allowing the patient home and monitoring her closely. In this case, the community midwife will provide close monitoring at home. The patient must have ready access to the hospital and must not be on her own. Appropriate counselling about the signs of deterioration and imminent eclampsia should be offered before she is allowed home. In some units, this is not an option as the disease is known to progress very rapidly to eclampsia without any warning. If the patient's blood pressure is high (consistently above 150/100 mmHg) then treatment with an antihypertensive, such as methyldopa, will be instituted. In addition to maternal monitoring, fetal monitoring in the form of regular cardiotocographs, fetal kick charts and Doppler velocimetry of the umbilical and middle cerebral arteries will be performed.

If the disease remains mild, pregnancy should be allowed to progress to term and labour should be induced if there are no contraindications to a vaginal delivery. If the disease is severe, however, the patient should be delivered. How and where she is delivered will depend on several factors. These include the presentation, the state of the cervix and the fetus, and the wishes of the patient. If the cervix is unfavourable and there is deterioration in the maternal condition, delivery by Caesarean section would be the best option. However, in the absence of any obvious deterioration in maternal condition or a contraindication, a vaginal delivery with epidural analgesia in labour should be the option of choice, provided the cervix is favourable.

The management of this patient must be tailored to suit her needs. Inpatient management on an outpatient basis may be suitable but the danger of rapid progression to eclampsia and its attendant complications need be recognized before accepting such an approach.

2. A 32-year-old primigravida with pre-eclampsia at 39 weeks' gestation has just had a fit in labour. Justify your management of this patient.

Common mistakes

- Take a history and do a physical examination
- Observe the fit and then exclude other causes of fits
- Deliver by Caesarian section
- Offer general anaesthesia
- Intravenous hydrazalline/labetalol
- Investigate and manage accordingly

A good answer will include some or all of these points

- Stop the fits – magnesium sulphate ($MgSO_4$) i.m. 4g stat then 2 g then every four hours
- Control airway
- Control blood pressure
- Intravenous line and take bloods for full blood count (FBC), blood group and safe, urea and electrolytes (U&E), liver function test (LFT), uric acid
- Indwelling catheter – fluid input/output
- Monitor fetus
- Maintain – i.v. magnesium sulphate?
- Assess cervix – vaginal deliver?
- Caesarian section if unfavourable
- Epidural?
- Watch oxygen saturation levels and central venous pressure (CVP)
- HDU/ICU care
- Any clotting problems?
- Counselling after

Sample answer

This an obstetric emergency and its management must involve the most experienced clinicians in the unit. These include an obstetrician, an anaesthetist and a midwife. Management should aim for maximum safety to the mother and the fetus. The airway must be secured to ensure that the patient is breathing. This could be achieved by turning the patient onto her left side and inserting a Guedel's mouthpiece, or another mouthpiece, which will prevent the tongue from falling back and blocking the airway or its being bitten during another fit. Any fits should be stopped by the administration of intravenous (i.v.) magnesium sulphate ($MgSO_4$) 4 g slowly over a period of 10–15 minutes. Randomized controlled trials have shown conclusively that this regimen is not only more effective in stopping convulsions but is associated with fewer side-effects (both to the mother and fetus) than intravenous diazepam in the management of eclampsia. With the administration of this drug, an intravenous line should be secured and bloods collected for a full blood count (FBC), urea and electrolytes (U&E), creatinine and uric acid levels, group and safe, liver function test (LFT) and fibrinogen and fibrinogen degradation products (FDPs). An indwelling urethral catheter will facilitate monitoring of urinary output, especially as eclampsia may be complicated by pre-renal renal failure. Overloading the patient with fluids may also result in pulmonary oedema – one of the causes of maternal mortality in this complication. A strict fluid input/output chart may therefore provide early warning signs, especially if there is significant imbalance between input and output.

The blood pressure should be controlled, as failure to do so may result in cerebrovascular accidents. The first option to achieve this will be a fast-acting antihypertenive agent. The choice will be between hydrallazine, nifedipine or labetalol. To use nifedipine, the patient must be able to swallow, although it may be administered sublingually. The best drug for this patient would be hydrallazine, this is fast-acting and can be given intravenously. It may have to be repeated to lower the blood pressure. The disadvantage of hydrallazine administration this way is that the rapid drop in blood pressure it induces may cause significant fetal hypoxia.

Once a patient has had an eclamptic fit, she is likely to fit again unless the cause of the fit is removed. The ultimate treatment, therefore, is delivery of the baby. However, before this is achieved, the mother must be stabilized as contractions may provoke further fits. She should therefore be given a continuous infusion of magnesium sulphate and monitored for toxicity by magnesium levels, knee reflexes, urinary output and respiratory rate. Once she is stable and her blood pressure is controlled, the baby must be delivered. The best means of delivery is vaginal unless there are contraindications. The cervix should first be assessed, and if it is favourable, the fetal membranes should be ruptured and syntocinon commenced to initiate contractions. Where the cervix is unfavourable, a Caesarean section is preferable to a difficult, and possibly failed, induction. It is important to keep stress to a minimum in this patient as this may precipitate further fits.

The most common complications of eclampsia include renal failure, circulatory overload, disseminated intravascular coagulation (DIC) and HELLP syndrome. Very close monitoring of the patient will identify early warning signs of these complications. A central venous line will minimize the risk of circulatory overload. It may also be necessary to transfer the patient to a high dependency or intensive care unit if she deteriorates or there are no facilities for optimum monitoring. Once the clinical symptoms have improved, time must be set aside to offer supportive counselling and a detailed explanation of the complication, the management and implications for any future pregnancies.

3. What steps will you take to improve the outcome of pregnancy in a 27-year-old known hypertensive, in her first pregnancy, booking for antenatal care at 10 weeks' gestation?

Common mistakes

- Refer her to a physician
- Routine screening for antenatal clinic
- Take a history and do a physical examination
- Treat cause of hypertension
- Offer dietary advice
- Refer patient to tertiary centre

A good answer will include some or all of these points

- Assess disease – any associated complications?
- Medication – switching to less teratogenic agents
- Screening for indicators . . .
- Complications of hypertension
- Severity of hypertension
- Pregnancy complications
- Intrauterine growth restriction (IUGR)
- Pre-eclampsia
- Control of blood pressure – medication
- Involvement of physicians
- Monitoring of fetal growth
- Monitor renal function
- Delivery
- Role of uterine artery Doppler scans + aspirin?

Sample answer

Hypertensive disorders constitute some of the most common complications of pregnancy. They include pregnancy-induced hypertension and pre-eclampsia. Various risk factors predispose patients to these complications. These include family history, obesity, pre-existing hypertension, renal diseases or previous pre-eclampsia. This patient is already hypertensive and therefore has an increased risk of developing these complications in her pregnancy. The outcome of her pregnancy could be significantly improved by minimizing the complications of this condition.

The initial step would be to assess the severity of the hypertension. If the patient's blood pressure is very high and she is not on regular medication, she needs to be placed on an antihypertensive agent. This must be after consultation with a physician. Drugs with known teratogenicity (for example, ACE inhibitors) should be avoided. If the patient is already on medication, this must be reviewed and changed to a less teratogenic agent if necessary.

Hypertension may be due to several causes. If the cause is known, appropriate screening must be offered to ensure that there is no deterioration in this situation. The renal and cardio-vascular systems need to be examined and investigated thoroughly for evidence of involve-ment secondary to the hypertension. The fundi should also be examined as they may indicate the severity of the disease.

The complications of hypertension in pregnancy include intrauterine growth restriction (IUGR) and pre-eclampsia. Steps need to be taken to screen for these complications, as their early detection will ensure appropriately timed intervention to minimize their sequelae. Ultrasound scan of the fetus to exclude anomalies will be performed as routine, but if the patient's antihypertensive drugs were teratogenic, then she must be screened for the specific anomalies which may result. In addition, a uterine artery Doppler scan at 20 and 24 weeks' gestation may indicate the risk of the patient developing pre-eclampsia. Later in pregnancy, serial growth scans and liquor volume estimation will identify abnormal fetal growth. Unfortunately, IUGR cannot be prevented, but early identification and necessary intervention will prevent the complications of intrauterine fetal death and severe intrauterine hypoxia.

During pregnancy, tight control of the patient's blood pressure and regular screening for proteinuria will be necessary to reduce the risk of IUGR and pre-eclampsia. It is essential to involve physicians in the care of the patient throughout the pregnancy, even more so if her blood pressure is difficult to control. Renal function should be monitored regularly and whenever necessary, her drug requirements should be reviewed. This is especially important in view of altered physiology during pregnancy. In the first trimester, vomiting may require more frequent administration of antihypertensive drugs, whereas in the second trimester dosages may be reduced in view of the physiological drop in blood pressure.

The timing of delivery will depend on the control of the patient's blood pressure and associated complications. In the absence of any complications, pregnancy should be allowed to go to term. However, when complications occur, appropriate measures need to be taken, including delivery. The method of delivery will be determined by several predominantly obstetric factors.

The role of aspirin in the management of this patient is controversial. If uterine artery Doppler scans are abnormal, she is certainly at a greater risk of pre-eclampsia. However, by the time the uterine Doppler scans are undertaken it may be too late for aspirin to be of any benefit. It may, therefore, be advisable to start the patient on aspirin at 10 weeks' gestation and await the results of the uterine artery Doppler scans. If the scans are normal, the aspirin could be discontinued. Overall, the outcome of this pregnancy will be improved if there is close monitoring of the mother and fetus to ensuring that any complications are identified early and the appropriate treatment is instituted.

4. A 26-year-old is admitted at 30 weeks' gestation with pre-eclampsia. Justify your subsequent management.

Common mistakes

- Assuming that the patient has severe pre-eclampsia
- Delivery by Caesarian section
- Discussing the complications of pre-eclampsia
- Assessing the state of the cervix and delivery at 30 weeks' gestation without justifying why
- Monitor mother and fetus – being non-specific

A good answer will contain some or all of these points

- Common complication of pregnancy associated with significant fetal and maternal mortality and morbidity
- Severity determines subsequent management
- Very severe disease – evidenced by symptoms and signs and abnormal blood investigations – deliver
- Consider steroids to improve fetal lung maturity
- Control blood pressure if necessary – 24-hour ambulatory blood pressure monitoring (ABPM)
- Mild to moderate disease
- Monitor mother – blood pressure, full blood count (FBC), urea and electrolytes (U&E), liver function test (LFT), coagulation profile, urine output
- Monitor fetus – CTG, Doppler scan, fetal growth – ultrasound scan, biophysical profile
- Delivery if deterioration
- If not, induce at 38–39 weeks' gestation
- Analgesia – epidural preferable
- Thromboprophylaxis

Sample answer

Pre-eclampsia is a common complication of pregnancy associated with significant maternal and fetal morbidity and mortality. To a large extent, the management of this patient is determined by the severity of the disease. The ultimate treatment, however, is delivery. The severity of the disease is determined by associated symptoms and or changes in biochemical and haematological indices.

In the management of this patient, the first important step is to determine the severity of the disease. For very severe disease, delivery may be the treatment of choice, whereas for milder disease, a more conservative approach may be adopted until better fetal maturity is attained. The presence of symptoms and signs of severe disease must first be excluded. These include headaches, nausea and vomiting, visual disturbances (visual spots, scotomas), right hypochondrial or epigastric pain and a feeling of restlessness and irritability. Increased tendon reflexes and the presence of ankle clonus are also signs of severe disease.

Biochemical and haematological derangements vary with the severity of the disease. These must be excluded from the blood investigations. It is important to recognize that the absence of these derangements does not necessarily exclude severe disease. By implication, their presence does not also necessarily imply very severe disease. The clinical picture must, therefore, provide the ultimate guide to her treatment.

The derangements include thrombocytopenia, low fibrinogen and high fibrinogen degradation products (FDPs), raised alkaline phosphatase and transaminases, raised uric acid creatinine and urea.

As this patient is only 30 weeks pregnant, early delivery is likely. A course of dexamethasone (12 mg i.m.)12 hours apart should be offered to reduce the risk of respiratory distress syndrome. The mother should be monitored closely by means of four-hourly blood pressure measurements, or more frequently if the disease is severe. Frequent urinalysis would be necessary after the initial quantification of urinary protein. This may be done by a combination of urinary dipstick or 24-hour urine protein estimation. A 24-hour blood pressure profile will also give a better idea of the severity of the disease. If the patient's blood pressure is above 150/100 mmHg, she will be commenced on an antihypertensive agent, such as methyldopa. However, if the blood pressure is persistently above 160/110 mmHg, a very fast-acting antihypertensive agent, such as hydrallazine, labetalol or nifedipine, may be offered. This must be given against the backdrop of a sudden fall in blood pressure, which may cause fetal hypoxia.

Fetal monitoring is essential in the management of this patient. An ultrasound scan will define fetal growth, especially as intrauterine growth restriction (IUGR) is a common complication of pre-eclampsia (especially one of early onset such as this patient). During the growth scan, liquor volume should be quantified and, if facilities are available, umbilical and middle cerebral artery Doppler scans should be performed. These indices will provide more information on fetal well-being and when combined with a biophysical profile will provide a comprehensive means of fetal monitoring. In the presence of any significant disease or fetal compromise, monitoring should be repeated and delivery timed appropriately. If there are no features of fetal compromise and the mother is stable, fetal monitoring could be by means of kick charts, regular CTGs, Doppler scans and fetal biophysical profiles.

The timing of delivery will depend on several factors. If the disease is severe and delivery is desired at this gestation, this would preferably be by Caesarean section as the cervix is less likely to be favourable unless the patient is in labour. If there are no fetal or maternal indications for delivery, the pregnancy should be allowed to continue and labour be induced at 38–39 weeks, or earlier if clinically indicated. During labour, an epidural anaesthetic would be excellent to control pain and blood pressure. Thrombo-prophylaxis should be offered to this patient for a least five days after delivery.

5. Mrs BOC is 36 years old, in her first pregnancy, at 38 weeks' gestation. She attended the antenatal clinic and was found to have a blood pressure of 160/120 mmHg and two plusses of protein. She has had a headache associated with nausea and vomiting over the past two days. Critically appraise your management.

Common mistakes

- Take a history and physical examination
- Treat with magnesium sulphate – no details
- Antihypertensives – which ones
- Refer to tertiary centre – no reason
- Uterine artery Doppler scan to monitor pregnancy
- Ultrasound scan for fetal growth and Dopper scans – why?

A good answer will include some or all of these points

- Diagnosis – pre-eclampsia
- Options – admit to the ward? Or delivery suite? Why?
- Benefits of admission – investigate for severity – bloods etc.
- Examine for sign of severity – why?
- Treat hypertension – which drug to administer and when to treat?
- Nifedipine? Hydrazaline? Labetalol? Methyldopa?
- $MgSo_4$ – why?
- Deliver – how?
- Examine/assess cervix?
- Caesarean section or vaginal delivery?
- Monitor fetus – how and benefits
- Monitor mother – biochemistry, fluid balance etc.

Sample answer

The diagnosis in this patient is pre-eclampsia. This complication is common in pregnancy and is associated with a high perinatal mortality and maternal morbidity and mortality. The ultimate treatment of pre-eclampsia is delivery. In this patient, there is superimposed onto the raised blood pressure and proteinuria, headaches, nausea and vomiting. These are signs of disease severity. She must therefore be admitted to the labour ward. The advantage of this is that the patient would be monitored closely and intervention instituted early if necessary. Admitting her to the ward will delay a thorough assessment and, ultimately, the time for a decision to be made on when and how to deliver the baby. In most units there are no doctors on the wards and admission may therefore delay an immediate assessment.

After admission, various biochemical and haematological investigations must be performed.

These include a full blood count (FBC), urea and electrolytes (U&E), liver function test (LFT), coagulation screen (FDP Fibrinogen) and serum uric acid and creatinine. These investigations will provide an assessment of the severity of the disease and also serve as a baseline for subsequent comparative tests to monitor progression of the disease or response to treatment. In more severe forms of pre-eclampsia, these indices may be significantly deranged.

It is necessary to institute treatment for the hypertension. This will depend on the drug of choice in the unit. Methyldopa is the antihypertensive agent most commonly used in pregnancy. However, it may not be able to control the blood pressure quickly enough. Sublingual nifedipine may therefore be the drug of choice. In its absence, intravenous (i.v.) labetalol or hydrallazine may be used. The slow-release form of nifedipine is preferred as the other type may reduce the blood pressure very quickly and make the patient uncomfortable, and also cause fetal hypoxia. For a patient who is used to a high blood pressure, caution must be exercised in rapidly dropping her blood pressure, as this may cause dizziness and other side-effects of hypotension. Monitoring the blood pressure should, therefore, be more frequent during the initial phase of treatment.

The severity of the disease must be established by examining for signs such as hyper-reflexia, ankle clonus, right hypochondrial tenderness and altered sensorium. The fact that these signs are absent in this patient does not exclude severe disease. Severe changes in the biochemistry and haematological indices will also indicate severity. Again, it is not uncommon for a patient with severe disease to have no significant changes in these indices. The most appropriate management must be tailored to the individual's needs and not the symptoms, signs and investigations.

Magnesium sulphate should be administered to prevent progression to eclampsia if the disease is judged to be severe. The Magpie trial demonstrates that such treatment significantly reduced the risk of developing eclampsia in patients with severe pre-eclampsia.

Fetal well-being has to be monitored as there may be hypoxia, which will necessitate early delivery. This will depend on the severity of the disease. With fetal hypoxia, delivery must be effected as soon as possible. This is also the case with severe pre-eclampsia, when delivery has to be effected as soon as possible. Ultrasound scan for fetal growth is not necessary in this patient, at this gestation, with such severe disease. In the interest of the mother, delivery is paramount even if there is no fetal hypoxia. However, where the disease is not severe, fetal monitoring would be undertaken to time delivery. Such monitoring can be by ultrasound scan for fetal growth, liquor volume assessment and Doppler velocimetry of the umbilical and middle cerebral arteries. Cardiotocography is useful but the frequency is difficult to define.

At 38 weeks, the patient should be assessed and the baby delivered. However, a second option is to manage her conservatively until she goes into spontaneous labour, thus bypassing an unfavourable cervix, associated with a difficult induction, a prolonged induction–delivery interval and therefore increased risk of complications. In this patient, if the cervix is unripe and induction is judged to be difficult and prolonged, Caesarean section would be the delivery method of choice. On the other hand, if induction was judged to be easy, a vaginal delivery would be the best option. Whatever the method of delivery, an epidural anaesthetic would be ideal for pain control. This lowers the blood pressure and minimiszes the risk of fitting. Caesarean section increases the length of hospital stay and patient immobility – all risk factors for thrombo-embolism. Adequate thromboprophylaxis, in the form of low molecular weight heparin (LMWH), should be given.

3

Medical disorders in pregnancy

1. Justify your management of a 28-year-old known epileptic on sodium valproate at 10 weeks' gestation.

2. A 33-year-old woman presented at 38 weeks' gestation with chronic cough, night sweats and right-sided chest pain. She is unemployed and has two other children with her at home. You suspect that she may have tuberculosis. Justify your management.

3. Critically appraise the screening for diabetes mellitus in pregnancy.

4. What steps will you take to improve the pregnancy outcome in an obese diabetic woman booking for antenatal care at six weeks' gestation?

5. A 26-year-old woman with cardiac disease Grade III is admitted in labour at 40 weeks' gestation. What steps will you take to minimize the complications of her cardiac disease?

1. Justify your management of a 28-year-old known epileptic on sodium valproate at 10 weeks' gestation.

Common mistakes

- Take a history and do a physical examination
- Elaborating on the past obstetric and medical histories
- Listing the complications of epilepsy in pregnancy
- Management to be transferred to physician
- Offer Caesarean section irrespective of any other indication or reason

A good answer will include some or all of these points

- Recognize that this is a common medical complication of pregnancy
- Pregnancy – effects on the disease
- Effects of the disease on pregnancy
- Management – ideally with physicians, general practitioner (GP) and midwife (team approach)
- Control of the disease
- Screen for fetal malformations
- Monitor control of epilepsy
- Intrapartum management
- Postnatal care

Sample answer

Epilepsy is a common medical disorder affecting about 0.5 per cent of all pregnant women. In most cases, the disease is known to exist before pregnancy although in some cases, it may be diagnosed for the first time in pregnancy. The disease has significant effects on pregnancy, and pregnancy has important implications for the disease, especially in the context of its control. Because of this, the management of this patient must aim to ensure tight control of her epilepsy and its associated complications in pregnancy.

At 10 weeks' gestation, if the patient is not already taking folic acid supplementation, this should be prescribed although it may be late for this to reduce the risk of fetal neural tube defects. The sodium valproate that this patient is taking is recognized to increase the risk of neural tube defects approximately 1–3 per cent. If her epilepsy is well-controlled on sodium valproate, there will be no need to change the medication. It is, however, important to monitor the levels of the drug in her circulation to ensure that adequate therapeutic levels are maintained. It may be necessary to increase the dose as pregnancy advances. This is because of the increased blood volume and binding proteins, which may reduce the concentration of the free valproate. If the medication is ineffective in controlling the epilepsy, it should be changed to a more effective drug after consultation with a physician.

The management of this patient should be within a team consisting of an obstetrician, her general practitioner (GP), a physician and a midwife. Members of the team must have an in-depth understanding of epilepsy and the possible complications that may occur in pregnancy. The role of the midwife is to ensure that any complications in the community are easily identified and dealt with. Dietary advice and general health measures should be offered, with special regard to what to do when fits occur. The patient's husband/partner must be educated and, if possible, emergency contact telephone numbers given to the couple.

Epilepsy is associated with an increased incidence of congenitial malformations. These include spina bifida, cleft palate and lips, dental hypoplasia and cardiac abnormalities. This patient should therefore be offered a detailed ultrasound scan at 18–19 weeks' and a cardiac scan at 22–24 weeks' gestation. Some of these fetal abnormalities may even be identified with early ultrasound scanning. An early ultrasound scan at 12–14 weeks' gestation may, for example, be able to identify most major neural tube defects. Once these have been excluded, fetal welfare should be monitored by serial ultrasound scans especially as intrauterine growth restriction (IUGR) is a recognized complication of epilepsy in pregnancy.

Once maternal epileptic control is satisfactory, the rest of the pregnancy should be managed as routine and the patient allowed to go into spontaneous labour unless there is an indication to induce labour. When, and how, to deliver the baby should not be determined by the disease itself unless her epilepsy becomes difficult to control. However, during labour, hyper-ventilation may precipitate fits and therefore the labour must be monitored closely. This is extremely important as the occurrence of fits during labour may be confused with eclampsia and unnecessary treatment may be instituted. Postpartum care must be supportive to minimize stress at home and in the hospital. Such stress may provoke further attacks of epilepsy. The incidence of epilepsy in children of mothers with epilepsy is higher than that of children of non-epileptic mothers. The parents therefore need to be counselled about this and advised to look out for early signs of the disease in their offspring.

2. A 33-year-old woman presented at 38 weeks' gestation with chronic cough, night sweats and right-sided chest pain. She is unemployed and has two other children with her at home. You suspect that she may have tuberculosis. Justify your management.

Common mistakes

- Not asked to discuss the differential diagnoses of tuberculosis, such as sarcoidosis
- Diagnoses of the differentials
- History of chronic cough, pulmonary embolism, cystic fibrosis, chronic bronchitis
- Not asked to justify suspicion of diagnosis if tuberculosis
- Irrelevant investigations, such as blood cultures, infection screen, stool culture, etc.
- No need to dwell on history
- JUSTIFY

A good answer will include some or all of these points

- Need to confirm the diagnosis
- How can this be done: chest X-ray (CXR) shielding abdomen – opacities in the upper right lobe; sputum for acid-fast bacilli; Mantoux test – tuberculin skin test
- Diagnosis confirmed: notifiable disease; involve chest physicians in her care; drugs (rifampicin and INH) or isoniazid and ethambutol with or without pyridoxine 50 mg daily; if not too ill, may be managed on outpatient basis in view of children. Otherwise, admit into an isolation unit. If any obstetric reason admit into an obstetric unit but barrier nurse
- Labour should be normal: inform paediatricians; baby to be given BCG (INH-resistant) if breastfeeding; isolate if mother is still AFB sputum positive or delivery less than two weeks after initiation of treatment; social services/contract tracing – children and family – notify general practitioner (GP); support to change social environment which promotes the perpetuation of the disease

Sample answer

Although the symptoms in this patient may be very typical of tuberculosis, it is important to confirm the diagnosis before proceeding with specific management. This can be achieved by a thorough clinical examination supported by ancillary investigations. General and chest examination may reveal signs of tuberculosis. Again, these may not be very specific as other differentials may present with similar features. Ancillary investigations that should be offered to confirm the diagnosis include a chest X-ray (CXR) (with the abdomen/fetus shielded) and a Mantoux test. This is safe in pregnancy and is the best means of detecting tuberculosis. The CXR may reveal opacities on the upper right lobe (the most common site of pulmonary tuberculosis) or other areas of opacities in the lungs. A Mantoux test will indicate the presence of tuberculosis antigens in the patient. This test may produce a false positive result with some other tropical diseases, such as leprosy, and in malnourished or immunosuppressed patients. Where the patient is producing sputum, this should be sent for acid-fast bacilli testing.

Once the disease has been confirmed, the public health department has to be notified as this is a notifiable disease. Subsequent treatment should be by a team consisting of a pulmonary physician, a general practitioner (GP), a health worker, a midwife, a paediatrician and an obstetrician. Her first-line treatment will be combination of rifampicin and isoniazid. The initial treatment may require hospital admission if the symptoms are severe. If this is necessary, she should not be admitted to an open ward. She should either be barrier nursed or admitted to an isolation unit until she is rendered sputum-negative. This will usually follow two weeks' treatment. The patient may resist admission because of her children, in which case she may be managed at home.

As part of her management, she must be educated on how the disease spreads, the need for better hygiene at home to minimize the risk of transmitting the infection to other members of the family (if they are not already affected) and advice on nutrition. If her living conditions are damp and dirty, appropriate support must be offered and advice given.

Provided she has been rendered sputum-negative, the rest of the pregnancy should be monitored as routine and labour allowed to follow the normal course. If, however, there is a suspicion of severe pulmonary compromise as a result of the infection, then second stage may be supported with an elective forceps delivery to avoid unnecessary pushing. If she has not been rendered sputum-negative (and goes into labour within two weeks of therapy) she should be barrier nursed. The danger at this stage will be to members of staff. However, after delivery, there is also the danger of transmitting the infection to the neonate. If the patient is to breastfeed, the baby must be given INH-resistant BCG and isolated for a week before the mother is allowed to breastfeed. During this time, expressed breast milk may be used to feed the baby. If she is not going to breastfeed, isolation is still required. The seven-day isolation period is to allow the vaccine to become effective. It is important that when the patient is admitted in labour the paediatrician is notified. Plans for the care of the baby should have been documented in the notes in case the medical staff on-call (when the patient is in labour) are different to those involved in her antenatal care.

An important part of the management of this patient must be to screen all contacts for the disease. Her children and contacts should be screened and be offered appropriate treatment. The role of the GP and health visitor in this regard is extremely important.

3.   Critically appraise the screening for diabetes mellitus in pregnancy.

Common mistakes

- Complications of diabetes mellitus in pregnancy
- How to perform a glucost tolerance test
- Management of diabetes in pregnancy
- Need for physician involvement
- Ultrasound scan for fetal abnormalities
- Management of neonatal complications

A good answer will include some or all of these points

- History – obstetric and family – reliability
- Maternal weight – obesity?
- Definition
- Race/age – reliability
- Obstetric risk factors/indications
- Fetal risk factors
- Other risk factors
- Methods
- Random blood-glucose/fasting blood-glucose
- Glucose tolerance test
- HbA1c

Sample answer

Diabetes is one of the most common medical disorders of pregnancy, associated with a high perinatal morbidity and mortality. One of the difficulties with this complication is that not all patients present with pre-existing disease. Indeed, some are recognized for the first time in pregnancy and some develop the disorder in pregnancy as a consequence of the diabetogenic effects of pregnancy. Screening for diabetes in pregnancy therefore assumes enormous significance if all cases are to be identified and managed appropriately to improve outcome. Unfortunately, screening still fails to identify all cases.

Screening for diabetes in pregnancy starts with a detail obstetric and family history. A previous macrosomic baby, unexplained stillbirth, congenital malformation (especially those common in diabetic pregnancies), polyhydramnios and a family history in a first-degree relative is associated with an increased risk of diabetes mellitus. Unfortunately, some of these risk factors are poorly defined. For example, the definition of fetal macrosomia depends on the population and the racial group. The use of a cut-off point of 4000 g, for example, may include too many women, whereas increasing it to 4500 g may exclude some cases. It is also not

45

uncommon to fail to identify close relatives affected with diabetes mellitus. Although a close relative is regarded as a first-degree relative, the exact role of second-degree relatives in increasing the risk of diabetes mellitus is unclear.

Maternal weight is another risk factor. Obesity is poorly defined. For example, in some units, this is regarded as weight over 90 kg at booking, whereas in others, a body mass index (BMI) of over 30 is the cut-off point. Such wide variation in standards suggest too many divergencies for the use of maternal weight as a screening tool. Race and age are also regarded as demographic risk factors. In some units, all those of Asian origin and women over the age of 35 years are considered at risk. It may be seen as discriminatory to label women from one particular ethnic group, or older women, as at-risk. Such risk factors are not universally acceptable and it is, therefore, not uncommon to have units which offer screening to all women defined by the above criteria, and others that do not. The rate of diabetess detection will therefore depend on the screening tools used.

During pregnancy, various risk factors may be identified and indicate the need for screening. These include glycosuria, polyhydramnios, macrosomia and recurrent infections, especially in the vulva and vagina. Glycosuria occurs in about four per cent of pregnancies because of reduced renal threshold. As a risk factor for diabetes, therefore, it is unreliable. A large number of women will therefore be offered further screening on account of this alone. Various attempts have been made to refine this indication, such as glycosuria on more than one occasion or in the early morning specimen of urine. Polyhydramnios is a late occurrence, as is fetal macrosomia. Congenital malformations, although occurring early, are often not identified until the second trimester. Although these may be identified in some patients with diabetes, identification is often late and the consequences would already have occurred. However, their presence must be regarded as an indication for second-stage screening.

Identification of at-risk groups is only the first step in the screening for diabetes mellitus. Following this, the definitive or second-stage screening must be offered. The most common form of screening is an oral glucose tolerance test. In the UK and most of Europe, this is with a 75 g glucose load. In the USA 100 g is used. This is undertaken after an overnight fast. The disadvantage of this form of screening is nausea and vomiting, which may be induced by the glucose. In addition, there is some disagreement on the diagnostic criteria. Currently, the fasting and 120 minutes glucose values are used for diagnosis. Whether venous or capillary blood is used for the test is another area of controversy.

Some attempts have been made to stratify this screening. Identifying patients, based on the above risk factors, has been shown to miss some cases of diabetes. To overcome this, it has been suggested that each patient be offered a random blood-glucose test and the value related to the time of the last meal. Where the value is <5.4 mmol/l, and the last meal was more than two hours previously, or the levels are <6.4 mmol/l within two hours of the last meal, then a full UT7 is undertaken. This however has remained controversial. Some have advocated a 50 g glucose load followed by a one hour blood-glucose test. This method will identify those who will further require a glucose tolerance test. Unfortunately, this regime is time-consuming and expensive, and is unlikely to be adopted by all units. Although HbA1c is used to monitor glycaemic control, it may be useful as a screening tool.

4. What steps will you take to improve the pregnancy outcome in an obese diabetic woman booking for antenatal care at six weeks' gestation?

Common mistakes

- Discussing screening for diabetes mellitus
- Discussing the diagnosis of diabetes and the classification in pregnancy
- Discussing the management of diabetes in general
- Being very vague and not discussing what you will do
- Advising the patient to lose weight

A good answer will include some or all of these points

- High-risk pregnancy – obese and diabetic
- Increased risk of pregnancy complications, fetal and neonatal complications
- Diabetic control: insulin (change oral hypogylycaemic agent to insulin); maintain BMs between 5.5 and 6.5; HbA1c <6.1 per cent; regular blood-glucose monitoring – four-hourly profiles; calorie restriction; folate supplementation
- Maternal complications: urinary tract infections – midstream urine samples (MSUs); hypertension/pre-eclampsia – checking blood pressure may be difficult, so use large cuffs; diabetic complications – hypoglycaemia, etc.
- Fetus – increased risk of congenital malformations and macrosomia: start on folic acid; anomaly scan
- Fetal growth – macrosomia more likely, although intrauterine growth restriction (IUGR) may occur; serial growth scans; abdominal palpation difficult; polyhydramnios needs to be excluded
- Labour: induced or spontaneous; cepahlo–pelvic disproportion; shoulder dystocia – precautions; neonatal complications – hypoglycaemia, respiratory distress syndrome (RDS), tetany, etc.

Sample answer

This patient, by virtue of her obesity and diabetes, is at an increased risk of complications antenatally, intrapartum and postpartum. These complications are both fetal and maternal. In order to improve the outcome of her pregnancy, there must be meticulous control of her diabetes, early recognition of complications and treatment and skilled care during the pregnancy.

The patient's diabetic control must be very tight. This is best achieved within a team of dedicated clinicians and midwives. There has to be a physician with an interest in diabetes mellitus, an obstetrician and her general practitioner (GP). Blood-glucose should be maintained between 5.5 and 6.5 mmmol/l. If the patient is not already on insulin, this must be instituted. Insulin offers the advantage of better diabetic control and, since it does not cross the placenta, is unlikely to have any teratogenic effects on the fetus. The patient's HbA1c should be less than 6.1 per cent. This tight control is monitored by frequent blood-glucose estimations – usually every four hours using BM stix. The patient must keep a personal chart of her insulin regimen and her BM values. At this early gestation, dietary advice must be offered. The patient should be placed on folic acid until the end of the first trimester.

Maternal complications that may occur include recurrent urinary tract infections (UTIs), hypertension, pre-eclampsia, hypoglycaemia and recurrent vulvo-vaginal infections. Early identification and treatment of these complications will minimize their consequences. Pre-eclampsia and hypertension may be difficult to treat. Using a standard cuff to measure her BP will produce erroneously high readings; a large cuff should therefore be used. Hypoglycaemia may be fatal to the fetus so educating the mother and her partner about this complication and ensuring that glucagon is readily available for its treatment is absolutely necessary.

The fetus is at an increased risk of congenital malformations, such as neural tube defects, cardiac, musculoskeletal and caudal regression syndrome. Early anomaly scans and traditional anomaly scans will identify some of these. It is important that a cardiologist undertakes an echocardiography to exclude major and minor cardiac malformations. Fetal macrosomia is a common complication of diabetes mellitus, especially when poorly controlled. During her antenatal care, therefore, she should have serial ultrasound scans for fetal growth. This is even more important in this obese patient in whom abdominal palpitations will be difficult.

Where diabetes is well-controlled, labour may be allowed to start spontaneously. However, in most units, it may be induced at 38 weeks' gestation. Because of fetal macrosomia, complications such as obstructed labour, failure to progress and shoulder dystocia should be identified early and managed accordingly. Once the baby is delivered, complications such as hypoglycaemia, hypothermia, respiratory distress syndrome (RDS), tetany, polycythaemia and jaundice may occur. These should be identified early and treatment instituted. If there is a possibility that the fetus may be delivered early, steroids (in the form of dexamethasone 12 mg 12 hours apart) must be given. The involvement of the paediatrician is crucial and must be from the time of admission of the patient to the labour ward.

In this patient, if all the adequate precautions are undertaken, the outcome of her pregnancy is likely to improve significantly.

5. A 26-year-old woman with cardiac disease Grade III is admitted in labour at 40 weeks' gestation. What steps will you take to minimize the complications of her cardiac disease?

Common mistakes

- Details of the American classification of cardiac disease
- Refer to physicians for management
- Central venous pressure (CVP) and Sangsten tubes
- Management to be controlled by anaesthetist
- Antibiotics for second stage
- Manage patient on the intensive care/high dependency unit only
- Causes of cardiac disease in pregnancy
- Investigate for the causes of cardiac disease in pregnancy

A good answer will include some or all of these points

- Definition of cardiac disease Grade III
- Implications of the disease for mortality and morbidity
- Complications of the disease in labour – risk of the disease: cardiac failure; fluid overload; risk of deep vein thrombosis (DVT)
- Teamwork – obstetrician, anaesthetist and experienced midwives
- First stage – normal, minimize oxytocin use
- Second stage – assisted delivery (forceps)
- Third stage – avoid intravenous (i.v.) ergometrine, monitor closely with pulse oximetry
- Postpartum management – watch out for risk of pulmonary oedema and fluid overload; may require HDU/ICU care
- Prophylaxis against venous thrombo-embolism

Sample answer

Cardiac disease Grade III is defined as heart disease with symptoms at rest. It is associated with a significant morbidity and mortality during pregnancy and labour. The management of this patient must be provided by a team consisting of an experienced obstetrician, an experience midwife and an anaesthetist. Complications that may occur include cardiac failure, death and venous thrombo-embolism. These complications are more likely to occur in the second and third stages and during the early puerperium. Fluid overload is the most common predisposing factor for these complications.

The diagnosis of labour must be confirmed in this patient. This is important, as the duration of labour must not be prolonged. Once the diagnosis is made, progress must be monitored closely. The rate of cervical dilatation and descent of the fetal head must be within the expected standards. The use of oxytocic agents needs to be considered carefully in consultation with senior obstetricians and anaesthestists. This is because of fluid retention associated with these agents. Fluid overload may subsequently lead to heart failure.

If the progress of labour is poor, oxytocic agents must be considered. They should be given through infusion pumps with very tight control of the dose administered. It may be advisable for a central venous pressure catheter to be inserted to monitor fluid input and therefore identify early fluid overload. In the second stage, delivery should be expedited by the use of forceps. This reduces the effect of the Valsava manoevre on venous return and, therefore, heart failure.

The third stage must be managed carefully. The use of i.v. syntometrine should be avoided as this would result in rapid venous return to the heart and subsequent heart failure. The only oxytocic agent that could be used for the third stage of labour is intramuscular (i.m.) oxytocin. There may be a case for the physiological management of the third stage. However, this must not be at the risk of postpartum haemorrhage and worsening maternal morbidity. The placenta should then be delivered by controlled cord traction.

The risk of venous thrombo-embolism is considered to be significant in this patient. This should be minimized by administering subcutaneous (s.c.) heparin/fragmin for approximately five days after delivery. Early mobilization of the patient is essential in this regard. Close monitoring of the vital signs during the puerperium is essential because increased venous return to the heart may result in cardiac failure.

4

Infections in pregnancy

1. Universal screening for human immunodeficiency virus (HIV) is better than selective screening. What are the advantages and disadvantages for the provision of such a service?

2. Justify your management of a 19-year-old primigravida who booked for antenatal care at 12 weeks' gestation and her hepatitis B screening has been reported as positive.

3. Justify the management of a woman at 37 weeks' gestation with herpes simplex type II infection.

4. A schoolteacher in her first pregnancy at 10 weeks gestation has been informed that one of her pupils has chickenpox infection. She is extremely worried. How will you set about trying to reassure her?

5. What steps will you take to minimize the risk of human immunodeficiency virus (HIV) transmission to the baby of a 28-year-old woman who is HIV positive?

1. Universal screening for human immunodeficiency virus (HIV) is better than selective screening. What are the advantages and disadvantages for the provision of such a service?

Common mistakes

- Discussing details of the criteria for a screening test
- History of HIV and its course once infection has occurred
- Benefits of screening
- Various laboratory test for the diagnosis of HIV
- Treatment of HIV

A good answer will include some or all of these points

- A viral infection that is increasingly becoming more common in the pregnant population
- Screening – why advantageous – ensures better outcome for the mother and fetus
- Universal screening: difficulties – resources – manpower for counselling, disclosure of results and consequences of a positive test; benefits – all of those infected identified; treatment offered and therefore outcome for the baby and mother better
- Selective screening – high-risk populations targeted, limited resources (manpower and other) better used: misses out others who are infected; danger of spreading the disease; cost – probably more effective; risk of alienating at-risk groups who may not attend for screening
- Conclusion – more likely that screening is becoming cheaper and therefore universal screening may be beneficial. Problem remains that of appropriate resources

Sample answer

Human immunodeficiency virus (HIV) is a retrovirus whose incidence is increasing in the sexually active population. It has significant consequences on patients and their unborn fetuses. It is recognized that early identification, institution of treatment and modification of the method of delivery and postnatal feeding significantly minimizes the risk of vertical transmission. Screening and identifying those who are HIV positive therefore affords the opportunity to deliver the strategy outlined above to improve outcome.

The question is how to screen for this infection. Universal screening ensures that all pregnant women are screened for HIV. The problem of marginalizing a particular group, either on the basis of lifestyle or race, does not arise. The difficulty with this approach is the large population that has to be screened. Appropriate screening must be accompanied not only by staff but by financial resources to support tests. Although laboratory tests may not be expensive, the need for adequate manpower for counselling before screening, and after identification of positive cases, will impose considerable strain on the limited resources within the National Health Service (NHS).

Selective screening targets at-risk groups, such as intravenous drug abusers, bisexuals, those from geographical areas with endemic rates of the disease and their consorts. This approach may result in better use of limited resources. It will also ensure that testing is concentrated in those likely to be HIV positive. The problem with this approach is that the infection is spread through heterosexual contact and therefore a significant proportion of those infected will be missed. In addition, by targeting the at-risk population there is always the danger of the screening programme being perceived as discriminatory.

The second approach, which operates in the UK at the moment, offers all patients an opportunity to be screened. Uptake of screening is increasing, but patients still have to opt-in. It is clear that a large proportion of infected women is missed during pregnancy, as has been demonstrated by anonymous pilot testing. On balance, therefore, the best approach is likely to be universal screening, resources permitting. The argument of cost is unlikely to be tenable considering the implications for a positive diagnosis not only for the woman and her unborn child but also for society as a whole. Until the stigma of testing is removed by offering universal screening, many people will continue to be reluctant to come forward for testing for fear of being stigmatized.

2. Justify your management of a 19-year-old primigravida who booked for antenatal care at 12 weeks' gestation and her hepatitis B screening has been reported as positive.

Common mistakes

- Outline the management of hepatitis B positive patients
- Outline the management of human immunodeficiency virus (HIV)
- Discussing lifestyle and risk factors for hepatitis B

A good answer will contain some or all of these points

- Hepatitis B – blood-borne and or sexually transmitted disease (STD). May therefore co-exist with other STDs. Further screening may be necessary or discussed
- Infectivity important, especially as regards staff: HbS, Hbc, Hbe antibodies and antigen. Presence of e antigen and absence of e antibody indicates very high infectivity
- Risk of transmission to the fetus, intrauterine growth restriction (IUGR) (not associated with congenital anomalies, therefore termination not an issue)
- Mother – acute symptoms – supportive treatment. Chronic – usually asymptomatic
- Monitor – fetal growth, liver function test (LFT). Inform paediatrician and infective disease counsellor
- Delivery – anticipate a normal vaginal delivery: neonate administer hepatitis B immunoglobulin (HBIG) within 12 hours; vaccinate within seven days; second dose one and six months later; HbsAg tested at 12–15 months
- Family members – counselled

Sample answer

Hepatitis B is a blood-borne infection, which may also be sexually transmitted. It may therefore co-exist with other sexually transmitted diseases (STDs). The first step in the management of this patient will therefore be to exclude other STDs, from serology and swabs taken from the endocervix, the urethra and rectum. Before initiating these investigations, appropriate counselling must be offered. In the presence of other STDs, the genito-urinary medicine (GUM) physician should be involved in her care.

This patient is at risk of transmitting the infection to hospital staff. This depends to a large extent on infectivity, therefore this must be ascertained. If not already requested, hepatitis serology consisting of hepatitis B surface antigen and antibodies, hepatitis core antigen and antibodies, and e antigen and antibodies should be checked. The infectivity state is high if the patient has hepatitis e antigen but no e antibodies. If the patient has e antibodies, her infectivity is not high. Whatever the state of infectivity, the patient remains a risk to the hospital staff.

There is no recognized treatment for hepatitis during pregnancy. However, there is a risk of the virus being transmitted to the fetus *in utero*. Such a fetus is at risk of intrauterine growth restriction (IUGR). There are no recognized congenital malformations associated with hepatitis B and therefore the infection is not generally considered an indication for termination of pregnancy.

If the mother has acute symptoms, treatment will be mainly symptomatic and supportive. This is usually in the form of analgesics and ensuring that she is generally well-nourished and rests properly. In view of the risk of IUGR, the fetus must be monitored with growth scans serially from 24 weeks' gestation. In most cases, fetal growth is normal and delivery is normal at term.

The course of the disease in the mother is unpredictable. There may be progression with significant deterioration in liver function test (LFT). The mother should, therefore, be monitored by means of serial LFTs (probably every month). In most cases, there are no alterations in these. Although the fetus may not be infected *in utero*, the mother may transmit the disease to her newborn child. In addition, fetal infection acquired *in utero* may progress if appropriate steps are not taken after delivery to minimize this.

When delivery is planned, or anticipated, the neonatologist must be notified. Ideally, this should happen antenatally so that a management plan is agreed and documented in the patient's notes. The infection control counsellor must also be notified to initiate screening for other infections after appropriate counselling.

After delivery, the neonate should be given hepatitis B immunoglobulin (HBIG) within 12 hours. Seven days later, appropriate hepatitis vaccination should be offered. A second dose is offered within one to six months of the first immunization. At 12–15 months of age, the child should be tested for Hbs Ag. Since this infection may be transmitted to other members of the family, appropriate counselling and screening should be discussed and offered. It is in this regard that expert counsellors need to be involved. There is also the need to continue monitoring the antigen levels in the mother long after delivery, as chronic carrier status may persist and increase her risk of liver cirrhosis.

3. Justify the management of a woman at 37 weeks' gestation with herpes simplex type II infection.

Common mistakes

- Take a good history and perform a physical examination
- Detail sexual history
- Viral screen and human immunodeficiency virus (HIV) testing – without counselling
- Treat for other sexually transmitted diseases (STDs) – without having screening for these
- Deliver by Caesarean section
- If membranes ruptured, Caesarean section immediately
- No place for vaginal delivery

A good answer will include some or all of these points

- Common viral infection – sexually transmitted
- Need to exclude other STDs as they tend to co-exist
- Risk of infection – transmission to the fetus – usually during labour
- Consequences – pneumonia, meningitis, poor feeding, chorioamnionitis, mental retardation, neonatal seizures and death
- Is it recurrent (chronic) or primary (acute infection) diagnosis?
- Immunosuppression of pregnancy may result in systemic symptoms, such as fever, myalgia, malaise and aseptic meningitis
- Main problem is how to deliver: intact membranes – active disease – Caesarean section; recurrent (chronic) disease – allow vaginal delivery – why?; ruptured membranes – less than four hours – Caesarean section, more than four hours - vaginal delivery; chronic (recurrent) – no lesions at the time of delivery – can active lesions really be excluded?; monitor the fetus – notify the neonatologist and watch out for early signs of infection in the neonate; contact tracing

Sample answer

Genital herpes infection is commonly due to herpes simplex type II. This is a common viral infection, which is transmitted sexually. The main problem with this infection in pregnancy, especially at this gestation, is that of transmitting the infection to the fetus and its consequences on the neonate.

The diagnosis of herpes infection in this patient will alter the management of her pregnancy, especially the method of delivery. It is therefore important to establish whether she has had herpes all along or this is the first time the diagnosis has been made. If she has chronic herpes, her management will be different. In patients with chronic disease, vaginal delivery is possible. It has been argued that in these patients, because of the antibodies that they produce, the baby is offered some protection and therefore acquiring the virus during delivery does not pose significant consequences on the neonate. Others argue that since there is no guarantee that the neonate would have received the antibodies from the mother *in utero*, in the presence of active lesions, the babies should be delivered by Caesarean section. Contemporaneously, those with chronic infections are allowed to deliver vaginally.

If the patient has been diagnosed for the first time, she should have a planned delivery by Caesarean section depending on the timing of the delivery in relation to the time of the diagnosis (as the risk of vertical transmission is significant). This will depend on whether or not the patient presents with prematuire rupture of fetal membranes. If the membranes ruptured more than four hours before the baby is delivered, there are no obvious benefits from delivery by Caesarean section on the basis that the virus would have ascended into the uterus and infected the fetus. If, however, the patient presents within four hours of the membranes rupturing, the baby should be delivered by Caesarean section.

At 37 weeks it is possible that by the time of delivery all active lesions from the genital tract would have healed. A vaginal examination should therefore be performed at 39 weeks' gestation to locate active lesions before a decision is made about the mode of delivery. In the presence of active lesions and intact membranes, or rupture within four hours of presentation, a Caesarean section should be performed. The diagnosis of active disease by such a method is unreliable. The absence of lesions does not exclude active disease. The neonatologist must be notified and the newborn observed closely for early signs of infection. These may manifest as feeding difficulties, clinical features of pneumonia or meningitis. Since this is a sexually transmitted disease (STD), all efforts must be made to exclude other STDs and, where possible, contact screening and treatment should be considered and offered.

4. A schoolteacher in her first pregnancy at 10 weeks gestation has been informed that one of her pupils has chickenpox infection. She is extremely worried. How will you set about trying to reassure her?

Common mistakes

- Take a good history and do a physical examination
- Screen for risk factors for varicella
- Listing the possible congenital malformations associated with chickenpox infection
- Offer termination of pregnancy
- Refer to a virologist
- Admit and treat with acyclovir

A good answer will include some or all of these points

- Common viral infection, spread by droplets
- Could have had infection without knowing
- May cause congenital malformations but usually mild
- Need to check antibodies to determine whether previously exposed to virus – confer life-long immunity
- If antibody present, IgG crosses the placenta and therefore protects baby
- Determine time of exposure to the virus – may have been at the time child not infective
- Timed paired blood samples for antibodies
- Reassure and offer anomaly scan
- Watch for any signs of disease and pneumonia which could be severe and associated with mortality in pregnancy

Sample answer

Chickenpox is a viral infection that is common among children. It is highly infective and transmitted by droplets. The virus is teratogenic and may cause complications in pregnancy, ranging from miscarriages to mild and serious congenital malformations. Fortunately, these malformations are uncommon. Although there is a subpopulation of adults who cannot recall being infected, a large proportion of them have antibodies suggesting previous infection, Previous chickenpox offers lifelong immunity and the antibodies, which are IgG, are capable of crossing the placenta and protecting the fetus.

In this teacher, therefore, it is important to establish whether she has had an infection with chickenpox before. If she has not, her antibodies must be checked. If these are positive, she should be reassured and the pregnancy allowed to continue without any further intervention. If, however, she has not been exposed before and she is antibody-negative, she is obviously at risk of *in utero* transmission of the virus. An important question, therefore, must be the time of exposure to the infected child. If the exposure was not during the vesicle and crusting stage, she is not at risk of the infection as this is the time during which the virus is shed from the infected person.

If the time of exposure is uncertain, paired serum samples should be collected from the patient and sent for antibody measurement. If the antibody titre is rising, or IgM antibodies are present, she has been exposed and is infected. Assuming that she is infected, the most appropriate counselling must be offered. The fetus is at risk of congenital malformations, most of which are minor and it is often not possible to identify them antenatally. However, the patient should be offered a detailed ultrasound scan at 18–20 weeks' gestation to exclude anomalies associated with varicella-zoster virus (VZV) infection. Although total and specific IgM may be detected in fetal blood by 19 weeks, it is not recommended unless there are sono-graphic features suggesting infection. In the presence of these antibodies, termination of the pregnancy should be considered.

It has been suggested that all sonographic abnormalities manifest within 20 weeks of maternal infection and therefore follow-up scanning may be arranged at 30 weeks. In the absence of any obvious abnormalities, the pregnancy should be allowed to continue and, after delivery, the baby should be assessed by a neonatologist, concentrating on the neurological system – especially the eyes. Although it is uncommon at this gestation, the risk of severe pneumonia occurring in pregnancy should always be born in mind and any symptoms of pneumonia should be treated aggressively. If the patient develops any symptoms of life-threatening disease, acyclovir should be considered. There is a place for administering varicella-zoster immunoglobin (VZIG) if she is non-immune.

5. What steps will you take to minimize the risk of human immunodeficiency virus (HIV) transmission to the baby of a 28-year-old woman who is HIV-positive?

Common mistakes

- Take a history and do a physical examination
- Exclude other sexually transmitted diseases (STDs)
- Counselling about protective sexual intercourse (use condoms)
- Barrier nursing

A good answer will include some or all of these points

- Transmission to the fetus – vertical – transplacental, during delivery and breastfeeding
- Transmission influenced by viral load
- Procedures which increase the risk of feto-maternal haemorrhage will increase the risk of transmission
- Antiviral treatment – monitor by viral load and CD4
- Offer Caesarean section
- Avoid breastfeeding
- Treat neonate
- Avoid invasive procedures such as amniocentesis, chorionic villus sampling (CVS) and external cephalic version (ECV). May be a place to offer first-trimester nuchal translucency (NT) and biochemical screening – associated with an 85 per cent detection rate compared to 65 per cent with biochemical screening and amniocentesis at 14–16 weeks' gestation

Sample answer

Human immunodeficiency virus (HIV) infection is a blood-borne viral infection, which is transmitted sexually, through blood products or via shared needles. It is more common in homosexuals, intravenous drug users and those from endemic areas. The disease is transmitted vertically to the fetus during pregnancy; transplacentally, during labour and in the neonatal and infant periods through breastfeeding.

If untreated, this HIV-positive woman has a risk of approximately 25–30 per cent of transmitting the virus to her fetus *in utero*. During breastfeeding, the risk is of the order of 50–60 per cent. Once the fetus or baby is infected, there is a high morbidity and mortality. Reducing the transmission risks *in utero* and after delivery is therefore essential. The first step to minimize the risk of transmission is to reduce the viral load in the mother. This is done by offering the mother combination antiviral treatment. The most commonly used antiviral treatment is AZT. Given during pregnancy, it reduces the viral load in the mother and therefore the risk of transmission to the fetus from 25–30 per cent to eight per cent. The treatment must be offered with expert advice from an HIV specialist – usually a genito-urinary medicine (GUM) consultant. The treatment should be monitored with the patient's viral load and her CD4 count.

In this patient, any procedure that may increase the risk of feto-maternal haemorrhage should be avoided unless it is not practicable to do so. Procedures such as amniocentesis, chorionic villus sampling (CVS) and external cephalic version (ECV) should therefore be kept to a minimum. If the patient requires prenatal diagnosis, the least invasive test should be offered. It is in precisely this type of patient that prenatal diagnosis by a combination of nuchal tranlucency (NT), PAP1 and inhibin in the late first trimester may be more appropriate. This will reduce the numbers being exposed to invasive testing.

Delivery by Caesarean section has been shown to significantly reduce the risk of vertical transmission to the fetus. The patient should therefore be offered an elective Caesarean section. In addition, she should avoid breastfeeding. The baby should be offered antiviral drugs for six weeks starting eight to 12 hours after birth. These measures will significantly reduce the risk of vertical transmission.

5

Isoimmunization

1. Critically appraise prohylaxis against Rhesus (D) isoimmunization.

2. Critically appraise the management of a 26-year-old woman in her first pregnancy with Rhesus (D) antibodies (32 IU/l) at 26 weeks' gestation.

3. Anti-D prophylaxis has significantly reduced morbidity and mortality from Rhesus (D) isoimmunization. There are, however, still many cases of isoimmunization occurring during pregnancy. How may this be remedied?

1. Critically appraise prohylaxis against Rhesus (D) isoimmunization.

Common mistakes

- Forgetting the first trimester
- Ignoring the recent recommendations from the Royal College of Gynaecologists (RCOG) about prophylaxis
- Detailing the management of a Rhesus-isoimmunized pregnancy
- Elaborating on other types of isoimmunization

A good answer will include some or all of these points

- Anti-D has reduced the incidence of HDN
- Recommendations
  - Selective
  - Rhesus-negative women – indications for prophylaxis
  - Bleeding >12 weeks, abdominal pain after delivery – difficulties with these recommendations
- Ideally, Kleihauer testing should be performed before administration of anti-D
- Also recommended after amniocentesis, chorionic villus sampling (CVS), fetal blood sampling and external cephalic version (ECV)
- Problems with selective prophylaxis
  - Failed administration
  - Failure of sensitization
  - Silent sensitization
  - Inadequate doses
  - Strict adherence to 72 hours when it is relatively effective within 10 days
- Recent recommendation about routine prophylaxis
  - 28 and 34 weeks – 500 IU
- Problems
  - Cost implications
  - Still miss out some silent sensitizations
  - Reluctance by patients to accept because of the fear of new variant Creutzfeldt–Jakob disease (CJD), human immunodeficiency virus (HIV) and hepatitis
- Monoclonal anti-D may overcome this

Sample answer

The advent of anti-D in the 1960s resulted in a significant reduction in perinatal morbidity and mortality from Rhesus isoimmunization. Prophylaxis against isoimmunization has been the key to this reduction. This prophylaxis has been to a large extent governed by standard recommendations. Very recently, these recommendations were modified by a Consensus Group consisting of obstetricians and haematologists.

The traditional recommendations were selective. Anti-D was given after a sensitizing event. These events included miscarriages, invasive diagnostic procedures, antepartum haemorrhage, external cephalic version (ECV), fetal blood sampling and after delivery. Recently, the criteria for prophylaxis in the first trimester have been modified. Women with a slight bleed before 12 weeks' gestation are no longer required to have anti-D. The difficulties with these modifications lie in their implementation. How is a mild bleed defined and what happens to patients who have repeated bleeds? The rationale for restricting this early group is the fact that significant feto-maternal haemorrhage is unlikely before 10 weeks' gestation. Ideally, these women should have a Kleihauer test and, where this is positive, anti-D should be given. Another consideration is that since anti-D is expensive, offering it at a time when it is least likely to be useful is not cost-effective. The consequences of this are that women who require anti-D by virtue of repeated bleeds and abdominal pain (but who have a high pain threshold) will be missed. In addition, those who are uncertain of their last menstrual period (LMP), whose pregnancies are therefore dated inappropriately, will not receive anti-D. An ideal situation would include scanning to date pregnancies accurately – but this is only possible when patients present to hospital. Since some of them do not and their general practitioners (GPs) are likely to follow recommendations, it is possible that sensitized women will appear as a result of this policy.

Since Kleihauer testing is not routinely done in every patient, the dose of anti-D administered (especially in the latter stages of pregnancy) may not be enough and therefore sensitization may still occur. Adminstration is often recommended within 72 hours of the sensitizing event, yet it is recognized that some protection is available within 10 days of the event. The guidelines fail to address this enigma and therefore when patients present late, anti-D may not be offered.

The recent recommendation that all pregnant Rhesus-negative women should be offered anti-D at 28 and 34 weeks' gestation, irrespective of a sensitizing event, recognizes the fact that failure to prevent isomimmunization in some patients is related to silent feto-maternal haemorrhages. Since anti-D remains in the circulation for six weeks, administration of 500 IU at these gestations will cover the period where feto-maternal haemorrhages are likely to be significant. The problem with this recommendation is that, nationally, only very few units have implemented it. This is because of costs. There are also patients who would not accept anti-D because it is a human product and also because of the risk of new variant Creutzfeldt–Jakob disease (CJD). These problems may be overcome with the advent of monoclonal anti-D.

Although prophylaxis has successfully reduced the incidence of sensitization, failure to administer anti-D, or to administer the correct dose, and failure to protect despite administration, continue to result in affected pregnancies. Although more recent recommendations have attempted to address some of the reasons for these failures, there remain several obstacles to complete implementation and so isoimmunization will persist.

2. Critically appraise the management of a 26-year-old woman in her first pregnancy with Rhesus (D) antibodies (32 IU/l) at 26 weeks' gestation.

Common mistakes

- Take a history and physical examination
- Refer to high-risk unit for further management and (end answer here)
- Discuss the pathogenesis of sensitization
- Discussing the reasons for the sensitization
- Deliver by Caesarean section

A good answer will include some or all of these points

- The antibodies are significantly high. Primigravida, there must have been a sensitizing event. Exclude from history, although it will not alter management
- The risk of haemolysis in fetus is high
- Further investigations are required to ascertain the severity of the disease on the fetus
- Two approaches – fetal blood sampling and amniocentesis
- From fetal blood – determine haemoglobin (Hb), blood group, presence of antibodies, bilirubin and reticulocytes. From amniotic fluid, OD450 and safety lines
- Ultrasound scan and MCA Doppler scan to determine cut-off values for peak systolic velocities
- Intrauterine transfusion – intraperitoneal or intravascular?
- Delivery
- Administration of dexamethasone
- Management in a unit with expertise
- Future pregnancies

Sample answer

The antibody levels in this primigravida are significantly high. This level is most likely to be associated with intrauterine haemolysis and severe fetal disease. Although it is uncertain how this patient was sensitized, it is possible that she either had a transfusion which she cannot remember or had a significant sensitization event in this pregnancy. This is possible but highly unlikely as first sensitization events are not often associated with such high levels. Whatever the cause of the sensitization, this is unlikely to alter the management of the patient. Similarly, determining the genotype of the putative father will not influence the management, as he may not be the biological father of the fetus.

The first step in the management of this patient is to ensure that the antibody levels are correct. It is therefore prudent to repeat them and also ask for titres. If there is evidence in the notes of levels in early pregnancy, a comparison will determine the rate of rise. Assuming that these levels are, indeed, correct and have risen very rapidly, further investigations of the severity of the disease on the fetus need to be undertaken. Such investigations and subsequent management must be in a unit with expertise for intrauterine transfusion. Referral to a tertiary fetal medicine unit is mandatory.

At the unit, either amniocentesis or a fetal blood sample will be performed. Amniocentesis will allow the colour of the liquor to be assessed by naked eye. Optical densitometric analyses at fluid at wavelength of 450 nm will then be undertaken. These values will then be plotted on Liley charts and, where actions lines are crossed, the most appropriate action will be undertaken. The advantages of amniocentesis include ease of the procedure and lower complication rates. However, this procedure does not allow the determination of the blood group of the fetus (although by use of modern molecular biology techniques, this is now possible), the quantified level of bilirubin in the fetus and its haemoglobin. However, where the site of sampling fetal blood is difficult to reach, this procedure provides an acceptable alternative. Fetal blood samples, on the other hand, may be obtained at the cord insertion – a free loop of the cord of the intra-abdominal portion of the umbilical vein. Fetal blood sampling is a very skilled invasive procedure associated with a preterm labour rate of three to four per cent and may be complicated with haemorrhage and haematoma formation, which could be fatal, especially if the arteries in the cord are compressed. At 26 weeks' gestation such a complication, necessitating immediate delivery, may be associated with a poor outcome. However, it provides an opportunity to determine the fetal haemoglobin (Hb), blood group, bilirubin levels, the presence of antibodies and reticulocytes, which indicate how the fetal erythropoietic system is responding to the haemolysis.

After this investigation there may be a need to transfuse the fetus. Such a transfusion may be performed intraperitoneally or intravascularly. If this is necessary, calculations of the volume of blood required will be determined by various factors, including gestational age, fetal haematocrit or the level on the Liley charts. The aim of transfusion is to completely replace the fetal blood with Rhesus-negative bloods and therefore erythropoiesis.

Very recently, the need for invasive procedures in the investigations of these fetuses has been superseded by the use of Doppler velocimetry of the middle cerebral artery to predict which fetuses will require intrauterine transfusion. Significant changes in systolic velocity frequencies are used to gauge severity of disease and therefore need for transfusion. In addition, close monitoring of the fetus by means of serial ultrasound biometry and Doppler scan studies will be required. The timing of delivery will depend on several factors, such as worsening fetal haemolysis, a successful transfusion and associated complications (for example, polyhydramnios and preterm labour). In the absence of any complications, the pregnancy should be prolonged as far as possible. The best approach to delivery will be determined by various obstetric and fetal factors at the time of delivery. A Caesarean section, however, is highly likely as this ensures minimal stress to the fetus. At the time of delivery, blood must be available as this baby will require exchange blood transfusion.

Following delivery, adequate counselling should be offered on the management of subsequent pregnancies. The blood group of the patient's partner should be determined if it is not already known. If he is heterozygous for Rhesus D, determination of the fetal blood group early in pregnancy (from amniocentesis for example) may eliminate the need for further close surveillance. For subsequent Rhesus-positive pregnancies, the onset of fetal haemolysis is likely to be earlier than 26 weeks. Invasive testing should therefore begin at about 24 weeks. For women who have been severely affected, donor insemination is an option that may be worth considering.

3. Anti-D prophylaxis has significantly reduced morbidity and mortality from Rhesus D isoimmunization. There are, however, still many cases of isoimmunization occurring during pregnancy. How may this be remedied?

Common mistakes

- Discussing anti-D prophylaxis – when and how it is administered
- Risk factors for sensitization
- Screening for Rhesus D in pregnancy

A good answer will include some or all of these points

- Identify why there is failure of prophylaxis: failed administration; inadequate dose; silent feto-maternal haemorrhage
- Overcoming the reasons for failure: patient/GP/midwife education – communication of results and importance; strict adherence to Royal College of Gynaecologists/National Institute for Clinical Excellence (RCOG/NICE) guidelines; administration even after 72 hours and up to 10 days – offers protection in up to 75 per cent of cases; larger doses (determined by Kleihauer test/flow cytometry)
- RCOG/Consensus Group recommendation – routine prophylaxis at 28 and 34 weeks (500 IU): poor implementation (not widely implemented yet) – expense – unavailable anti-D – New variant Creutzfeldt–Jakob disease (CJD) – fear from patients (if human anti- D); monoclonal antibodies
- Recognition of the effects of other antibodies and effective screening

Sample answer

The persistence of sensitization against Rhesus disease occurs for four main reasons. These are: failure to administer anti-D; administration of inadequate doses; late administration; and silent feto-maternal haemorrhages. Until all these are remedied, Rhesus sensitization will continue to occur.

There are several approaches to overcome persistent sensitization. The first is the education of patients, midwives, general practitioners (GPs) and all those involved in the care of pregnant women. Communication of blood group results to patients ought to be accompanied by leaflets explaining the implications of being Rhesus-negative and imploring them to ensure that anti-D is given whenever there is a sensitizing event in any pregnancy. Second, there must be mechanisms to guarantee strict adherence to guidelines on the administration of anti-D. Included in these guidelines should be an explanation of the rationale for this practice and that, where the 72-hour limit has been missed, prophylaxis should still be given as it offers some protection within 10 days of the sensitizing event. Where possible, Kleihauer testing or flow cytometry should precede all anti-D administration and larger doses given if required.

This may not be necessary in the first trimester since the 250 IU often administered is enough to neutralize 4 ml of fetal blood and the volume of fetal blood at this gestation is not significantly more than this.

The Royal College of Gynaecologists (RCOG)/Consensus Group recommendations about routine administration of anti-D at 28 and 34 weeks' gestation should be implemented. For effective implementation, adequate resources must be provided. Poor implementation has been blamed on inadequate finances to fund anti-D. For those objecting to human-derived anti-D, monoclonal anti-D should be made available. The risk of acquiring new variant CJD from anti-D is considered to be extremely small. Better education will therefore minimize the chances of rejection on this basis. Although Rhesus isoimmunization may soon become uncommon, other rarer types of isoimmunization are becoming more common. These must be recognised and efforts made to identify and prevent them in the same fashion as Rhesus isoimmunization.

6

Abnormal fetal growth

1. A 26-year-old primigravida presents at 26 weeks' gestation with severe intrauterine growth restriction (IUGR) confirmed on ultrasound scan. Justify your management.

2. What factors will determine the mode of delivery of a severely growth restricted fetus in a primigravida?

3. A 30-year-old primigravida attended for her routine anomaly scan at 20 weeks' gestation. Ultrasound scan revealed a viable fetus of appropriate gestation with anhydramnios. She denies a history of spontaneous rupture of fetal membranes. Critically appraise your management of this patient.

1. A 26-year-old primigravida presents at 26 weeks' gestation with severe intrauterine growth retardation (IUGR) confirmed on ultrasound scan. Justify your management.

Common mistakes

- Take a history and perform physical examination
- Do an ultrasound scan to confirm gestational age
- Serum screening for Down syndrome
- Deliver by Caesarean section
- Monitor fetus regularly (no details of monitoring)
- Refer to tertiary unit for management
- Fetal blood sampling before deciding when to deliver
- Prognosis is too poor, therefore do nothing unless she goes into labour

A good answer will include some or all of these points

- Definition of severe IUGR – most cases aetiology is unknown
- Assess fetal health to establish baseline – amniotic fluid index (AFI), Doppler scan of UmA, MCA, biophysical profile
- Investigate for possible causes of IUGR
- Involvement of paediatrician – why?
- Administer steroids – why?
- Timing of delivery – how?
- Delivery – when and how?
- Further management
- Severely compromised with very poor prognosis – conservative management may be an option

Sample answer

Severe intrauterine growth restriction (IUGR) will be diagnosed if the abdominal circumference is below the third centile and there is associated oligohydramnios. This is associated with severe morbidity and mortality. Prematurity superimposed on this complication is associated with an even poorer prognosis. In most cases, the aetiology is unknown but even in those with known aetiologies, at 26 weeks' gestation, management presents several dilemmas.

The first step in the management of this patient will be to assess the fetal health and thereby establish baseline indices for subsequent comparisons and also to determine whether to deliver or manage conservatively. In some cases, some of these indices would have been established during the ultrasound scan. Assuming that these are not available, then they should be elicited. These indices include quantification of amniotic fluid (that is, amniotic fluid index, AFI), Doppler velocimetry of the umbilical and middle cerebral arteries and biophysical profilometry. During scanning, structural malformations need to be excluded, although with severe IUGR (especially when associated with oligohydramnios) this may be difficult. The next step would be to investigate for the possible cause(s) of the IUGR. Checking the maternal blood pressure and urine samples will identify pre-eclampsia. Other investigations include viral, protozoal and bacterial infection screening from a sample of blood from the mother, thrombophilia screening, lupus anticoagulant and anticardiolipin antibody levels, and an autoimmune profile. Where possible, a fetal blood sample should be obtained for blood gases (which will determine a co-existent hypoxia and the degree), karyotyping and infection screen.

This patient should be admitted to hospital. This will ensure bed rest and permit more comprehensive surveillance of the fetus and urgent delivery if necessary. Monitoring will include at least twice-daily cardiotographs (CTGs), four-hourly maternal blood pressure measurements, daily urinalysis (if the patient is pre-eclamptic), twice-weekly biophysical profiles and growth scans every 10–14 days. A course of dexamethasone (two doses) should be given to help reduce the risk of respiratory distress syndrome (RDS).

As part of her management, the patient must be seen by a paediatrician for counselling about survival and handicap rates at this gestation, and for details of how the baby will be managed after delivery. The mother should also be encouraged to visit the neonatal unit to familiarize herself with the facilities and staff. Seeing a ventilated preterm baby in an incubator will help her understand and relate better to her baby when it is born.

The timing of delivery will be determined by the monitoring parameters and other associated complications. Assuming that the fetus is chromosomally normal and there are no lethal structural abnormalities, this will be determined by the CTGs, Doppler scans and biophysical profile indices. If there is reversed end-diastolic flow or the biophysical profile score is low (four or below) delivery should be considered. The method of delivery is likely to be Caesarean section, as a vaginal delivery for this already compromised fetus will be associated with a poorer prognosis. The type of Caesarean section will also depend on a several factors. At this early gestation, the lower segment is unlikely to be well-formed. A classical Caesarean section, or a modified one, is the likely operation of choice. This must take place where there are neonatal intensive care facilities and the paediatrician should be present at delivery. If these facilities are absent in the unit, the fetus is best transferred *in utero*. If there is absent or reversed end-diastolic flow on the umbilical artery Doppler scan, the neonatologist should be informed as this is associated with an increased risk of necrotizing enterocolitis (NEC). The placenta should be sent for histology as this may provide some clues as to the cause of the IUGR. The recurrence risk of IUGR is high, therefore knowing its cause will help in counselling and the management of any subsequent pregnancies. The patient must be counselled properly about the type of delivery and the implications for the next pregnancy. At 26 weeks' gestation, decisions about when to deliver are difficult.

Where there is severe fetal compromise and the outcome is thought to be poor, the decision on how to manage the pregnancy must be made after adequate counselling. In view of the severe difficulties with delivery at this early gestation, the associated significant maternal morbidity (if a classical Caesarean delivery) and implications for subsequent pregnancies, an option is to allow the fetus to be delivered vaginally or to die *in utero*. This is an ethical/moral dilemma and one that must be considered sensitively.

2.   What factors will determine the mode of delivery of a severely growth restricted fetus in a primigravida?

Common mistakes

- Take a history and do a physical examination
- Management will depend on past obstetric history – therefore obtain information about past obstetric history
- Discussing the details of monitoring of a fetus with intrauterine growth restriction (IUGR)
- Screening and Doppler scanning in IUGR
- Mode of delivery should be determined by the patient in conjuction with neonatologist

A good answer should include some or all of these points

- IUGR is a high-risk pregnancy and the outcome is influenced by the time of diagnosis and severity
- Late onset – better prognosis; milder forms better prognosis
- IUGR is due to several causes – some of which cannot be resolved with delivery
- The mode of delivery should offer the best outcome for the fetus and minimal risk to the mother
- Factors influencing mode of delivery
  - Gestational age at diagnosis – very severe and early diagnosis – Caesarean section best option; likely classical
  - Presentation – breech/transverse lie – Caesarean section/cephalic vaginal delivery if safe for baby and mother
  - Severity – determined by size and/or monitoring indices – no intrauterine compromise and monitoring indices normal – vaginal delivery
  - Associated complications – pre-eclampsia/ruptured membranes and infections/oligohydramnios, placenta position
  - State of the cervix
  - Wishes of the patient

Sample answer

Severe intrauterine growth restriction (IUGR) is associated with significant morbidity and mortality. The magnitude of these complications depends on the gestational age at which the diagnosis is made. The earlier the onset, the poorer the prognosis. The mode of delivery should offer the best outcome for the fetus and minimal risk to the mother.

Where the onset of IUGR is early (for example, occurring before the late second trimester) and the fetus is not significantly compromised (so as to have an extremely poor prognosis), the best option would be a Caesarean section. It is most likely that, at this early gestation, the lower segment will be poorly formed. This, compounded with oligohydramnios (a common association of severe IUGR), will make a standard lower-segment Caesarean section difficult. A classical Caesarean section or a modified lower-segment Caesarean section (such as Delee, U-shaped or a J-shaped incision on the lower uterine wall) would be more suitable. Although this is the best option at this early gestation, it must be remembered that maternal morbidity with this type of delivery is significant and that it also has a significant influence on subsequent pregnancies.

At a more advanced gestation, the lower segment may be formed in which case the Caesarean section would be for a breech presentation, a significantly compromised fetus which cannot withstand the stress induced by labour or associated complications such as preeclampsia, placental praevia or ruptured membranes with chorioamnionitis. If the fetus is not significantly compromised, there may be a place for a vaginal delivery. This will only be suitable if the cervix is ripe or ripening it will not be prolonged, the presentation is cephalic and there are no associated complications. Although this may be the safest option for the mother there is always the risk of progression to emergency abdominal delivery, which is associated with more morbidity than that following an elective Caesarean section. The decision to allow a vaginal delivery in a severely growth restricted pregnancy must, therefore, be made bearing in mind that a larger proportion of cases will require an emergency abdominal delivery.

Although attempts to deliver a live fetus seem to be the best approach in the management of this primigravida, if the fetus is considered to be severely compromised and with a very poor prognosis, there may be a case to allow it to die *in utero* and opt for a vaginal delivery. The other option would be to induce a vaginal delivery knowing that the outcome will be uniformly poor. Such a decision has to be made with appropriate counselling from obstetricians and paediatricians. Whatever the case, the mode of delivery should be determined only after counselling the patient and taking her wishes into consideration alongside the state of the fetus and its long-term outcome.

3. A 30-year-old primigravida attended for her routine anomaly scan at 20 weeks' gestation. Ultrasound scan revealed a viable fetus of appropriate gestation with anhydramnios. She denies a history of spontaneous rupture of fetal membranes. Critically appraise your management of this patient.

Common mistakes

- Take a history and do a physical examination to exclude 'causes' of spontaneous rupture of fetal membranes and oligohydramnios
- Listing all the causes of oligohydramnios/anhydramnios
- Management will depend on the degree of oligohydramnios
- Discussing the methods of diagnosing spontaneous rupture of fetal membranes
- Terminate the pregnancy
- Delivery should be by Caesarean section
- Screen for abnormal Doppler scans
- Failing to critically appraise your answer
- Induce labour at 28–34 weeks' gestation

A good answer will include some or all of these points

- Anhydramnios at this early gestation is associated with a poor prognosis (related to pulmonary hypoplasia) unless it can be corrected
- Definition of anhydramnios – complete absence of liquor
- Most likely causes – renal agenesis or obstruction to outflow. Other causes – congenital infections/chromosomal abnormalities
- Spontaneous rupture of fetal membranes – history has been excluded but not very reliable. Speculum examination may be necessary – not reliable if anhydramnios
- Tertiary level ultrasound scan (by fetal medicine expert if available) – not reliable (anhydramnios – acoustic window absent)
- Amnioinfusion – will enable better imaging. However, risk of infection and miscarriage
- Karyotyping – placental biopsy – mosaicism, most likely to be normal. Unlikely to influence management
- Renal artery imaging – with colour/power Doppler – absence will confirm diagnosis
- Renal agenesis/abnormalities – incompatible will life – termination
- No obvious abnormality, amnioinfusion – liquor maintained, serial monitoring/repeat amnioinfusion and deliver when appropriate. May be able to assess lungs
- Involve neonatologists

Sample answer

Anhydramnios is defined as complete absence of liquor amnii around the fetus. At this early gestation, the prognosis is poor unless it can be corrected. This will depend largely on the cause, which in most cases is not compatible with survival. The most likely causes are renal agenesis, obstruction to urine outflow and rupture of fetal membranes. In some cases it may be due to chromosomal abnormalities or other structural abnormalities.

The first step in the management of this patient is to attempt to establish the cause of the anhydramnios. Since she has denied the history of rupture of fetal membranes, her notes should firstly be reviewed to establish whether she has had previous ultrasound scans that revealed normal liquor. A booking ultrasound scan is the most likely one and this is unable to correctly predict anhydramnios as during the early gestation there is no significant production of liquor amnii. However, it might have identified possible aetiological factors.

Although the history has been denied, it is essential to undertake a speculum examination and perform a test to exclude rupture of fetal membranes. With anhydramnios, this is likely to be negative. If it is positive, it will suggest a possible premature rupture of fetal membranes, although this is unlikely to influence the management. The tests used for this are recognized to have false negatives and positives and may, therefore, not provide conclusive evidence for or against spontaneous rupture of fetal membranes.

The absence of liquor means that detailed ultrasound scanning will be difficult. The detailed scan should therefore be organized in a tertiary centre where level three ultrasound is available. It may be necessary to undertake an amnioinfusion in order to facilitate this procedure. However, amnioinfusion is associated with the risks of chorioamnionitis and spontaneous miscarriages. Sometimes this procedure may rectify the anhydramnios and allow the pregnancy to progress to viability. It is, however, rare in cases of anhydramnios and more likely where there is oligohydramnios.

Since renal agenesis is a common cause of this complication, demonstrating the presence of kidneys may help in the management. The presence of kidneys may support repeated amnio-infusions provided there are no other abnormalities that are incompatible with life. The use of colour Doppler scanning to delineate renal arteries may be useful. It must be remembered that where there is renal agenesis, the adrenal arteries may be confused with renal arteries.

Since chromosomal and metabolic abnormalities may also be responsible for this complication, karyotyping should b discussed and offered. The best approach is in this case is placental biopsy (chorionic villus sampling, CVS). This is unlikely to alter the management. In some cases, where termination is offered CVS may be done before termination.The problem of placental mosaicism is a recognized difficult of this method of karyotyping.

In the absence of any karyotypic or structural abnormality, repeated amnioinfusions may be associated with a relatively good prognosis provided the infused saline is retained. The neo-natologist should be informed and involved in the care of the neonate from such management. However, at this very early gestation, pulmonary hypoplasia and pressure deformities are most likely, and after delivery the neonate would most probably succumb to hypoplasia of the lungs. Where the prognosis is considered to be poor, termination of pregnancy should be offered and following this, an autopsy is needed to confirm the antenatal diagnosis and exclude the presence of other abnormalities that could be combined to constitute a syndrome with an obvious risk of recurrence.

7

Epidemiology, social obstetrics, drugs in pregnancy

1. What steps will you take in advising an alcoholic to give up alcohol at six weeks' gestation?

2. Justify the steps you will take in persuading a 20-year-old woman, in her first pregnancy, who smokes 30 cigarettes a day to give up smoking in pregnancy.

3. A 22-year-old mother of two attends for antenatal care at 30 weeks' gestation with her partner and their two children. You observe that the children are rather subdued and also during your examination, you elicit tenderness over the left lower loin, which is also bruised. You suspect domestic violence. What subsequent steps will you take in her care and why?

1. What steps will you take in advising an alcoholic to give up alcohol at six weeks' gestation.

Common mistakes

- Discussing details of the management of the patient in pregnancy
- Identification of fetal alcohol syndrome by ultrasound or other means
- An alcoholic – no need to ask how much she drinks
- Why are you an alcoholic? Why do you have to drink so much? (Be sensitive in your approach)
- Advice to consult general practitioner (GP), social workers, etc. for information on how to stop drinking!! How realistic is this?
- You need to be specific – not just say alcohol is associated with features of fetal alcohol syndrome (FAS), etc. Be specific

A good answer will include some or all of these points

- The approach must be sensitive, supportive, empathic and non-judgemental
- The problems of teratogenicity and alcohol ≥15 units/week
- Involvement of social workers
- Social and other background information – from patient or other people – problems possibly associated with the drinking will be identified and, once resolved, are more likely to be associated with success in stopping drinking
- Organizations – Alcoholics Anonymous, other support/help groups, pamphlets about alcohol and pregnancy
- Staff – GP, midwives, family, friends, social workers
- Maternal dangers of alcohol – liver failure, heart failure, encephalopathy, anaemia, vitamin B12 deficiency

Sample answer

Excessive alcohol in pregnancy is associated with a significant perinatal morbidity and mortality, and maternal morbidity. Patients who overindulge are often not aware of their excesses. The approach to counselling this patient must therefore be sensitive, supportive, empathic and non-judgemental. It is important that the patient is not antagonized from the outset. Once she develops confidence in the clinician, the process becomes easier and the results are much better.

The first stage in counselling is to make sure that the patient is aware of the existence of a problem. There may be initial denial but persistence and supportive counselling will eventually result in acknowledging that there is, indeed, a problem. The next stage in the counselling will be to educate the patient on the possible consequences of excessive alcohol on the fetus. Alcohol teratogenicity therefore has to be discussed. These consequences include congenital cardiac anomalies, microcephaly, micro-opthalmia, intrauterine growth restriction (IUGR), impaired intellect, neurodevelopmental delay, skeletal anomalies, etc. These problems arise where alcohol intake is more than 80 g/day (eight units per day = eight glasses of wine or four pints of lager/day). Furthermore, the consequences of alcohol on the mother need to be discussed. These include liver failure, heart failure, encephalopathy, anaemia, vitamin B deficiency – leading to Wernicke–Korsakoff's encephalopathy and gastro-intestinal disturbances, such as gastritis and pancreatitis.

An important step in the counselling of this patient is to seek expert support and help. This will be from social workers who may provide home support for her and any children she may have. Her partner needs to be counselled as well. Often, they too are alcoholics and failing to involve them in the counselling process will be counterproductive. It is important to obtain some social and other relevant background information about the patient. This may provide clues as to why she drinks. For example, it may be related to childcare, abuse from partner or family, rejection by society or other deepseated problems. Identification and resolution of these problem(s) may suddenly result in a change in attitude.

Organizations such as Alcoholics Anonymous or other support groups locally or nationally and contacts with other women who have had similar problems may provide support. They may also provide information pamphlets about alcohol and pregnancy, which will reinforce the discussion on teratogenecity and the consequences of alcohol on the mother. The GP, the midwife, friends and family should be involved if possible. It may be easy for the patient to relate to them than to doctors at the hospital. Once a breakthrough has been achieved, this has to be followed up by frequent positive re-enforcement and encouragement. Relapse is easy and therefore the counselling must not only concentrate on pregnancy but must make provisions for continuing support after delivery.

2. Justify the steps you will take in persuading a 20-year-old woman, in her first pregnancy, who smokes 30 cigarettes a day to give up smoking in pregnancy.

Common mistakes

- Take a history and examine patient
- Refer to physician
- Offer alternate cigarettes
- Advantage – reduce the risk of pre-eclampsia

A good answer will contain some or all of these points

- Smoking produces nicotine and carboxyhaemoglobin. These cross the placenta and circulate within the fetus. Consequences – intrauterine growth restriction (IUGR), intrauterine fetal death, hypoxia
- Neonatal mortality and morbidity
- Cot death
- Reduced intelligence
- Early death in the neonatal period
- Consequences of smoking on maternal health

Sample answer

Smoking in pregnancy is associated with a high perinatal morbidity and mortality, and maternal morbidity. The first step in persuading this woman to give up smoking is to educate her on the consequences of smoking, first on her baby, and then on herself. The next step will be to offer support and alternative means of giving up smoking.

Smoking produces nicotine and carboxyhamoglobin, which cross the placenta into the fetal circulation. The consequences of this combination include hypoxia, intrauterine growth restriction (IUGR), long-term neurodevelopmental disability, poorer intellect and cot death in the neonatal period. In addition, the fetus may develop polycythaemia, which may be complicated by neonatal venous thrombosis and associated mortality.

The consequences of smoking on the mother include chronic lung disease, placental abruption, hypertension and venous thrombo-embolism (VTE). Long-term consequences include lung cancer and arterial disease, heart failure, heart attacks and chronic obstructive airway disease. Although not a direct effect, the cost of purchasing cigarettes is high and this affects the patient's expenditure on other more important household goods.

Counselling on these consequences may not be enough to stop the patient from smoking. If she is motivated enough, she may still lapse occasionally. It is therefore important to consider the use of nicotine patches and gum, which may provide some fallback whenever there is a craving for a cigarette. The patient's partner or family members who smoke must be counselled as well and their role in supporting the smoking highlighted to them. The dreaded problem of sudden infant death syndrome (cot death) has been associated with smoking during and after pregnancy. Providing this information to the patient may persuade her to stop smoking.

It must be remembered that patients will cite friends who have smoked and had normal pregnancies. The definition of 'normal' is vague and the patient must be informed that the absence of a congenital abnormality does not mean a healthy baby. Often, smoking will have important but less obvious consequences that only manifest later in life. Lastly, the process must involve experts who are devoted to supporting and counselling such patients. These may be a support group, a midwife whose role is to counsel women to give up smoking in pregnancy or social workers.

3. A 22-year-old mother of two attends for antenatal care at 30 weeks' gestation with her partner and their two children. You observe that the children are rather subdued and also during your examination, you elicit tenderness over the left lower loin, which is also bruised. You suspect domestic violence. What subsequent steps will you take in her care and why?

Common mistakes

- Take a history about domestic violence from the patient and her partner
- Involve social workers, so that the children can be taken away to safety
- Confront the husband and ask him to stop
- Offer more frequent visits to the hospital and ensure that the midwife sees patients weekly

A good answer will include some or all of these points

- A difficult problem – requiring sensitivity, confidence-building and a non-threatening approach
- During examination, meticulously record all the suspected areas – being careful not to make them too obvious in the patient's hand-held notes as the partner may have access to them
- Need to identify when to discuss with patient without the risk of further violence. Confidentiality must be assured to ensure that the patient co-operates: in the clinic; after admission; at home by midwife or social worker
- Look for risk factors – alcohol, drug abuse, loss of job, impending divorce or separation, unplanned pregnancy
- Involve social workers to obtain more information and to help in the management when confirmed
- Notify the appropriate authority if necessary
- Once confirmed, is there violence towards the children? Who is the guilty one – mother or father? Are the children's lives in danger? Is unborn child at risk – may need to be on the at-risk register. Are the children on an at-risk register?
- May need to notify police

Sample answer

Domestic violence is a difficult problem to diagnose and manage. It requires sensitivity, tact, confidence-building with the patient and professional advice from those with expertise in the management of these patients. Once this is suspected, the management must be tailored to confirming this diagnosis before appropriate counselling could be offered.

The only way the suspicion may be confirmed will be from interviewing the woman. Certainly, this cannot be done in the presence of her partner. It may be possible, however, to create an opportunity to interview the patient on her own in the clinic but this must be done carefully as the partner may be suspicious. In fact, in most cases, the partner dominates and is commonly the one who speaks for the patient. If there is sufficient evidence to make this most likely, an alternative could be to admit the patient and interview her during the admission. During the interview, the patient needs to be certain that information provided will be treated in the strictest confidence and such an assurance should be provided voluntarily, otherwise the patent may not volunteer any information.

Additional information should be obtained from the patient during the interview. The aim of this is to identify other risk factors for domestic violence, such as alcohol, drugs, depression, stress – especially at work (this is more likely if the partner has just lost his job), the pregnancy was unplanned or there are extraneous factors, such as impending separation or divorce.

The physical examination should be meticulous and all suspicious areas documented carefully as they may be used as evidence. It will be difficult to examine the children in the clinic but social workers should be involved. They will visit the family and use their special skills to acquire the information. If the children are considered to be at risk, attempts must be made to protect them. The social workers will explore the possibility of the unborn child being at risk. It may also be that the children are on an at-risk register. If so, steps must be taken by the social workers to either remove the children from the care of the parents or remove the violent partner from the home.

If the suspicion is confirmed, various authorities need to become involved. The obstetric complications of domestic violence are preterm labour and placental abruption (if there is trauma to the abdomen). The patient must be educated on the warning signs of these two complications. She should also be educated on the need to report early if there is any trauma to the anterior abdominal wall.

Domestic violence is difficult to manage and unless the patient is willing to co-operate, it may be difficult to diagnose and managed properly. It is important, too, to remember that although the violence may be coming from the partner, it may also stem from the patient.

8

Abnormal presentation

1. External cephalic version (ECV), performed at 36 weeks' gestation, is not justified. Debate this statement.

2. Justify your management of a mother of three, at 38 weeks' gestation, with an unstable lie.

1. External cephalic version (ECV), performed at 36 weeks' gestation, is not justified. Debate this statement.

Common mistakes

- Discussing the process of external cephalic version (ECV)
- Complications of ECV
- Differences between ECV at 36 and 37 weeks' gestation
- Failing to debate (debate means – advantages, disadvantages and conclusion)

A good answer will include some or all of these points

- Advantages: easier; higher success rate at the time of ECV – more liquor and smaller baby; bypass preterm breech delivery before 37 weeks' gestation
- Disadvantages: large number of pregnancies will be offered ECV; some will undergo spontaneous version after ECV; complications – increased morbidity and neonatal complications
- Conclusions – on balance not advisable

Sample answer

Breech presentation at 36 weeks' gestation occurs in about five to seven per cent of singleton pregnancies. External cephalic version (ECV) has been shown to reduce the prevalence of breech presentation at term and, therefore, the need for Caesarean section for breech presentation in labour or at term. The timing of this procedure has significant bearings on the numbers presenting at term.

Although most experts recommend that ECV be performed at 37–38 weeks' gestation, it is accepted that it can also be performed at 36 weeks. At this gestation, the procedure is easier because there is more liquor around the fetus and therefore the chances of success are higher. It is also considered to be easier as the fetus is smaller. For pregnancies that may go into spontaneous labour before 37 weeks' gestation (preterm), performing ECV at this early gestation ensures that such patients present in labour with cephalic presentation. This will inevitably reduce the complications associated with preterm breech delivery.

However, there are significant disadvantages to performing ECV at this gestation. Although it may be easier and more likely to succeed, it may be argued that approximately 20–25 per cent of breech presentations at 36 weeks' gestation will turn spontaneously into cephalic presentation at term. These pregnancies, therefore, do not require intervention. Performing the procedure at 36 weeks' gestation will involve a larger population of patients. ECV is associated with complications, such as preterm labour, placental abruption and cord entanglement, all of which may necessitate immediate delivery. At 36 weeks' gestation, the risks of prematurity are still significant and, therefore, undertaking this procedure just because of an increased success rate, but with an increased risk of prematurity and its complications, may not be the ideal trade-off.

The timing of ECV should be influenced by the chances of success, associated complications and the number of patients requiring this procedure. On balance, although 36 weeks may be associated with a higher success rate, it is not the ideal time for this procedure. It should be performed at a gestational age when most cases that would have undergone spontaneous version have done so. In addition, it should be undertaken when fetal maturity is considered to be sufficient in case emergency delivery is necessary. On this basis, therefore, 36 weeks does not appear to be the best time for ECV. The best time for this procedure should be at 37 or more than 37 weeks' gestation.

2. Justify your management of a mother of three, at 38 weeks' gestation, with an unstable lie.

Common mistakes

- Offer elective lower-segment Caesarean section
- Offer a classical Caesarean section
- Discussing the complications of cord prolapse
- Advantages and disadvantages of external cephalic version (ECV)
- Different types of Caesarean section

A good answer will include some or all of these points

- Unstable lie considered a high-risk pregnancy
- May be complicated by ruptured membranes – cord or hand prolapse, difficult Caesarean section
- Admission into hospital?
- Advantages – monitored daily
- Rupture – immediate access to surgery and possible risks
- Disadvantage – patient away from family
- Expensive to hospital
- Management at home?
- Alternative to inpatient management
- Easy access to hospital
- Education on the complications
- Timing delivery
- ECV
- Stabilization indication
- Caesarean section if fails
- Caesarean section – emergency or elective
- Rupture membranes
- During version

Sample answer

Unstable lie at term is considered a high risk because of the potential problems of prelabour rupture of fetal membranes which may be accompanied by cord or hand prolapse. The management of such a patient is therefore aimed at minimizing potential complications. In some cases, the fetus reverts to longitudinal lie and these complications may not be applicable. Unfortunately, it is difficult to predict which pregnancies will revert spontaneously. Management of the pregnancy must, therefore, be on the assumption that this will not occur and thus these potential complications must be minimized.

The ideal management in most cases is to admit the patient to hospital. The cause of the unstable lie must be excluded. Causes include placenta praevia, pelvic tumours (such as ovarian cysts, uterine fibroids) and congenital malformations of the uterus. These may easily be excluded by an ultrasound scan. In the presence of these factors, a planned elective Caesarean section at 39 weeks' gestation will be the management of choice as the fetus is unlikely to revert to a longitudinal lie and, even if it did, a vaginal delivery would still be contraindicated.

However, where the causes have been excluded (as is the case in a majority of patients) the patient should be admitted to hospital until fetal lie is stabilized or the baby is delivered. The problem arises if the patient has other children at home (as has this woman) or refuses hospital admission. A detailed explanation of the reasons for offering hospital admission should be given to the patient. Where she refuses admission, it is essential that her concerns are addressed. There is a place for managing the patient at home provided she is within easy reach of the hospital and has been counselled to report immediately there are contractions (irrespective of how mild they are), any vaginal bleeding or suspicion of ruptured membranes. However, if she is not within easy reach of the hospital, admission is likely to be the only option.

Her subsequent management will consist of daily palpation of the fetal lie. Once the lie has been become longitudinal and remains so for at least 48 hours and, especially where the head is engaged, she should be allowed home and the spontaneous onset of labour awaited. However, if fetal lie remains unstable, external cephalic version (ECV) may be offered and, if this is successful and the lie remains stable, again she could be allowed home. The other option is to offer the patient stabilization induction at 41 weeks' gestation. This involves external version into a longitudinal position followed by syntocinon. Once adequate uterine contractions have been established, fetal membranes should be ruptured and labour allowed to progress as normal. In some cases, if the cervix is favourable, the membranes should be ruptured after version (with the fetus held in the longitudinal position) during the rupture. Once the liquor has drained, the likelihood of the fetus changing its lie becomes very small. Contractions could therefore be initiated with syntocinon.

In the event that the fetal membranes rupture with the fetus in the transverse of oblique position, the first step must be to exclude cord prolapse. Thereafter, the fetus must be delivered by Caesarean section. This is one of the few recognized indications for classical Caesarean section. However, where the Caesarean section is performed soon after the membranes have ruptured (that is, before all the liquor has drained), a lower-segment Caesarean section may be possible, especially if the back of the baby is posterior.

9

Preterm labour/premature rupture of fetal membranes

1. Evaluate the options available for the management of a woman who has had two previous preterm deliveries, at 24 and 26 weeks' gestation, respectively.

2. Preterm delivery is one of the most important causes of perinatal mortality. Evaluate the methods available for the prevention of preterm labour.

3. A 37-year-old primigravida, with a history of infertility, presents at 23 weeks' gestation with premature rupture of fetal membranes. Critically appraise your management of the patient.

1. Evaluate the options available for the management of a woman who has had two previous preterm deliveries, at 24 and 26 weeks' gestation, respectively.

Common mistakes

- Take a history and perform a physical examination
- Assume that she is pregnant
- Refer to tertiary centre
- Offer a cervical cerclage
- Admit for bedrest until delivery
- Induce labour at 34 weeks' gestation
- Offer prophylactic antibiotics
- Screen for cervical infections

A good answer will include some or all of these points

- Preterm labour is the most common cause pf perinatal mortality and morbidity
- The risk of recurrence in this patient is 30 per cent
- Management outside pregnancy – diagnosis of cervical weakness (incompetence), improvement in nutrition and change in lifestyle
- Management during pregnancy
  - Diagnosis of cervical weakness
  - Treatment of cervical weakness
  - Use of tocolytic agents
  - Use of steroids
- Place of confinement
- The role of biochemical testing for preterm labour
- Conclusion

Sample answer

Preterm labour is the most common cause of perinatal morbidity and mortality. It occurs in about five to ten per cent of all pregnancies. The recurrence risk in this patient is considered to be of the order of 30 per cent. Her management will depend on whether she is pregnant or not, and gestation.

Additional information about the preterm labours may suggest the cause. This must be obtained by questioning the patient. Classical cervical weakness (incompetence) will present with painless contractions, which may be accompanied by rupture of fetal membranes and quick vaginal delivery. The presence of such a history in this patient suggests this as the cause of the preterm deliveries. Although some experts may insist on confirmation by transvaginal ultrasound scan, in the classical case, this is unnecessary before the insertion of a cervical cerclage.

Outside pregnancy it may be possible to diagnose cervical weakness. The two traditional methods are hysterosalpingography (HSG) and retrograde cervical dilatation. The former is painful and uncomfortable, and there is the added risk of ascending infections. Similarly, retrograde dilatation may introduce infections. The two methods are intrusive and unreliable. For the diagnosis of cervical incompetence to be made, the cervix should be able to take a size 7 mm Hegar dilator without analgesia. The appearance of coning on HSG will also be diagnostic.

An important part of the management of this patient if she is not pregnant is to educate her to alter her lifestyle. Factors such as smoking, stress, alcohol, recreational drugs and poor diet all increase the risk of preterm labour. It may be necessary to involve other disciplines in this regard. Screening for infections such as bacterial vaginosis is useful, although it does not imply that this was the cause of her preterm labours. Similarly, infections of the urinary tract must be excluded.

During pregnancy, every effort must be made to identify asymptomatic bacteruria and bacterial vaginosis – all of which are treatable and recognized causes of preterm labour. The presence of beta-haemolytic streptococcus will influence her management in labour but will not necessarily influence the prevention of preterm labour. Ensuring that lifestyle changes introduced during pre-pregnancy are maintained is essential in pregnancy.

During the early second trimester, the patient will be offered serial cervical length and internal cervical os diameter assessment by transvaginal ultrasound scan. If the cervix becomes shorter, or is dilating, a cervical cerclage will be inserted. However, on the basis of her previous history, some authorities may insert a cervical stitch at 14–16 weeks. The advantage of this is that it ensures that the cervix is not changing significantly prior to the stitch. If the cervix becomes too short or is dilated, the insertion may be difficult and accompanied by complications which may precipitate preterm labour.

Admission for bedrest could be offered from 24 weeks. There is no scientific evidence that this is effective but it has a psychological effect on the patient. Steroids must be considered in view of her past history. She should be offered two doses of dexamethasone (12 mg i.m. 12 hours apart) at 24 weeks. Although subsequent weekly administration has been standard practice, the fear of neurodevelopmental damage to the fetus and intrauterine growth restriction (IUGR) has virtually condemned this practice. In the absence of any risk factors, adequate rest must be ensured, especially around 24 weeks. Tocolytic agents have almost no role in the management of this patient.

If she presented in preterm labour, the use of tocolytic agents may prolong the pregnancy and therefore outcome. There is some evidence to suggest that various biochemical markers, such as fibronectin, salivary oestriol and tenascin, may be used to predict which pregnancies will go into preterm labour. These are, however, not very predictive and therefore are only available as research tools. Preterm labour is likely to recur in this patient. Her management should therefore aim to minimize the risk of recurrence by identifying the cause and also instituting treatment that is effective and acceptable.

2. Preterm delivery is one of the most important causes of perinatal mortality. Evaluate the methods available for the prevention of preterm labour

Common mistakes

- Description of the procedures of cervical cerclage
- Stating that cervical cerclage is not of any proven benefit
- Inaccurate facts
- Detailed discussion on the causes of preterm labour
- Listing the causes of perinatal mortality
- Discussing the management of preterm labour

A good answer will include some or all of these points

- Identification of at-risk group
  - Previous preterm labour – recurrent risk – $\times 1 = 15$ per cent, $\times 2 = 20$–30 per cent
  - Lifestyle factors – low socio-economic group, smoking, drugs
  - Vaginal infections – bacterial vaginosis
- Education to minimize the risk factors, for example smoking, etc.
- Treatment of conditions which may lead to iatrogenic preterm labour
- Early identification of such conditions and preventing progression which may lead to preterm labour, for example pre-eclampsia
- Other systemic diseases, for example diabetes mellitus, etc. – good control?
- Infection screen – urine for asymptomatic bacteruria, high vaginal swab (HVS), ECS for bacterial vaginosis, beta-haemolytic streptococcus
- PROM – antibiotics? ORACLE
- Cervical weakness (incompetence) – ultrasound scanning and cerclage. Diagnosis outside pregnancy – hysterosalpingraphy (HSG) and cervical retrograde dilatation with Hegar's dilators
- Biochemical – fibronectin, oestriol, tenascin and prophylactic tocolytic agents?
- Multiple pregnancy – selective fetocide/fetal reduction
- Polyhydramnios – amnioreduction

Sample answer

Preterm labour accounts for about 33 per cent of all perinatal deaths. It occurs in about five to ten per cent of all pregnancies. The aetiology is unknown in a large number of cases. In some, however, this is iatrogenic; commonly secondary to other maternal complications of pregnancy, such as pre-eclampsia. Prevention of preterm labour is therefore an important part of perinatal medicine if its impact on morbidity and mortality is to be reduced.

Prevention of any condition must start with the identification of the at-risk group. Previous preterm labour is the single most predictive risk factor for recurrence. The risk of recurrence is 15 per cent after one preterm labour and this rises to 30 per cent after two and to 45 per cent after three. Other risk factors include lifestyle factors, such as smoking, recreational drugs, alcohol and low socio-economic class. Maternal systemic diseases, such as diabetes mellitus, and cardiorespiratory conditions increase the risk of preterm labour. Some of these risk factors can be identified from a detailed history from the patient. Although a physical examination may identify some risk factors, this is unlikely to be effective.

A cheap and effective means of preventing preterm labour must be to educate patients to change their lifestyles, for example stopping smoking and the use of recreational drugs. In addition, improvement in nutritional status and treatment of infections and systemic disease will significantly minimize the risk of preterm labour. Identification of infections is easy and effective. Routine urinalysis of samples from all pregnant women will identify those with asymptomatic bacteruria. Screening for diabetes mellitus and bacterial vaginosis will also identify others at risk. Once those at risk have been identified, appropriate treatment would significantly reduce the risk. Conditions amenable to treatment include urinary tract infections (symptomatic and asymptomatic) and genital tract infections (especially bacterial vaginosis).

The use of uterine artery Doppler scanning in patients at risk of pre-eclampsia may identify a subgroup of patients who may benefit from prophylactic aspirin and, in some cases, anti-coagulants to reduce the risk of pre-eclampsia. In addition, close monitoring of these patients will identify this complication early and afford an opportunity for treatment to reduce its severity and therefore the need for early delivery. Serial ultrasound scanning of the cervical length and canal in the at-risk group will identify those at risk of preterm labour. Such an investigation should be offered to all those with mid-trimester miscarriages, previous surgery on the cervix, multiple pregnancies and premature rupture of fetal membranes. The use of antibiotics in those with preterm rupture of fetal membranes has been shown to prolong pregnancy by a few days (ORACLE 2001). In patients with intact membranes presenting with preterm labour, however, this has not been shown to be beneficial.

The use of biochemical markers, such as fetal fibronectin (FFN), salivary oestriol and tenascin, for the prediction of preterm labour is associated with poor predictive values. However, these may be used in conjuction with other tests, such as cervical scanning. ffN, for example, may be able to identify a subgroup of patients likely to go into preterm labour and better monitoring of these patients may prolong pregnancy. However, these methods are expensive and require complex calculations of ratios. Therefore, most are not available as a clinical aid to predict preterm labour.

Although polyhydramnios and multiple pregnancy are not common causes of preterm labour, these are well-recognized, and selective fetocide and amnioreduction have been shown to reduce the risk of preterm labour. The latter is more common in pregnancies of higher order – usually above two.

Although preterm labour is predictable in some groups of patients, it is often unpredictable in a large majority. It is therefore not possible to offer some of these screening tools to the general population because of logistical and manpower limitations. Screening and targeted treatment, therefore, can only be to a selected group of patients.

3. A 37-year-old primigravida, with a history of infertility, presents at 23 weeks' gestation with premature rupture of fetal membranes. Critically appraise your management of the patient.

Common mistakes

- Repeating the question
- Being very pedantic in your answer
- Performing repeated high vaginal and endocervical swabs
- Terminating the pregnancy because viability has not been achieved – the only option!

A good answer will include some or all of these points

- Appreciate anxiety and provide supportive care
- Monitor
  - Four-hourly temperature, pulse and respiration (TPR) – advantages and disadvantages
  - High vaginal swabs (HVS) – daily, weekly or low vaginal swabs?
  - C-reactive protein
  - Serial full blood counts (FBCs)
  - Cardiotographs (CTGs)? When do you start and how reliable?
  - Ultrasound – why and when. Cervical length, liquor volume, cord compression, fetal anomalies?
- Neonatologist involvement at tertiary centre
- Steroids – weekly? Value of repeated administration, any side-effects?
- Antibiotics? Any value? ORACLE results
- Tocolysis is indicated – any value?
- Amnioinfusion – any value?
- Treatment of the amniorrhexis – blood patch? Fetoscopic mesh insertion? How valuable and successful?
- Delivery – when and how
- Monitoring – inpatient versus outpatient

Sample answer

In the management of this patient, it is imperative to appreciate the degree of anxiety she must have and to offer her supportive care. This will be generated from the previous history of infertility and her age. Empathy should therefore be an important part of her management. She needs to be admitted to start with and subsequent management (at least at the outset should be on an inpatient basis).

The most common complications that may occur in this patient are preterm labour, chorioamnionitis and significant oligohydramnios, leading to pulmonary hypoplasia. This fetus is one week from viability and, taking into account her reproductive history, it would be unreasonable to offer her a termination at this gestation on account of the potential risks. This is unlikely to be acceptable and may arouse antagonism from the patient and her partner.

Initial investigations to be performed to establish a baseline for subsequent comparisons include a full blood count (FBC) (specifically the white cell count (WCC) and differentials), a C-reactive protein and a high vaginal swab for microscopy, culture and sensitivity during confirmation of the rupture. Unfortunately, these parameters are not very sensitive in predicting choroamnionitis. For example, C-reactive protein is unreliable, although serial levels showing a consistent rise will be suggestive of infection but not necessarily from the uterus. Similarly, a rise in WCC, which is not uncommon in pregnancy, may also be indicative of infection anywhere in the body. However, serial values showing significant changes will raise suspicions of chorioamnionitis unless other sources of infection can be identified. The FBC and C-reactive proteins need to be repeated at least twice-weekly.

Early maternal manifestations of chorioamnionitis are pyrexia, tachycardia and tachypnoea. These may be identified by four-hourly temperature, pulse and respiratory (TPR) rate recordings. These need to be performed on this patient even if she is to be managed on an outpatient basis. In addition to these, daily palpation of the lower abdomen for tenderness and examination of a pad for the colour of liquor and its smell will help in identifying early chorioamnionitis. Unfortunately, these signs may not always be present with infections. The value of serial vaginal swabs is limited, as frequent introduction of the swabs in the vagina may increase the risk of ascending chorioamnionitis. Some argue that low vaginal swabs may be useful but these may only yield normal lower genital tract flora of no clinical significance. The diagnosis of beta-haemolytic streptococcus will, however, influence management.

An ultrasound scan in this patient will quantify liquor volume, assess fetal growth and afford an opportunity for Doppler studies of the umbilical and other fetal vessels. Serial ultrasound scans will allow for estimation of the liquor volume but, more importantly, will enable a visual subjective assessment of the lung volume and fetal breathing which is associated with a better prognosis. In the absence of liquor the prognosis is poor and under these circumstances amnioinfusion must be considered. Problems with this procedure include infections and failure to achieve any satisfactory residual volume as it may leak out as soon as it is infused. This is not only a tedious process for the clinician but it is uncomfortable to the patient and may not be successful.

Neonatologists must be involved in the management of this patient. They will provide information about the chances of survival at different gestational ages, the neonatal course and management, and possible complications. Timing delivery must also be decided in close liaison with neonatologists.

Steroids should be administered (dexamethasone given in two doses of 12 mg i.m. at 12 hours apart). This will accelerate lung maturity. Although mostly given after 24 weeks' gestation, there is a case for offering them to this patient. Whether this is followed by weekly booster is increasingly becoming controversial in view of recent publications suggesting an association with neurodevelopmental disability and intrauterine growth restriction (IUGR). Tocolytic agents may be used if the patient starts having contractions, but these have not been shown to significantly prolong pregnancy. The recently concluded MRC ORACLE trial concluded that prophylactic antibiotics in these patients do not only prolong pregnancy, but reduce perinatal morbidity. Erythromycin will therefore be offered to the patient after admission.

Various experiments suggest that the treatment of amniorrhexis by use of a blood patch or fetoscopic insertion of a mesh over the rupture site may improve outcome. In this patient, if this expertise is available, these options must be considered. A controversial issue is whether to manage the patient as an inpatient or as an outpatient. The advantage of inpatient care is close monitoring and early intervention when necessary. In addition, bedrest can be enforced. Nowadays, some sensible and well-motivated patients may be able to monitor themselves at home and, with the help of midwives, undertake all the serial monitoring offered in the hospital. In this patient, in view of the very high risk, on balance it may be advisable to monitor her as an inpatient. Cardiotocography (CTG) is an important part of fetal monitoring, especially as cord compression may occur with oligohydramnios. At this very early gestation this will not be instituted as an abnormal trace is difficult to interpret and, in addition, adopting a more proactive approach may not be the best option. The timing of this monitoring will therefore remain controversial. However, it may be started between 25 and 26 weeks – gestational ages at which a Caesarean section may be considered if there is need to do one.

The timing and mode of delivery depends on several factors. These include gestational age, the availability of neonatal intensive care (NICU) facilities and the perceived chances of survival. If there are no NICU facilities, *in utero* transfer is the best option. At the lower end of the gestational age spectrum delivery is difficult and Caesarean section may be the only option if the baby is to be given the best chances of survival. However, if survival is not possible, after appropriate counselling, a vaginal delivery may be allowed. The management of this patient therefore poses several problems which must be addressed together or individually.

10

Anaesthetic disorders in pregnancy

1. Mendelson's syndrome is a recognized cause of maternal mortality and morbidity. What steps are normally taken to minimize this complication in pregnancy/labour?

2. How may complications of epidural analgesia be recognized and how may they be avoided?

3. Briefly outline the advantages and disadvantages of epidural and general anaesthesia (GA) in labour.

1. Mendelson's syndrome is a recognized cause of maternal mortality and morbidity. What steps are normally taken to minimize this complication in pregnancy/labour?

Common mistakes

- Should be managed only by anaesthetist
- Discussing the management of Mendelson's syndrome
- Process of induction – unnecessary details (drugs etc.)
- Minimizing Caesarean section rates

A good answer will include some or all of these points

- Definition of condition
- Increased risk in pregnancy – why?
- Measures to minimize complications: diet; antacids; empty stomach: epidural/regional preferred to general anaesthesia (GA); cricoid pressure; cuffed endotracheal tubes; extubation in lateral position
- Early recognition and treatment

Sample answer

Mendelson's syndrome or 'aspiration pneumonia' is a chemical pneumonitis that is common in labour or during operative deliveries and has a high morbidity and mortality. The risk of this complication is higher in pregnancy because of the physiological changes occurring. These include slowed gastric emptying, displacement of the stomach into the thorax by the gravid uterus and therefore the removal of the protective oesophago-gastric sphincter.

Measures that may be taken to minimize this complication range from preventative to early diagnosis and treatment. Preventative measures must guard against vomiting and aspiration. This complication most commonly occurs at the time of induction of general anaesthesia (GA). Avoiding or reducing the rate of GA in obstetric units will significantly reduce the risk of this complication. Although it may occur during the administration of regional anaesthesia, the risks are not as high as during GA. Where an operative delivery is planned, as in the case of elective Caesarean section, or anticipated, an empty stomach is essential. However, although this may be practicable for elective cases, it is not feasible in patients during induction of labour. However, during this process, a light diet should be provided as it is easier for this to be absorbed. Overnight fasting ensures that the stomach is empty before surgery.

The use of antacids has become universal in labour and before surgery. During labour, every patient should be given an antacid, such as sodium citrate. This neutralizes the acid in the stomach and reduces the risk of chemical pneumonitis should the patient vomit and aspirate. For those undergoing surgery, this is administered in the form of an H_2-antagonist (Zantac) overnight and on the morning of surgery. For emergency Caesarean sections, sodium citrate should be given before induction of GA. A combination of this and anti-emetics, such as metoclopramide will significantly reduce the risk of vomiting and therefore aspiration. In some cases of emergency Caesarean section, intravenous H_2-antagonists may be administered.

An important procedure to minimize the risk of aspiration is the application of cricoid pressure during intubation. This helps to prevent vomiting and aspiration. A cuffed endoctracheal tube prevents aspiration even if the patient vomits. A suction machine, readily available, will ensure that all vomit is sucked out of the patient's mouth and throat. Vomiting and aspiration can occur during extubation. This should therefore be performed preferably with the patient in the lateral position and head down with readiness to suck if there is any vomiting.

Once this complication has occurred, early recognition and prompt treatment will minimize the consequences. Recognizing that this complication can occur in normal labouring women is vital. Early symptoms include tachypnoea, cyanosis and rhonchi in the chest. Treatment must include steroids, antibiotics and, if necessary, ventilation. A combination of these measures will reduce the risk of this complication and minimize the consequences when it occurs.

2. How may complications of epidural analgesia be recognized and how may they be avoided?

Common mistakes

- Discussing the indications for epidural anaesthesia
- Details of how epidurals are performed
- Counselling patients about complications
- Ensure that appropriate instruments are available

A good answer will include some or all of these points

- Most effective form of analgesia in labour
- Offered for Caesarean section as well
- Complications: unblocked segments; weakness of the legs; postpartum pain; retention of urine; hypotension; dural tap; intrathecal injection of local anaesthetic; spinal block; others
- Recognition and avoiding them

Sample answer

Epidural analgesia is increasingly regarded as one of the most effective and popular forms of analgesia during labour and Caesarean section in the UK. This trend is related to the increased safety attributed to this technique and the seemingly fewer complications that occur with its use. However, despite the increasing use and demonstrated safety, there are recognized complications, some of which may be associated with mortality or severe morbidity.

These complications include weakness of the legs, unblocked segments, postpartum pain, retention of urine, hypotension, dural tap and intrathecal injection of local anaesthetic agents. Fortunately, most of these are uncommon. An unblocked segment is said to occur in about 10–15 per cent of patients. This is easily recognized by persistent pain with each contraction. This pain tends to be located especially in the groin region. It can be ameliorated by changing the position of the patient and increasing the level of the block or the concentration of the anaesthetic agent. Occasionally, the epidural may have to be re-sited.

Some weakness of the legs is expected with most epidurals. However, where there is muscle paralysis the leg may become very weak. When the patient complaints of this, it can be treated by administering a weaker concentration of the local anaesthetic agent. Postpartum pain is often described as excruciating pain in the perineum and especially at the episiotomy site. This may only be treated with local or mild systemic analgesic agents. Urinary retention may occur during labour or afterwards, when the epidural has worn off. Often, this is because the loss of sensation during the epidural causes distension of the bladder and subsequent loss of the sensation to void. If this is prolonged, the patient may suffer from urinary retention after the epidural has worn off. It should be treated with catheterization and in some cases the catheter should remain *in situ* for at least 24 hours.

Hypotension is a common complication of epidural anaesthesia. This may cause fetal hypoxia and bradycardia associated with decelerations. This is due to reduced venous return to the heart. An epidural anaesthetic blocks the sympathetic and sensory nerves to the lower limbs, causes vasodilatation and pulling of blood into the lower limbs. This is recognized by a drop in maternal blood pressure and fetal bradycardia. To prevent this, a preload is often advised. When it occurs, the mother should be placed on her left side and intravenous (i.v.) fluid administered. Very rarely, vasopressors may be used.

Another uncommon but potentially fatal complication is intrathecal injection of the local anaesthetic. The greatest risk of this complication is that of complete spinal paralysis with complete apnoea or signs of respiratory insufficiency. Urgent intervention is required to prevent mortality. This takes the form of intubation and ventilation. A clinician experienced in resuscitation should therefore be available when an epidural is being sited. A more common complication is an accidental dural tap/puncture. This occurs in about one to two per cent of all cases. It is recognized from the passage of cerebrospinal fluid (CSF) through the needle, which is larger than spinal needles. The patient may complain of headache. Treatment is either by means of a blood patch or infusing a ringer-lactate solution into the epidural space with the patient confined to bed for three or four days.

Epidural analgesia is recognized to be associated with backache in the long term. This is unlikely to be recognized at the time of siting the epidural and these patients may benefit from physiotherapy and analgesics.

3. Briefly outline the advantages and disadvantages of epidural and general anaesthesia (GA) in labour.

Common mistakes

- Listing the contraindications for either epidural or general anaesthesia (GA)
- Describing in details how to site an epidural anaesthetic
- Details of other methods of pain relief in labour
- Differences between spinal and epidural anaesthesia
- Details of the mobile epidural
- Failing to outline the advantages and disadvantages of both forms of anaesthesia

A good answer will include some or all of these points

- General anaesthesia – advantages: quick to administer; patient relaxed and asleep; surgeon and staff less tense; disadvantages: during induction blood pressure rises and increases the risk of cardiovascular accident (CVA), risk of aspiration higher as well; recovery risk of aspiration; risk of chest infections; recovery from anaesthesia longer; requires pain relief postoperatively; can only be offered during operative delivery
- Epidural – advantages: patient awake; partner available during delivery; risk of aspiration reduced; postoperative recovery shorter; used for analgesia for the immediate postoperative period; used for pain relief during labour; disadvantages: backache; dural tap; no guarantee that it will work; prolongs first and second stage and therefore increases operative deliveries; where rapid intervention is required, may not be suitable; where there is massive haemorrhage, patient and partner anxiety may affect staff

Sample answer

Epidural analgesia and anaesthesia are increasingly becoming the most potent forms of pain relief in labour, and anaesthesia for operative deliveries, respectively. With the evolution of obstetric anaesthesia as a discipline, most good units in the UK have epidural rates of over 30 per cent. The increasing use of this form of pain relief is mainly due to the advantages it confers over other forms of pain relief, but there are also several disadvantages.

The main advantages of epidural compared to general anaesthesia (GA) include the lesser risk of aspiration, quicker mobility after surgery (and therefore a lower risk of venous thrombo-emboloism, VTE), faster postoperative recovery (with some patients eating soon after surgery), continuous use of the epidural anaesthetic for postoperative pain relief, the opportunity for the partner or family member to be present at the time of delivery and, for the patient herself, an opportunity to cherish the very moment of delivery. These are advantages compared to GA for operative deliveries. For pain relief in labour, epidural anaesthetics offer prolonged and effective pain relief, and easy conversion to potent anaesthesia for surgery if necessary. In hypertensive patients, epidural anaesthesia lowers the blood pressure and therefore reduces the risk of CVAs and fits. Disadvantages include the potential for a dural tap, which may be complicated by headaches, prolonged backache and infection in the spine. Occasionally, it may inadvertently become a spinal block, which may be total, requiring immediate ventilation of the patient. Other disadvantages include the potential psychological distress complications of surgery may cause to the patient and her partner or relative, and the pressure their presence or awareness of these complications, may have on staff. When used for pain relief, epidural anaesthesia may cause a delay in the first and second stages of labour and be associated with an increase in the rate of assisted vaginal deliveries.

GA, on the other hand, has advantages such as rapid administration whenever there is the need to act quickly, better relaxation and the potential to paralyse the patient, and absence of the external pressure on staff from the patient or her partner. However, GA is associated with the following disadvantages: a rapid rise in blood pressure during induction (which may precipitate a stroke in a hypertensive patient); increased risk of aspiration (Mendelson's syndrome) during induction and waking up from anaesthesia; increased risk of chest infections; the need for additional pain relief during recovery from surgery; and slower post-operative recovery. The risk of venous thrombo-embolism (VTE) is higher because of the slower recovery. It cannot be used for pain relief during labour and requires a more experienced anaesthetist to administer.

11

Intrauterine and intrapartum stillbirth

1. A 25-year-old schoolteacher has just had a stillbirth. She refused to have an autopsy on the baby. She has returned to the clinic for follow-up. Summarize your approach to her care.

2. A patient returned for a postnatal follow-up visit following the delivery of an intrauterine fetal death. The postmortem examination showed that the fetus died from multiple severe congenital malformations. How will you counsel her?

3. How will you counsel a couple whose baby died in the neonatal period from an autosomal recessive condition?

4. A 32-year-old patient who had a neonatal death two years ago is now 20 weeks into her second pregnancy. Her previous pregnancy had been uncomplicated but at 37 weeks' gestation, she had a prolonged labour which was followed by a failed ventouse and forceps and then an emergency Caesarean section of a very asphyxiated baby who died one week after delivery, from intracranial haemorrhage. She wishes to be delivered by an elective Caesarean section at 36 weeks' gestation. Debate the advantages and disadvantages of her decision.

1. A 25-year-old schoolteacher has just had a stillbirth. She refused to have an autopsy on the baby. She has returned to the clinic for follow-up. Summarize your approach to her care.

Common mistakes

- Blame her for not having had a postmortem
- Refer to perinatologist
- Take a history and offer investigations (which and why?)
- Offer chorionic villus sampling (CVS)/amniocentesis in next pregnancy – for what?
- Discuss prepregnancy counselling and dietary control (about what)
- Refer to geneticist

A good answer will include some or all of these points

- Difficult problem – there may be no answer (no explanation for the stillbirth)
- Offer support and empathy
- Summarize the events that culminated in the delivery of the stillbirth
- Go through investigations that were performed – ensure that results are available
- Arrive at conclusions if possible
- Counsel about next pregnancy
- Refer to other experts if necessary
- Document plan in notes and write to general practitioner (GP)/midwife in community

Sample answer

The occurrence of an intrauterine death is a tragedy and counselling demands skill, empathy and a through understanding of the pathology involved in the situation. Often, this latter part is provided by a postmortem examination. Where this is declined, as in this case, extreme care must be exercised in not blaming the parents for the inability to provide answers. The reasons for this are twofold: first, there is no guarantee that an autopsy would have provided an answer, and second, blaming the parents may worsen their grief.

When counselling this patient, the first approach would be to ensure that adequate sympathy is offered and support provided, with obvious demonstration of empathy. It would be advisable to briefly go through the sequence of events that resulted in the delivery and to be positive about the aspects of the pregnancy and delivery of which she was part. For example, if the patient permitted some investigations to be undertaken, this would be praised. However, it is important to be factual and therefore the lack of an autopsy should also be discussed. That this might not have provided an answer anyway is an important supportive statement.

The results of infection screen on the fetus, mother and any other blood tests from the mother and father have to be discussed in detail, and all abnormalities pointed out, with the implications discussed. Often, nothing abnormal is found. Such negative findings need to be stressed positively, especially in relation to the recurrence of this complication. If the results are thought to have contributed to the death of the fetus, this must be approached sensitively. It is essential that the means of preventing or minimizing the cause of the abnormality, if available, are introduced at this stage. It would reassure the couple that, although it happened last time, with adequate treatment this would be unlikely to occur again. In the unlikely event that the implications of the abnormal result are unknown, the patient must be informed of this and efforts made to obtain further information for her.

In most cases, there will be no obvious cause for the stillbirth. If there is one, the risk of its recurrence must be discussed. In addition, the possibility of prenatal diagnosis, where there is an obvious cause of death, should be considered and discussed. Plans for the next pregnancy should also be discussed and documented in the patient's notes. In some cases, it may not be possible to identify the exact syndrome involved, especially where external examination findings identified possible features of a syndrome. Referral to a geneticist may therefore be necessary. This process is incomplete without writing to the patient and her general practitioner (GP) with plans for her management in a subsequent pregnancy. Where there is a cause, and there are other experts better equipped to deal with it, the patient should be referred for counselling. Counselling should not be seen as a single-visit process. The patient should be encouraged to seek support and offered further appointments if considered necessary.

2. A patient returned for a postnatal follow-up visit following the delivery of an intrauterine fetal death. The postmortem examination showed that the fetus died from multiple severe congenital malformations. How will you counsel her?

Common mistakes

- Discussing chorionic villus sampling (CVS) or amniocentesis
- Discussing how to manage a woman whose baby has been diagnosed as having congenital abnormalities
- You have not been told that the congenital malformations are recurrent or are chromosomal
- Need to start trying immediately as Down syndrome risk increases with age!!
- No one has said the baby had Down syndrome

A good answer will include some or all of these points

- Need for empathy
- Use of appropriate language
- Importance of preparation for the visit – may be need to research on malformations
- Take the patient through antenatal events
- Explain and relate antenatal findings, if any, and autopsy findings and differences, if any
- Other investigation results – (discuss normal and abnormal)
- Any other obvious explanation for the malformations, such as epilepsy, diabetes mellitus, drugs, etc. – discuss
- Does the patient and her partner need to see a geneticist?
- Help with grieving process – Stillbirth and Neonatal Deaths Society (SANDS), etc.
- Recurrence risk – if known
- Prepregnancy advice – diet, etc.
- Plan for next pregnancy
- Detailed scan – at tertiary level
- Karyotyping in pregnancy
- Neonatologist involvement

Sample answer

When counselling the patient empathy must be demonstrated. The language and communication used should be appropriate to ensure that comprehension is maximum. It is important to prepare for the visit by gathering all the investigations performed on the mother and fetus beforehand. If there are any results that are difficult to interpret, these must be clarified with the appropriate authorities, or information about them sought from the literature, before seeing the patient.

The first step is to express sympathy and then take the patient through any antenatal events that you feel are essential. An explanation of the results of investigations and their implications is then offered. It is not necessary to offer details of some investigations, for example details of how the autopsy was conducted. There may be other explanations for the stillbirth. Conditions such as diabetes, epilepsy and its drug treatment, and other teratogenic drugs, which might be implicated should be identified and discussed in detail.

Information should then be provided about support groups if necessary. Groups such as SANDS would provide telephone counselling and information leaflets about how to cope with a stillbirth. Occasionally, the patient and her partner may have to be referred to another expert (for example, a geneticist) for counselling about recurrence risks and the possibility of pre-natal diagnosis. If the risk of recurrence is known, it should be discussed.

After counselling about the stillbirth, details about the next pregnancy should be discussed and documented. A plan for the identification of these abnormalities must be clearly documented and explained to the patient. If these are associated with a chromosomal abnormality, prenatal karyotyping should be discussed. The options of amniocentesis and chorionic villus sampling (CVS) would be discussed, but details would be unnecessary at this stage. Where necessary, a neonatologist should be involved so as to discuss the potential problems of babies with such malformations when they are born alive. If necessary, prepregnancy dietary advice should be offered. Counselling of patients like this is easier where the cause of the stillbirth is known. Where it is unknown, it is more difficult to come to terms with it. However, counselling is incomplete without communication with the patient's general practitioner (GP), who will offer support in the community. The midwife ought to be involved in this process and all information relevant to the diagnosis of the cause should be passed on to the midwife and the GP.

3. How will you counsel a couple whose baby died in the neonatal period from an auto-somal recessive condition?

Common mistakes

- Enquire about any previous normal child – this history should be obtained from the couple – what is the relevance of this?
- The recessive condition must be identified – is this not obvious?
- Offer termination in the next pregnancy and discuss surrogacy or adoption as their only option
- Quoting/regurgitating what the general approach is from textbooks
- Failing to focus your answer on this couple

A good answer will include some or all of these points

- Recessive condition – both parents are carriers and are unaffected
- Risks of: having and affected child – 25 per cent (one in four) – having a carrier child – 50 per cent (one in two) – having a normal child – 25 per cent (one in four)
- The condition is likely to be a lethal one (unless there was mutation) – therefore is it lethal? Is that information available?
- Is the condition known (is it defined?) – test both parents to confirm that it is not a mutation
- If prenatal diagnosis is possible, discuss options – chorionic villus sampling (CVS)/amniocentesis, etc.
- If prenatal diagnosis not possible – any obvious markers on ultrasound that may help identify condition? If none, parents must understand risks involved
- Prenatal diagnosis available – affected – termination of pregnancy
- Pre-implantation diagnosis – available?
- Other option – egg donation, artificial insemination with donor sperm and adoption

Sample answer

An autosomal recessive condition is one, which will only manifest if homozygously present in the offspring. This couple must each carry the recessive trait, although it is possible that a mutation could result in the expression of a recessive condition.

When counselling this couple, the first step will be to discuss the inheritance pattern of the condition. The risk of having a normal child if both parents are carriers is 25 per cent (one in four); having an affected child is 25 per cent (one in four) and having a carrier child is 50 per cent (one in two). The condition is likely to be lethal since the baby died from it. There may, of course, be mutations, which may reduce the severity of the disease but this cannot be predicted.

It is important to ascertain that the condition has been defined and that both parents have been tested to confirm that they are carriers. An important aspect of counselling is to discuss prenatal diagnosis. The options will include chorionic villus sampling (CVS) and amniocentesis. If prenatal diagnosis is not possible, are there any possible soft markers on ultrasound and how soon can they be identified. It may be possible to diagnose this condition with ultrasound (if there are obvious markers). If it is not possible to diagnose the condition, from either amniocentesis or CVS or from ultrasound scan, the parents must be informed of the chances of having an affected baby. If this is possible then termination may be offered for an affected fetus. It may also be necessary to refer the couple to an unit where there are facilities for making a diagnosis. The recent advances in molecular biology techniques have increased the number of conditions that can be diagnosed pre-implantation. If this option is available, the couple should be counselled appropriately and referred to the most relevant unit.

The last options for them will include artificial insemination with donor sperms, GIFT or *in vitro* fertilization (IVF) with donor eggs or adoption where the couple are unwilling to take any chances or cannot afford other options. The counselling should ideally involve clinical geneticists.

4. A 32-year-old patient who had a neonatal death two years ago is now 20 weeks into her second pregnancy. Her previous pregnancy had been uncomplicated but at 37 weeks' gestation, she had a prolonged labour which was followed by a failed ventouse and forceps and then an emergency Caesarean section of a very asphyxiated baby who died one week after delivery, from intracranial haemorrhage. She wishes to be delivered by an elective Caesarean section at 36 weeks' gestation. Debate the advantages and disadvantages of her decision.

Common mistakes

- Discussing how to monitor the pregnancy – advantages and disadvantages of consultant-led care versus midwifery care, hospital versus community care
- Refer patient to a specialist unit
- Failing to debate
- Simply outlining how you will manage her
- Involving a psychiatrist

A good answer will include some or all of these points

- Traumatic experience – needs to be avoided. Appropriate counselling pivotal to a successful (psychological) outcome
- Delivery at 36 weeks' gestation
  - Psychological benefit to the patient (37 weeks when last complication occurred not reached)
  - Risk of respiratory distress syndrome (RDS) and transient tachypnoea of the new-born (TTN) (associated with complications of neonatal intensive care unit (NICU) admission, for example iatrogenic infection and chronic lung disease)
  - Cervix unripe therefore likely to be a Caesarean section or a difficult induction with risk of uterine rupture
- How to deliver – Caesarean section – morbidity and mortality associated with it (infections, etc.)
  - Subsequent pregnancies – delivery by Caesarean section recommended, venous thrombo-embolism (VTE)
  - Advantages – avoids fear of repeat traumatic experience
  - Planned and therefore unlikely to go into spontaneous labour
- Conclusion – timing and counselling, empathy and support. Reassurance about planned delivery and closer monitoring with specific instructions – most likely to result in good outcome

Sample answer

This patient has been through a very traumatic experience, which should be avoided in the current pregnancy. She needs to be reassured that everything will be done to avoid a repetition of the previous pregnancy, although a cast iron guarantee cannot be given. It may even be necessary to offer counselling from a clinical psychologist.

Her demand for elective delivery by Caesarean section at 36 weeks is a sensible and logical one. This will obviously be of an important psychological benefit to the patient. However, while it will reduce her anxiety and fear of reaching 37 weeks' gestation, delivering at this gestation is associated with possible neonatal complications. These include transient tachypnoea of the newborn (TTN) and respiratory distress syndrome (RDS), all of which are likely to require admission into the neonatal intensive care unit (NICU). Such an admission may be associated with nosocomial infections acquired on the unit. The proportion of babies with long-term chronic lung disease delivered at 36 weeks' gestation is higher that that at 37–38 weeks. Delivering by Caesarean section is also associated with maternal morbidity and possibly an effect on subsequent pregnancies and general health in later years. The advantages of delivery by Caesarean section at this gestation include the avoidance of uncertainty about the delivery and complete prevention of the psychological fear which will certainly grip her around the time of her last experience, and more so when she goes into labour. Although planning to deliver at this early gestation may seem logical, there is also the possibility that she may go into spontaneous labour before this time. If that were to happen, the fear and anxiety related to her last experience will become evident.

The other option would be to induce and hope for a vaginal delivery at 36 weeks' gestation. At this gestation, the cervix is unlikely to be ripe. In addition, an early induction is more likely to be protracted and the longer the interval between induction and delivery, the more anxious the patient will be. Therefore this is not an option.

In the management of this patient, although the decision to deliver early is a reasonable request, appropriate counselling, empathy and support, coupled with reassurance that a planned delivery and closer monitoring may minimize the psychological trauma of her last experience and allow the pregnancy to progress beyond 36 weeks' gestation. An elective Caesarean section is not unreasonable, but this could be planned for 38 weeks or later, with the proviso that if the patient went into labour before then, an emergency Caesarean section could be performed. A vaginal delivery is not unrealistic, but the stress associated with this may be difficult for the patient to cope with.

12

Labour, including induction – normal/abnormal

1. Induction of post-term pregnancies at or before 42 weeks is associated with a significant reduction in perinatal mortality. Debate the statement.

2. Evaluate the different manoeuvres you will apply to the management of shoulder dystocia.

3. What measures will you take to minimize the risk of uterine rupture at induction in a woman who has had a previous Caesarean section and how will you recognize it?

4. Critically appraise the methods of induction of labour of an uncomplicated pregnancy at 41 weeks' gestation in a grande multipara.

5. A primigravida was admitted in spontaneous labour at 40 weeks' gestation 14 hours ago. Fetal membranes had ruptured spontaneously 12 hours before admission. Her cervix was 3 cm on admission. The cervix has remained at 8 cm for the last four hours and, in addition, she now has a pyrexia of 37.8 °C. The fetal heart rate is, however, normal. Justify your management of this patient.

1. Induction of post-term pregnancies at or before 42 weeks is associated with a significant reduction in perinatal mortality. Debate the statement.

Common mistakes

- Listing the indications for induction
- Details of the different methods of induction – oral prostaglandins, vaginal, Foley's catheters etc.
- How to date pregnancies to reduce the number of inductions at 42 weeks' gestation
- Complication of induction of labour
- Stating that inductions should only be done at 41 weeks

A good answer will include some or all of these points

- Induction at this gestation is common (most common indication for induction of labour)
- Perinatal mortality rises after 42 weeks' gestation
- To save one death, need to induce 500 pregnancies
- Complications of induction – increased Caesarean section (theoretical rather than real), postpartum haemorrhage, prolonged hospitalization and risk of venous thrombo-embolism (VTE)
- Disadvantages – intervention
- Failure to date pregnancies properly means improper inductions
- Pressure on staff – parental demands/expectations
- Neonatal encephalopathy decreased after 41–42 weeks' gestation
- Cerebral palsy increased especially in primigravidas (if induced before 41 weeks)
- Meconium staining associated with decreased cord arterial pH. Meconium aspiration syndrome increased after 42 weeks
- Dystocia increased with delivery after 42 weeks' gestation
- Emergency Caesarean section increased – for failure to progress and fetal distress
- Benefits of induction
- Decreased risk of perinatal death
    - Meconium liquor
    - Increased risk of neonatal jaundice
    - Caesarean section rate not increased (Hannah *et al.*, 2000)
- Women's view
- Attitude of care-givers
- Practical consideration – paid maternity leave

Sample answer

Induction of labour is a common obstetric intervention on delivery suites. The most common indication is 'postdates' (pregnancies beyond 40 weeks' gestation). The induction rate for this indication varies from 10 per cent to 20 per cent, depending on the unit. The rationale for these inductions is the increased risk of stillbirth and complications which may result in peri-natal death, including a failing placenta.

Perinatal mortality falls to a trough between 38 and 40 weeks' gestation and then starts to rise after 41 weeks' gestation. Induction at or before 42 weeks' gestation is said to be at the time when the perinatal mortality is beginning to rise, but is not high enough to warrant immediate delivery. Cardozo et al. (1986), in a randomized trial, demonstrated that, in order to reduce one perinatal mortality at or before 42 weeks' gestation, at least 500 inductions have to be performed.

Although there are those who argue against induction and regard it as an unnecessary inter-vention, parents are increasingly demanding intervention at term. Such incessant demands put undue pressure on staff who, in most cases, are inclined to give in to these demands, especially in the context of the blame culture and the increasingly litiginous environment in the UK.

Inductions are associated with prolonged hospitalization, a higher postpartum haemor-rhage rate and dysfunctional labour. A large proportion of patients end up having their labours augmented. The use of oxytocic agents in women undergoing induction of labour is significantly higher than that in those undergoing spontaneous labour. This is associated with postpartum haemorrhage and neonatal jaundice. In the past it has been argued that Caesarean section rates were higher in those who had inductions, but modern approaches to induction of labour have significantly reduced the Caesarean section rate. However, the consequences of hospitalization (increased risk of deep vein thrombo-embolism, VTE) remain higher in this group. For some patients, interference with the natural process is often unacceptable and considered unnecessarily intrusive.

Although induction of labour at or just before 42 weeks is associated with a lower perinatal mortality and morbidity, the consequences of induction of labour on resources are tremendous. There needs to be a balance between the pro-active induction group and those advocating conservative management. With adequate monitoring of fetuses, pregnancies may be allowed to go to 44 weeks. The problem is that there is currently no reliable method of monitoring postdate pregnancies and, until this is available, this will remain a thorny issue. On balance, therefore, all pregnancies at or around 42 weeks' gestation should be induced unless the parents opt for a conservative approach, in which case, adequate intensive fetal surveil-lance is required.

References

Cardozo L et al. Prolonged pregnancy: the management debate. *BMJ* 1986; 293: 1059–1063.
Hannah ME, Hannah WJ, Hewson SA et al. Planned Caesarean versus planned vaginal birth for breech presentation at term: randomised multicentre trial. *Lancet* 2000; 356: 1375–1383.

2. Evaluate the different manoeuvres you will apply to the management of shoulder dystocia.

Common mistakes

- Causes of shoulder dsystocia
- Complications of shoulder dystocia
- Prevention of shoulder dystocia
- Risk factors for shoulder dystocia
- Refer to senior colleague
- Take a history
- Review notes for risk factors for shoulder dystocia

A good answer will include some or all of these points

- Complication of macrosomic babies – uncommon in normal-sized babies
- Morbidity and mortality high and so, too, is litigation
- Management – obstetric emergency
- Successful delivery – episiotomy
- Manoeuvres: McRoberts; all fours; corkscrew; hand in vagina; suprapubic pressure; symphysiotomy; Zavenelli's procedure
- Conclusion

Sample answer

Shoulder dystocia is an obstetric emergency that all staff on the delivery suite must understand, and have in-depth knowlege of the different manoevres in its management. Although it can be anticipitated in those with fetal macrosomia and diabetic pregnancies, most often it occurs without any warning signs. Once diagnosed, the first and most important step is to call for help. Junior staff must request immediate senior help and an anaesthetist and paediatrician should be present or summoned.

The first step is to ensure that an adequate episiotomy has been made. If one has already be made, it should be extended. It must be recognized that, although shoulder dystocia is mainly a problem of the bony pelvis, a generous episiotomy will allow for better manipulation and therefore easier delivery.

The most commonly used manoeuvre is McRobert's technique. This involves hyperflexion and abduction at the hip joints. Ideally, this should be undertaken by two operators. This enlarges all the pelvic dimensions through straightening of the lumbosacral angle and superior rotation of the symphysis pubis, and with suprapubic pressure, allows delivery of the shoulders. It is thought to be successful in over 80 per cent of cases. This manoeuvre is easy to apply and is successful in most cases.

Another manoeuvre involves turning the patient to the lateral position or on to all fours. This allows for easy manipulation and effective delivery. By adopting these positions, the pelvic dimensions are increased slightly and allow mild dystocias to be overcome. In severe instances, however, this is unlikely to be successful. Although effective in some cases, it may be difficult turning a labouring patient to these positions.

Where these fail, other manoeuvres have to be applied. The first of this is the lateral suprapubic pressure with the patient in the lithotomy position and maximum abduction at the hip joints. Here, an assistant applies lateral suprapubic pressure behind the anterior shoulder and the accoucher simultaneously applies backward traction on the fetal neck. The aim is to push the anterior shoulder into the pelvis in an oblique fashion. It results in the adduction of the shoulders and the bisacromial diameter. The pressure should be continuous for about 30 seconds and, if this is unsuccessful, it should be abandoned and the next manoeuvre embarked upon.

This is the cockscrew manoeuvre and involves internal rotation of the shoulders away from the anterior posterior position. The operator inserts a hand into the vagina posteriorly and moves it up to the posterior aspect of the anterior shoulder. This is then pushed from behind into an oblique position. This may not succeed in which case the posterior shoulder should be rotated through 180°. This allows it to be disimpacted whilst permitting the trapped anterior shoulder to enter the pelvis. Further rotation will then bring down the other shoulder and the delivery will be effective. These manoeuvres require confidence and skill, especially during inserting the hand and undertaking the rotation. Often, they are undertaken after others have failed and the concerns of delay in delivering make them more complicated.

Another option is to deliver the posterior shoulder, which is already in the pelvis and then rotate the fetus and deliver the other shoulder. Here, the operator inserts a hand vaginally, flexes the elbow and shoulder and bring the forearm across the chest of the baby to deliver. If the anterior shoulder does not follow, the baby is rotated to allow it to be delivered.

Where all the above methods fail, more uncommon methods may be used. These are the Zavanelli's replacement of the head or symphysiotomy. The former involves the risk of annular detachment of the uterus. In good hands, the latter is associated with a good outcome provided care is taken to avoid damaging the urethra and the hip joints.

Shoulder dystocia is one of the common causes of litigation in obstetrics. It is associated with significant injury to the baby and mother and only timely intervention and careful application of one of these manoeuvres will result in a good outcome. Even when they are judiciously applied, the risk of trauma remains.

3. What measures will you take to minimize the risk of uterine rupture at induction in a woman who has had a previous Caesarean section, and how will you recognize it?

Common mistakes

- Discussing methods you will undertake preinduction (decision has already been made about induction)
- Avoid adding too many variables, for example breech presentation, previous classical Caesarean section – you ought to know that these will be classified as contraindications for induction
- Do you cross-match blood or group and safe?
- Classical Caesarean section – will not be induced (this is considered by some as criminal or gross negligent practice)
- Do not mention anything no longer regarded as contemporaneous practice
- No need to go into the details of the induction process, for example delay syntocinon for 22 hours, etc.

A good answer will include some or all of these points

- There are two parts to the question and each carries equal marks
- Need to exclude contraindications (assume they have been excluded)
- Ruptured uterus is more commonly caused by hypertonic contractions, malpresentation or feto-pelvic disproportion
- Only induce for correct reason
- Induction – with prostin extreme caution needed
- Caution with number of prostins per day – may need to limit them
- When in established labour
- Must avoid hyperstimulation
- Palpation? Cardiotocography (CTG) – not reliable
- Intrauterine pressure tip catheter best – but why not commonly used?
- Syntocinon – non-judicious use must be avoided
- Progress in labour – good contractions, cervical dilatation and exclusion of feto-pelvic disproportion. Hyperstimulation – intravenous (i.v.) ritodrine
- Recognition: bradycardia; abdominal pain/shoulder tip pain; maternal hypotension and tachycarda; vaginal bleeding; fetal parts easily felt per abdomen or presenting part receding into the abdomen

Sample answer

Ruptured uterus is a recognized complication of induction of labour, especially in women with a previous Caesarean section. Because of this complication, controversy remains about the induction of labour in women with a scar on the uterus. Although a recent report from the USA (Lyndon-Rochelle 2001) quotes a risk of uterine rupture of 16 following VBAC and syntocinon, there is overwhelming evidence that the judicious use of oxytocic agents in these patients will result in successful inductions with no significant risk of uterine rupture.

The first step to minimize the risk of rupture is to recognize the risk factors for its occurrence and, if possible, to avoid them. These include hypertonicity/hypertenic contractions, malpresentations, feto-pelvic disproportion and the type of scar on the uterus. In general, a classical Caesarean section will be considered a contraindication, whereas a complicated previous Caesarean section, especially one where there was postoperative infection, may be a relative contraindication. Multiple prostaglandins are more likely to result in hypertonia and therefore a limit should be put on the number of prostins to be used.

Once the patient is in labour, avoiding the injudicious use of syntocinon will minimize the risk of overstimulation. This can only be achieved by titrating the dose of syntocinon against carefully monitored uterine contractions. Where hyperstimulation occurs, intravenous (i.v.) ritrodine may be given to counteract it. Uterine contractions should be monitored objectively to ensure that their strength and frequency are within normal limits. The ideal method is by means of an intrauterine pressure tip catheter, but these are rarely used. Continuous fetal monitoring will offer a better objective estimation of the frequency and duration of contractions. Palpation of contractions may complement this method of monitoring, but this should not be the only method of monitoring contractions in this high-risk group.

An important aspect of any labour is progress. This should be monitored and charted carefully and any early signs of obstruction or disproportion recognized, and the induction abandoned for an abdominal delivery. Similarly, if progress is poor, induction should be discontinued in favour of a Caesarean section.

Irrespective of the above precautions, ruptures will occur. The early signs of rupture must therefore be recognized. These include a sudden bradycardia, abdominal pain breaking through an epidural, vaginal bleeding, maternal hypotension, tachycardia, receding fetal head, easily palpable fetal parts and shoulder tip pains. In most cases, the sudden and non-recovering bradycardia is the first sign, especially in those with epidural anaesthesia. However, the other signs may occur together or in isolation. Once rupture is suspected, the management is laparotomy.

Reference

Lyndon-Rochelle M, Holt VL, Easterling TR, Martin DP. Risk of uterine rupture during labour among women with a prior cesarian delivery. *N Eng J Med* 2001; 345: 3–8.

4. Critically appraise the methods of induction of labour of an uncomplicated pregnancy at 41 weeks' gestation in a grande multipara.

Common mistakes

- Take a history and do a physical examination to determine
- Complications of previous labour
- Methods of delivery in previous pregnancies
- Birthweights of babies
- Contraindications to a vaginal delivery
- Discussing the benefits of awaiting spontaneous labour and suggesting inductions should be delayed
- In view of the parity, precautions must be undertaken
- Listing the complications of induction of labour in this woman

A good answer all include some or all of these points

- A grande multipara is at a greater risk of uterine rupture and precipitate labour
- Assumption made – no contraindications for a vaginal delivery
- Options
- Artificial rupture of fetal membranes alone – if cervix is favourable (may not be). Onset of uterine contractions may be delayed with the risk of chorioamnionitis
- Least likely to be associated with increased risk of hypertonia and therefore rupture
- Artificial rupture of fetal membranes + syntocinon – only if favourable. Syntocinon, if used injudiciously, may result in rupture. Syntocinon infusion can be stopped if hyper-stimulation
- Prostaglandins – unripe cervix. Initiate contractions, mobilize. Risk of hypertonia and rupture. Unable to control once administered. Intravenous (i.v.) ritrodrine may counteract hypertonia
- Lamineria tents – mechanical, dilatation of the cervix. Insertion may be uncomfortable
- Foley's catheter – balloon to dilate cervix and release endogenous prostaglandins. Same as for the lamineria tents
- Oestrogens – outdated

Sample answer

A grand multiparous woman is one who has had at least five (although there appears to be a move to reducing this to four by some experts) deliveries after 24 weeks' gestation. By virtue of this high parity, this patient is at an increased risk of uterine rupture, precipitate labour and postpartum haemorrhage during labour, especially one that is either induced or augmented. Postdates is one of the common indications for induction of labour. Various methods are available for this labour, ranging from simple artificial rupture of fetal membranes to the use of a combination of surgical and medical methods. It has to be assumed in this patient that there are no contraindications to a vaginal delivery, otherwise she would not be undergoing an induction.

Where the cervix is unfavourable for artificial rupture of fetal membranes, a membrane sweep may be followed by spontaneous onset of labour. Randomized trials have shown that sweeping the membranes and even massaging the cervix results in the onset of labour in a large proportion of patients, especially multiparous women. In this grande multipara, this may be an effective option. Its main advantage is that is allows labour to start spontaneously and this may be at the expense of waiting for a few days. Since the patient is at only 41 weeks' gestation, this method provides significant advantages as she could wait for a few days before further intervention.

The second option is artificial rupture of fetal membranes where the cervix is ripe. A ripe cervix is one with a Bishop's score of at least six. If the membranes are ruptured, the patient may go into spontaneous labour. She may, however, require syntocinon to initiate contractions or augment labour. Artificial rupture of fetal membranes alone is less likely to be associated with hypertonic contractions and therefore is associated with no increased risk of uterine rupture. However, because it may require syntocinon, the risk remains high with this combination. In addition, waiting for contractions to start spontaneously may increase the risk of ascending infections, although this is rare.

Prostaglandins (PGE$_2$) and misoprostol are the most effective agents for the induction of labour in this patient. This is especially where the cervix is not favourable for artificial rupture of fetal membranes. One of the advantages of prostaglandins is that the patient is not confined to bed during the early phase of induction. Apart from ripening the cervix, the patient is more likely to go into spontaneous labour with prostaglandins. However, these may induce hypertonic contractions, which may result in uterine rupture in this grande multiparous woman. Once administered, it is difficult to control the absorption rate. Therefore the only means to overcome hyperstimulation is by the administration of intravenous (i.v.) sympathomimetics agents. These agents (whether given orally or vaginally) are associated with systemic side-effects, such as vomiting and diarrhoea.

Mechanical methods of induction, which could be used in this patient include Foley's catheter – usually with a 30 ml balloon. The catheter is inserted into the cervical canal and the balloon inflated and left *in situ* until it falls out. This will happen when the cervix is sufficiently dilated, and at this stage, the patient either goes into spontaneous labour or the membranes are ruptured and syntocinon initiated if necessary. This method is cheap, available to all units and effective. It may be difficult to insert the catheter and some patients may find this extremely uncomfortable. Other hygroscopic devices, such as lamineria tents, offer the same advantages as the Foley's catheter, except that they may be more expensive. Although 17-beta-oestradiol has been used in the past, this is rarely used contemporaneously.

5. A primigravida was admitted in spontaneous labour at 40 weeks' gestation 14 hours ago. Fetal membranes had ruptured spontaneously 12 hours before admission. Her cervix was 3 cm on admission. The cervix has remained at 8 cm for the last four hours and, in addition, she now has a pyrexia of 37.8 °C. The fetal heart rate is, however, normal. Justify your management of this patient.

Common mistakes

- Do a physical examination to identify the cause of the pyrexia
- She has an obstructed labour and should be delivered by Caesarean section (you cannot make this diagnosis without justifying it)
- Criticizing the management of patient so far – not really asked to do this
- Involve anaesthetist and paediatrician in the decision to deliver
- Discussing the methods of delivery with the patient and giving her the options so she can make a decision on how to be delivered

A good answer will include some or all of these points

- Two problems – prolonged spontaneous rupture of fetal membranes and slow progress in labour
- Most likely cause of the pyrexia – chorioamnionitis
- Most likely cause of the prolonged labour – dysfunctional labour
- Review partogram – frequency, duration of contractions
- Examine abdominally – fetal head (proportion palpable per abdomen)
- Examine vaginally – to exclude disproportion and imminent obstruction
- Give parental antibiotics
- Rehydrate and start syntocinon if no contraindications for vaginal delivery
- If disproportion – Caesarean section with care re extension and bladder damage
- Spontaneous vaginal delivery (SVD) – risk of postpartum haemorrhage and puerperal endometritis – continue with antibiotics
- Neonate – paediatrician

Sample answer

There are two problems concering this patient – prolonged rupture of fetal membranes and slow progress in labour. The two may be related and possibly be responsible for her pyrexia. Her management must, therefore, focus on these problems.

The most likely cause of the pyrexia is chorioamnionitis, although it could be related to an epidural and significant dehydration. If the patient has had epidural anaesthesia, and is possibly dehydrated as a result of prolonged labour, an increase in intravenous (i.v.) fluids will be associated with lowering her temperature. However, in this scenario, this is unlikely to happen. Treatment for chorioamnionitis should therefore be instituted. An intravenous broad-spectrum antibiotic should be administered parenterally.

The patient's partogram needs to be reviewed to ascertain the frequency of uterine contractions and their duration. This will reveal whether contractions are adequate, in which case another cause of the slow progress should be excluded, or dysfunctional labour is responsible. Unfortunately, manual palpation and recording of contractions are not objective enough and therefore these can only provide a guide rather than objective means of assessing the contractions.

An abdominal examination will provide information about the lie of the fetus, the descent of the presenting part and the presence of features suggestive of obstruction, such as Bandl's ring. A pelvic examination will exclude feto-pelvic disproportion from palpation of the suture lines and assessment of the pelvis. Again, this is a subjective assessment and one that may not be reliable. Cervical dilatation and the station of the fetal presenting part should be confirmed at this stage.

After administration of i.v. antibiotics and fluid to rehydrate the patient, if disproportion has been excluded and she has dysfunctional labour, syntocinon should be initiated. Where there is evidence of disproportion (significant moulding and a tight-fitting head), a Caesarean section should be performed. The danger of this procedure is an extension into the vagina and postpartum haemorrhage. The neonatologist should be notified at the time of delivery, so that he or she can attend and start the neonate on prophylactic antibiotics. Because of the chorioamninotis and prolonged labour, the patient is at increased risk of endometritis, deep vein thrombosis (DVT) and postpartum haemorrhage. Adequate precautions must therefore be taken after delivery.

13

Intrapartum care and complications of labour

1. Comment critically on the manoeuvres used in the management of the after coming head in a breech delivery.

2. Mrs BB is 27 years old. She is mentally subnormal. In her first pregnancy, she refused intervention but fortunately had a normal delivery, which was complicated by a retained placenta that was delivered spontaneously with a postpartum haemorrhage of 800 ml. She presented in labour at 41 weeks' gestation with spontaneous rupture of fetal membranes and regular uterine contractions and, again, refuses a vaginal examination and any form of intervention. Identify the potential problems with the management of this woman and outline how you will deal with them.

3. Evaluate your options for the management of a primigravida with a ruptured uterus induced by oxytocic agents and prostaglandins.

4. What steps will you take to reduce the risk of cord prolapse and how will you manage it when it occurs?

5. A 27-year-old teacher, in her second pregnancy, wishes to deliver at home. Her first pregnancy was uncomplicated and she had a four-hour normal delivery of a 3.5 kg male infant. How will you counsel her?

1. Comment critically on the manoeuvres used in the management of the after-coming head in a breech delivery.

Common mistakes

- Take a history and do a physical examination
- Establish the indications for breech delivery
- Extolling the virtues of delivery all breeches by Caesarean section (Canadian trial)
- Ultrasound scan to estimate the diameter of the fetal head
- Ensure that the pelvis is adequate
- Pelvimetry – radiological/clinical
- Examine the patient to ensure that she is fully dilated

A good answer will include some or all of these points

- Most breech presentations are now delivered by Caesarean section (Canadian trial and Royal College of Obstetricians and Gynaecologists (RCOG) recommendations)
- After-coming head could be difficult to manage
- Complications – usually of cord compression and trauma to the fetus and mother
- Three common approaches to management: Burns–Marshall technique; Mauriceau–Smellie–Veit manoeuvre; forceps to after-coming head
- Uncommon methods: symphysiotomy; Zavenelli technique; destructive operation; Caesarean section
- Conclusions

Sample answer

Breech delivery occurs in about two to four per cent of pregnancies at term. Recent evidence from the Canadian Randomized Trial and recommendation from the Royal College of Obstetricians and Gynaecologists (RCOG) are to offer patients elective Caesarean sections at term if external cephalic version (ECV) has failed, is contraindicated or is unavailable. This patient either opted for a vaginal breech delivery or was admitted in advanced labour and elected to proceed with a vaginal delivery.

The management of the after-coming head requires a good understanding of the mechanisms and processes of labour and the pelvic anatomy. There are traditionally three classical approaches. These include the Burns–Marshall technique, the Mauriceau–Smellie–Veit manoeuvre and the application of forceps. In some circumstances, however, these may not be successful and other options must therefore be considered.

The Burns–Marshall technique allows the breech to hang until the nape of the neck is visible. This allows the fetal head to descend into the pelvis. Either the operator or an assistant then grasps the fetal ankles and feet and raises the body/trunk above the mother's abdomen. A hand is placed over the perineum to prevent precipitate labour. The head is then delivered either with maternal effort or with some pressure from the suprapubic region. This technique is simple to apply, however, it may be associated with precipitate delivery of the head and intracranial haemorrhage – secondary to tentorial tears. By raising the trunk above the abdomen, hyperextension may result and make delivery complicated.

Application of forceps to the head after raising the trunk above the mother's abdomen allows gentle and better-controlled delivery of the head and therefore minimizes the risk of intracranial haemorrhage. However, during the application of the forceps, failure to recognize that the lowest part of the fetal head is, indeed, the smallest, and therefore prematurely straightening the forceps may cause undue pressure on the fetal head and may result in fractures. This complication is more common if forceps with short shanks are used. Prolonged interval between application and delivery may also result in un-necessary compression of the fetal head.

The third technique is the Mauriceau–Smellie–Veit manoeuvre. The operator places the fetus over one forearm and then inserts the middle finger of that hand into the baby's mouth and the index and ring fingers on the malar eminences. The second hand applies pressure downwards on the occiput of the fetus. Combining this pressure with downwards traction to the mandible allows delivery. Occasionally, an assistant may apply suprapubic pressure to assist the delivery. Exerting too much force on the mandible may result in dislocation or fracture of the mandible. Inserting the finger too far into the throat and exerting pressure may also result in the creation of a pseudo-diverticulum.

Although these techniques are effective in most cases, occasionally delivery is impossible. A symphysiotomy may therefore be performed. This is an uncommon procedure in developed countries and is associated with damage to the urethra and instability at the pelvic joints. It may also be complicated by symphysitis. Another manoeuvre, which is uncommon is pushing the baby back into the abdomen and performing a Caesarean section. The difficulty is pushing the fetus into the abdomen, as usually the uterus is contracting on the fetus. The risk of annular detachment of the uterus is quite high in this procedure. Craniotomy is an uncommon procedure but may be performed in cases where the fetus is dead and delivery is impossible, or if there is hydrocephalus. This operation is only performed as a last resort and parts of the bone may cause maternal injuries such as vesico-vaginal fistula.

2. Mrs BB is 27 years old. She is mentally subnormal. In her first pregnancy, she refused intervention but fortunately had a normal delivery, which was complicated by a retained placenta that was delivered spontaneously with a postpartum haemorrhage of 800 ml. She presented in labour at 41 weeks' gestation with spontaneous rupture of fetal membranes and regular uterine contractions and, again, refuses a vaginal examination and any form of intervention. Identify the potential problems with the management of this woman and outline how you will deal with them.

Common mistakes

- Outline details of the diagnosis and management of labour
- Complications of spontaneous rupture of fetal membranes
- Management of postpartum haemorrhage
- Refer patient to psychiatrist
- Ought to have made a plan before delivery, therefore substandard care
- Care of patient should be in specialized unit

A good answer will include some or all of these points

- Mentally subnormal, therefore potential issues of consent, communication and understanding
- In established labour (rupture of fetal membranes and contractions) – need to exclude cord prolapse
- Monitoring of labour and fetal heart rate
- Increased risk of retained placenta and postpartum haemorrhage
- Where an emergency arises – how to proceed

Sample answer

This patient poses problems with her management. These focus on consent to the various procedures to be undertaken during labour. If she is so subnormal that she cannot understand or has no insight into implications of any interventions, she cannot provide consent. It is expected that this would have been identified antenatally and necessary precautions taken to address this problem, but if there is no documentation, appropriate steps must be taken.

The patient's management should involve the most senior member of the obstetric, midwifery, anaesthetic and management team on duty. A relative who would have been with her throughout pregnancy, and her midwife, have to be present as they may provide support in a strange and perhaps frightening environment. Issues relating to consent about her care include assessment of progress of labour, monitoring of the fetus (first, to exclude cord prolapse), prophylaxis against retained placenta and primary postpartum haemorrhage (which are more likely to occur) and the necessary steps to take in the case of an emergency.

A close relative and the patient's midwife may be able to persuade her to allow the fetus to be monitored. In fact, they could encourage her to place the cardiotocograph (CTG) on her abdomen herself. Provided the fetal heart is normal and the patient is not in distress, labour can be allowed to continue without the need for vaginal examinations (provided cord compression has been excluded) and when there is anal dilatation she will start to push by reflex. This is more likely since she has had a normal delivery before. Administrators may have to seek permission from the courts to treat in her best interest if necessary. Such authority may allow for the forced administration of oxytocic agents to prevent postpartum haemorrhage and transfusion, if required. It should also make provisions for an emergency Caesarean section if it is thought necessary.

The postnatal care of the baby must be reviewed and confirmed if there are any instructions documented in the patient's notes. If there are none, clues could be gleaned from the care of her previous baby. If the baby was fostered or has been adopted, a similar approach must be followed unless there are relatives who can guarantee looking after the child. The baby may, therefore, be made a ward of court and cared for in the hospital until appropriate steps have been taken to ensure its care in the community. The care of the mother after delivery must also be planned. In this case, the midwife and social workers involved will offer the necessary support and provide the required care in the community. Although contraception may not be offered at this stage, it must be discussed and a plan made on how to prevent her from further pregnancies.

In the care of this patient, there should be adequate communication between social workers, psychiatrists, senior obstetricians and anaesthetists, paediatricians and midwives, and all the necessary decisions must be agreed upon. Discussions at all levels will ensure that all aspects are considered as deemed necessary.

3. Evaluate your options for the management of a primigravida with a ruptured uterus induced by oxytocic agents and prostaglandins.

Common mistakes

- Take a history and do a physical examination
- Review notes to determine whether she has had any surgery
- Do a 30-minute cardiotocograph (CTG) to monitor the fetus
- Only the consultant should manage such patients as she is very high risk
- Anaesthetist must insert a central venous pressure (CVP) monitor
- Input/output

A good answer will include some or all of these points

- Fetus still alive or not – laparotomy and deliver fetus
- Repair if rupture is clean (i.e. not ragged)
- Repair and tubal ligation
- Hysterectomy
- Most important step – resuscitation: intravenous (i.v.) access; anaesthetist; involve haematologist

Sample answer

Ruptured uterus is uncommon in primigravidas. Management will depend to a large extent on the time it is recognized and associated complications. For ruptures identified incidentally at Caesarean section, management will usually consist of delivering the baby and repairing the rupture. In this patient, it will be assumed that the diagnosis was made before surgery and/or delivery.

An important sign of uterine rupture is sudden fetal bradycardia and associated abdominal pain. If this is how the diagnosis was made in this patient, an immediate laparotomy must be performed – preferably under general anaesthesia (GA) to save the baby. This should be performed through the quickest means and, therefore, a midline subumbilical skin incision may be preferred to a Pfannenstiel incision. Where possible, this procedure should be performed by a skilled obstetrician; however, in the absence of one, delivery cannot be delayed but a senior obstetrician should be involved in the patient's management.

Haemorrhage from an unscarred uterus is more likely to be life-threatening. A second intravenous (i.v.) access should therefore be secured immediately the diagnosis is suspected. This could be shortly after the patient is under GA. Blood should also be cross-matched, and it may be necessary to have uncross-matched blood available. The involvement of an experienced anaesthetist, haematologist and obstetrician is an important part of the management of this patient. These would ensure that complications of the rupture, such as haemorrhage and the need for massive transfusion, are minimized.

Once the baby has been delivered, options are repairing the rupture alone, repairing and ligating the tubes or a hysterectomy. The decision has to be made based on the nature of the rupture. If it is a linear rupture, a simple repair is all that is necessary. In this primigravida, this must be the preferred option, but it must not be at the risk of losing her life. Confidential enquiries into maternal mortality state that delay in offering hysterectomy to patients was partly responsible for some mortalities from haemorrhage. Therefore, this option must only be considered if the risk to the mother's life is not considered to be significant.

Where there is very extensive damage to the uterus and it is perceived that it will not be able to carry another pregnancy after it has been repaired, tubal ligation will be necessary. Again, this decision must be made against the background of the patient's parity. In cases where the uterus has been extensively damaged and repair is not possible, a hysterectomy will have to be performed.

One of the most important aspects of this patient's management is postnatal counselling. Details of the events leading to the rupture must be discussed, as well as the type of treatment offered and its implications for subsequent pregnancies. If the rupture is linear and in the lower segment (and therefore mimics a Caesarean section scar) there is a place for allowing for a trial vaginal delivery in subsequent pregnancies, but the use of oxytocic agents must be avoided. In most cases, however, the rupture will be in the upper segment and this must be considered as a classical Caesarean section scar and subsequent pregnancies managed appropriately. It may be necessary to involve a psychologist in the counselling of this patient.

4. What steps will you take to reduce the risk of cord prolapse and how will you manage it when it occurs?

Common mistakes

- Forgetting that there are two parts to the question
- Listing all the causes of cord prolapse
- Assuming that the prolapse has occurred in labour or only in a singleton pregnancy
- Delivery by Caesarean section – the only option

A good answer will include some or all of these points

- Cord prolapse is an obstetric emergency – results in hypoxia and intrauterine fetal death if no immediate intervention
- Risk factors: polyhydramnios; preterm labour; abnormal presentation (breech, transverse lie); unengaged head; second twin – intrapartum
- Minimizing risk factors: polyhydramnios – defining causes, treating polyhydramnios and therapeutic reduction; unengaged head – avoid rupturing membranes unless necessary; prematurity – be aware of risk, especially when membranes rupture prematurely; management of second twin – avoid early intervention
- Management: early recognition on delivery suite – push presenting part away from the cord with hand in the vagina and retain it in place until delivery; rupture of fetal membranes – cord prolapse – is the fetus alive?; cervix fully dilated – fetus alive, vaginal delivery possible – ventouse; cervix not fully dilated or cervix dilated and vaginal delivery not possible – Caesarean section; twins – high head – membranes just ruptured – internal podalic version and breech extraction

Sample answer

Cord prolapse is an obstetric emergency that requires immediate delivery, otherwise the fetus will die from severe asphyxia. It occurs after spontaneous rupture of fetal membranes (prelabour, intrapartum or after delivery of a first twin). To reduce the risk of this complication, those at risk must be identified and appropriate steps taken to minimize the risk.

Risk factors for cord prolapse include polyhydramnios, preterm labour, premature rupture of fetal membranes, abnormal lie (oblique and transverse) and presentation (breech and shoulder), a high head (especially at term) and multiple pregnancies, especially in those undergoing a vaginal delivery.

The risk of cord prolapse may be minimized in some of the high-risk groups listed above, but in some it cannot. Where there is polyhydramnios, the cause should be found and, if possible, attempts should be made to reduce the liquor volume, especially where the patient is uncomfortable (in cases of acute polyhydramnios). The problem with this risk factor is that, in many cases, treatment is unable to reduce the liquor volume significantly and, therefore, the risk of cord prolapse. Other means of minimizing the risk factors include counselling high-risk patients on when to present (especially when they are contracting, bleeding or suspect rupture of fetal membranes). Rupture of membranes when the head is unengaged should be avoided if possible and induction of labour undertaken only when it is appropriate, especially where the head of the fetus is high.

Once the diagnosis has been made, the fetus must be delivered as soon as possible. For all scenarios other than twin delivery, a hand must be maintained in the vagina to push the presenting part away from the cord until the baby is delivered. The quickest method of delivery is Caesarean section. Asphyxia in these cases is often secondary to spasm of the vessels in the cord, and compression. By minimizing compression, most cases where the diagnosis is made early are not compromised. Where the diagnosis is made in a twin delivery, and the cervix is fully dilated, the cord can be pushed to one side and the baby delivered with a ventouse if the presenting part is cephalic. If it is breech and the membranes have only ruptured, it may be possible to do a breech extraction. Occasionally, the head may be too high to apply a ventouse. If this is the case a Caesarean section should be performed, but where the membranes have just ruptured it may be possible to undertake an internal podal version and a breech extraction. Where the cervix is not fully dilated, the same principles should apply as when managing cord prolapse in a singleton pregnancy. It is, however, possible to undertake a ventouse delivery when the cervix has reformed after the delivery of a first twin. The main problem is the delivery may be delayed and the fetus may be compromised.

5. A 27-year-old teacher, in her second pregnancy, wishes to deliver at home. Her first pregnancy was uncomplicated and she had a four-hour normal delivery of a 3.5 kg male infant. How will you counsel her?

Common mistakes

- Discourage her from a home delivery
- Details of the conduct of a normal delivery
- Complications of labour

A good answer will include some or all of these points

- Recognize that is an option in the UK
- Criteria for this option – uncomplicated pregnancy
- Advantages of a home delivery: home environment; no high-technology monitoring of fetus; personal midwife
- Disadvantages: no doctors available at short notice; if need for urgent intervention, may not have enough time; psychological/guilt feelings if outcome is poor; neonatologist unavailable
- Overall – perinatal mortality high
- If happy to take the risks – delivery should be allowed

Sample answer

Home delivery is an option that should be open to all uncomplicated pregnancies in the UK. In fact, the government White Paper on changing childbirth supports this option. Despite this support, it is still taken up by only a minority of women. Counselling of the patient should be objective and based on evidence rather on personal beliefs. Home births are supervised by either an independent midwife practitioners or hospital staff. The option will only be available to this patient if there are midwives who are prepared to supervise the delivery.

Assuming that a midwife is available, the advantages and disadvantages of home births need to be discussed. The main advantage of home confinement is that of 'demedicalization' of the birth process. In addition, the patient and her family are in their own environment where high technology is unavailable. Care is provided either by a named midwife or by an independent midwife practitioner. The patient is, therefore, likely to be delivered by someone she has seen throughout the pregnancy or by someone with whom she has built a rapport. This makes the experience more comfortable. Although there is a real desire to have a named midwife, for hospital delivery, practically, this is difficult to implement. It is therefore common for patients to have several midwives supervising their labour – and it is not unusual for some of them to be meeting the patient for the first time.

The disadvantages of home confinement include the absence of facilities for more intensive surveillance of the fetus. That said, the Dublin trial did not show any benefits from continuous fetal monitoring. If anything, there was an increase in the operative delivery rate. Since there are no high-technology facilities for monitoring, it may be difficult to recognize fetal distress early and to intervene. In this situation, intervention may be delayed whilst the patient is transferred to hospital. This disadvantage has been supported by evidence indicating that perinatal morbidity and mortality in those who are transferred to hospital from a planned home birth is significantly higher than that from planned hospital confinement. The absence of a neonatologist and facilities for ventilation is another disadvantage. This means that even if the baby were delivered normally, but started grunting or required immediate intubation and ventilation, this would be impossible.

Although adverse events are rare, the patient should be informed that whereas statistics may be acceptable when they do not apply to oneself, if there are complications, she must live with her decision. If she is fully aware of this, and is prepared to have the delivery at home, this option should be made available. The alternative is for her to have a hospital delivery (in a home-from-home unit, if available) with her named midwife and to be discharged home four to six hours after delivery.

14

Operative obstetrics

1. How will you counsel a 34-year-old teacher, in her third pregnancy, the previous two having been delivered by Caesarean section, who presents at 37 weeks' gestation requesting a vaginal delivery.

2. Do you agree that Caesarean section rates in the UK are too high?

3. You are about to perform an elective Caesarean section on a 28-year-old woman having her third baby. She requests that sterilization be performed at the time of surgery. How will you counsel her?

4. Critically appraise the management of a woman in her second pregnancy, the first having been delivered by emergency classical Caesarean section for transverse lie.

1. How will you counsel a 34-year-old teacher, in her third pregnancy, the previous two having been delivered by Caesarean section, who presents at 37 weeks' gestation requesting a vaginal delivery.

Common mistakes

- Offer sterilization
- Cannot delivery vaginally
- Decision can only be made by consultant so refer
- Discussing the operation of Caesarean section
- Quoting incorrect rates of uterine rupture

A good answer will include some or all of these points

- Traditional practice – after two Caesarean sections, elective Caesarean section
- Rationale – increased risk of uterine rupture
- Increasingly, women are being allowed to deliver vaginally (references, if any)
- Good evidence to indicate safe delivery in well-selected cases
- Why the previous two Caesarean sections – maybe for recurrent reasons, for example contracted pelvis, etc.
- Why does she want a vaginal delivery?
- Type of previous Caesarean section – if classical or inverted-T, unsafe for trial of vaginal delivery
- Allow vaginal delivery if no contraindications, but: cross-match blood or group and safe; hospital confinement; continuous monitoring in labour – cardiotocographs (CTGs) early detection of rupture
- Warn patient of potential risks of uterine rupture
- Emergency Caesarean section and other complications
- If goes past dates
- Induction – oxytocin or prostaglandins – relatively contraindicated
- Place of second opinion
- Exclude contraindications to vaginal delivery, such as abnormal presentation, fetal macrosomia, etc.

Sample answer

Standard practice after two or more lower-segment Caesarean sections is to recommend delivery by Caesarean section. This is based on the fact that the risk of uterine rupture during labour is significantly greater in these women. Increasingly, this approach has been questioned as there are no randomized trials to justify the reasoning behind this. Many practitioners are allowing a trial of vaginal delivery in well-selected cases after two lower-segment Caesarean sections, and the evidence emerging is in favour of such a pragmatic approach. However, before a patient is offered this choice, careful consideration must be given to her past obstetric history and the index of the pregnancy. It is only after appropriate counselling about the risks that this option should be allowed.

The first approach in counselling this patient is to establish why she wants a vaginal delivery. It may be her previous experiences or she might have read or heard about this option. The reasons for the previous two Caesarean sections should also be established from the notes and from the patient. If they were for a recurrent problem, such as contracted pelvis or a congenital malformation of the uterus, this option will be unsafe for her. If this was not the case, the types of Caesarean section performed should be ascertained from her notes. If either of them was a classical or an inverted-T Caesarean section, a trial of vaginal delivery would be considered unsafe. It is also important to establish that the Caesarean sections were not complicated by postoperative infections (especially the second one) which could easily have weakened the scar.

Assuming that there are no contraindications from the past obstetric history, the index of the pregnancy needs to be evaluated to exclude contraindications to a vaginal delivery. This evaluation will include abnormal lie, placenta praevia and abnormal presentation. In the absence of any of these, the patient should be counselled about the risk of a trial of vaginal delivery. The risk of uterine rupture is significantly greater than that in women with one previous Caesarean section or no scars on the uterus. The delivery should therefore take place only in the hospital where blood would be grouped and saved, an intravenous (i.v.) access will be secured during labour, there are facilities for continuous fetal monitoring and ready access to a theatre and experienced staff should the need for an emergency delivery arise because of a uterine rupture. In addition, the complications of emergency Caesarean section should be discussed, including the possibility of a hysterectomy were the uterus to rupture. Where there is a rupture, there may be fetal bradycardia, which may require very precipitate delivery when general anaesthesia (GA) would be the chosen form of anaesthesia.

Part of the counselling should include the problems that could arise when the pregnancy goes past term. Induction of labour with prostaglandins would be considered unsafe in this patient. If this were to happen, an elective Caesarean section would be the preferred mode of delivery. In addition, if the patient went into labour and required augmentation, syntocinon would be relatively unsafe because of the risk of rupture. Again, were this to be necessary, a Caesarean section will be the better option.

If there are contraindications to a trial vaginal delivery, or the patient is unprepared to accept these conditions, a second opinion should be sought. She should be referred to some-one senior or to another obstetrician. It is very likely that once her reasons for requesting a vaginal delivery have been addressed and information provided in an unbiased way, the patient will opt for the approach that is safest for her baby and herself.

2. Do you agree that Caesarean section rates in the UK are too high?

Common mistakes

- Discussing the indications for Caesarean section
- Arguing about the complications of Caesarean section
- Discussing patients' choice for Caesarean section
- Listing the procedure of Caesarean section

A good answer will include some or all of these points

- Incidence of Caesarean section is rising in the UK
- What is the nationally accepted Caesarean section rate? Any internationally acceptable rates – World Health Organization (WHO) rates?
- Why is the Caesarean section rate rising – obstetric/medical, social/patient choice and litiginous society
- What are the problems with a high Caesarean section rate – morbidity and mortality. Long-term medical complications, cost implications
- Other implications of a high Caesarean section rate – deskilling of junior doctors and other clinicians in vaginal delivery procedures

Sample answer

Caesarean delivery rates are rising in most developed countries. In some parts of the world, up to 50 per cent of women are delivered by Caesarean section. This is not only more expensive for the care provider but is associated with significant morbidity. In the UK, the Caesarean section rate has been rising gradually from less than 10 per cent in the 1970s to current rates of between 20 per cent and 35 per cent (depending on the unit). There is obviously some concern about this trend and, if it continues to rise at this rate, it is possible that within the next two decades over 50 per cent of women will be delivered by Caesarean section.

What is considered a high Caesarean section rate and who determines what the Caesarean section rate should be? This is an issue, which is difficult to address. By implication, therefore, an unacceptably high Caesarean section rate is difficult to define. The World Health Organization (WHO) has attempted to define what an acceptable Caesarean section rate should be. The rationale for this standard is unclear. A few studies from developing countries were used to arrive at the rate of about 10–15 per cent. Although this appears to be the acceptable rate to most in the UK, countries with such rates should be evaluated within that environment rather than on a global perspective.

An important question is why the Caesarean section is rising? Many reasons could be advanced for this. These include obstetric, medical, social and legal factors. Neonatal survival has improved significantly so that compromised fetuses at early gestations can be delivered safely now and nurtured to survive in modern neonatal units. A large number of Caesarean sections, therefore, are performed in early pregnancy when complications such as severe intrauterine growth restriction (IUGR) and pre-eclampsia require early delivery. In addition, increasing numbers of multiple pregnancies from ever-improving assisted conception techniques increase the rate of Caesarean section. Although the indications appear to be changing, the experience of medical staff has a significant effect on the rates of Caesarean section. The less experienced the medical staff, the higher the Caesarean section rates. Since training has been restructured to comply with the Calman timescale and the European Union working time directive, experience will continue to be eroded. Recent evidence and recommendations that all breech presentations at term should be delivered by Caesarean section is also responsible for the rising Caesarean section rates. In a society where litigation is becoming the norm, most obstetricians (junior and senior) are inclined to practise defensive obstetrics, which inevitably means more Caesarean sections. Although there are some women who admonish obstetricians for doing too many Caesarean sections, there is a larger number who elect to have Caesarean section deliveries for fear of uncertainties about vaginal delivery and the complications. It has been argued in the journals and national press that women should be allowed to chose their method of delivery. This social pressure imposes a significant stress on obstetricians who, for fear of litigation, increasingly allow Caesarean section on demand.

Caesarean delivery is associated with prolonged hospitalization and recovery, complications of surgery (for example, adhesions, venous thrombo-embolism (VTE), etc.), most of which have cost implications for the hospital and the family. Often, the management of subsequent pregnancies may be affected. However, it may be argued that since the average family size in the UK has been falling, a scarred uterus will not significantly influence the number of children families have. However, an increasing Caesarean section rate results in the deskilling of doctors in the art of vaginal delivery, especially where there are complications such as breech presentation and deep transverse arrest. Ultimately, all abnormal labours will be resolved by Caesarean section with its accompanying morbidity and mortality.

Although there are no nationally acceptable standards for a Caesarean section rate, the Sentinel Audit demonstrated that there are very wide variations in standards nationally. The rate of rise is alarming in some units. Since the factors responsible for this rise are not as dynamic as the rate, there must be intrinsic factors which may be minimized to reduce the rate of rise. This can only be done via national audits, such as the Sentinel Audit, and by re-education of patients, obstetricians and midwives.

3. You are about to perform an elective Caesarean section on a 28-year-old woman having her third baby. She requests that sterilization be performed at the time of surgery. How will you counsel her?

Common mistakes

- Discussing the merits and demerits of sterilization in general
- Stating that counselling can only be offered if the partner is present
- Making sweeping statements such as *'Reversals will not be done on the NHS' 'Sterilization is permanent' 'She will not be offered this procedure at this stage' 'It will be performed laparoscopically – at Caesarean section'*!!

A good answer will include some or all of these points

- When was the decision to have sterilization made? Before time of Caesarean section or at time of Caesarean section?
- Ideally should be long before Caesarean section (at least 2 weeks)
- Timing of decision – suboptimal
  - Emotional period
- Complications of the procedure
- Decision may be influenced by fear of Caesarean section, lack of support
- Offer interval procedure – three months and effective contraception
- Offer alternative – vasectomy/Mirena IUD
- If patient insists: counsel about failure rate
- Procedure itself – portion of tube to be removed
- High regret rate
- Increased risk of ectopic pregnancy and failure
- Low successful reversal rate

Sample answer

Sterilization is regarded as a permanent method of contraception, although under certain circumstances it can be reversed with a good chance of success if the procedure was undertaken with clips or rings. The decision to undergo this process must therefore be taken very carefully, especially as about a third of women sterilized live to regret the decision.

Sterilization during delivery is gradually being discouraged. This is because pregnancy is a very stressful time for most women and decisions could be influenced by experience during the pregnancy. In this patient, it is important to establish when the decision to undergo sterilization was taken. If it was made just before the time of the Caesarean section, it is unlikely to have been thought through carefully. Of course, the patient might have made this decision long before the pregnancy but only informed her carers before the Caesarean section.

Where the decision was made long before the Caesarean section, was documented in the notes and appropriate counselling offered, it could be performed provided all the options were discussed.

Where the decision was made only at the time of the Caesarean section, this must be questioned. However, if there is evidence that the patient is very certain about her decision, further counselling must be offered on the complications of the procedure and the difference between Caesarean section sterilization and interval sterilization. She should be offered the option of depo-provera for three months after the Caesarean section and an interval laparoscopic sterilization if she has not changed her mind at that time. Other contraceptive options, such as vasectomy and subdermal implants (Implanon or Norplant), should also be discussed. It should be emphasized that the failure rate following sterilization at Caesarean section is considered to be slightly higher than that after interval procedures with clips or rings, and that reversal is less likely to be successful with such procedures.

If the patient is certain or the decision was made long before the time of Caesarean section, counselling about the risks of failure, the complications of the procedure, the regret rate and increased risk of ectopic pregnancy should be offered. Where the decision is to undergo the procedure, a Pomeroy or modified Pomeroy will be the most common approach.

4. Critically appraise the management of a woman in her second pregnancy, the first having been delivered by emergency classical Caesarean section for transverse lie.

Common mistakes

- No place for a vaginal delivery
- Induction
- Repeat classical if cause of transverse lie present
- No need for routine antenatal care
- Any benefit in seeing her frequently on outpatient basis?
- Monitoring lie (not really relevant)
- Not asked to expound on the problems of Caesarean section (morbidity and mortality not really relevant)
- Indications for Caesarean section not relevant

A good answer will include some or all of these points

- Main danger – uterine rupture during pregnancy and labour (silent rupture not usually preceded by labour)
- At booking – consultant unit. Discuss plan of pregnancy care
- Admission
  - When and why? 24, 28, 32 weeks, etc.
- Frequent visits to the hospital? Why?
- Outpatient care? Why
- Delivery – when?
- 37–38 weeks – advantages and disadvantages
- Repeat Caesarean section – why, how, disadvantages and advantages. Bypasses emergency Caesarean section
- Spntaneous vaginal delivery – advantages/disadvantages
- Augmentation – not an option
- Use of oxytocic agents if vaginal delivery
- Sterilization?

Sample answer

Since Craigen's dictum that 'Once a Caesarean, always a Caesarean', many women with a previous Caesarean section have successfully been allowed to deliver vaginally. In fact, more than 70 per cent of women with a previous lower-segment Caesarean section will have successful vaginal deliveries in subsequent pregnancies. The situation with a classical Caesarean section, however, is different as the risk of uterine rupture is significantly high. This rupture may occur during pregnancy (silent rupture) or during labour. The risk of rupture in these patients is between 30 per cent and 50 per cent. The management of this patient should therefore take into consideration this risk.

If the patient had been counselled properly after the classical Caesarean section, she would be well-informed of the potential risk of rupture in this pregnancy. At booking, which must be in a consultant unit, the risks and implications should be discussed. The plan for the pregnancy should be discussed. This should include the need for admission for inpatient observation and the timing of delivery.

There is considerable debate about the need for antenatal admission. Some advocate admission from 24 weeks and others after 28 weeks. The rationale for this is the risk of silent ruptures. Those who advocate admission argue that if rupture occurs in the hospital, the chances of delivering a live baby are better than if it occurred at home. Early admission, however, may be stressful to a mother (who would leave her other child at home for a long time). If a rupture did occur at 24 weeks, the chances of the fetus surviving would be considerably lower. Therefore, it may not be advisable to admit at this early gestation. However, after 28 weeks this is more likely. Although admission may be offered to the patient, she may decline it. In this case, will she benefit from frequent hospital visits? There is no evidence to suggest that such visits will improve the detection of early rupture. It is important that she is counselled about the warning signs of rupture and made to report to hospital immediately should they occur. These include rupture of fetal membranes, abdominal pain, shoulder tip pain or if she starts contracting or is bleeding per vaginam.

The timing of delivery in this patient is another area of controversy. When should it be? It has been suggested that this could be somewhere between 37 and 39 weeks' gestation. If there have been no complications at 37 weeks, delivery would guarantee a viable matured fetus. However, there is an increased risk of transient tachypnoea of the newborn (TTN) and respiratory distress syndrome (RDS) at this gestation compared to delivery at 39 weeks' gestation. However delaying up to 39 weeks may risk uterine rupture and fetal death. Although there are advantages in delivering at 37 weeks, if the decision is to deliver at the latter date, the patient ought to be in hospital.

Delivery should be by a repeat Caesarean section, preferably by the lower segment. This has the advantage of reduced morbidity, although it leaves the uterus with an inverted-T scar. This does not increase the risk of rupture in a subsequent pregnancy. However, if there are contraindications to a lower-segment Caesarean section, a repeat classical incision should be made. After two classical Caesarean sections, sterilization should be considered in the interest of the mother. This should be discussed with the patient before surgery.

Where the patient requests a vaginal delivery, this must be discouraged. Although there are several reported cases of spontaneous vaginal delivery following classical Caesarean section, a 30–50 per cent risk of uterine rupture and the associated morbidity should discourage any woman from opting for such a delivery. Even if she went into spontaneous labour and wanted to continue, prostaglandins and oxytocic agents should be regarded as contraindicated.

15

Postpartum complications

1. Evaluate the methods of controlling severe postpartum haemorrhage at Caesarean section for placenta praevia.

2. A woman who has just had a vaginal delivery is bleeding profusely from the vagina. Evaluate your management options.

3. Justify the investigations you will perform on a woman six days after delivery presenting with a pyrexia of 38.6°C. She is breastfeeding and both breasts are normal.

4. The recent confidential enquiries into maternal mortality revealed that psychiatric disorders have become an important cause of maternal mortality. What steps will you take to minimize this preventable cause of maternal mortality?

1. Evaluate the methods of controlling severe postpartum haemorrhage at Caesarean section for placenta praevia.

Common mistakes

- Listing causes of postpartum haemorrhage
- Forgetting the fact that this is following Caesarean section
- Take a history and physical examination!
- Quickly examine the patient to ensure that she is haemodynamically stable
- Remove retained products of conception

A good answer will include some or all of these points

- Most likely cause of postpartum haemorrhage in this patient is bleeding from the lower segment
- This may be from large vessels or from placenta accreta or increta
- Methods of controlling the bleeding will therefore depend on the aetiology
- Bleeding from large vessels – under-run the vessels
- Uncontrollable – hebamate (prostaglandins) – unlikely to be effective
- Brace suture
- Internal iliac artery litigation
- Hysterectomy
- Uterine artery embolization

Sample answer

Postpartum haemorrhage is a recognized complication of placenta praevia. Anticipation of this complication is essential in reducing morbidity and mortality from it. The most likely source the haemorrhage in such patients is the placental bed in the lower segment. The haemorrhage may be recognized at the time of surgery or immediately after.

At the time of surgery, the haemorrhage may be from the placental bed after it has been removed. In some cases the placenta may either be an accreta or an increta in which case partial separation will be associated with hamorrhage. The first approach to controlling the haemorrhage at this time is under-running the bleeding vessels. This is effective in some cases. The advantage is that it is done under direct vision ensuring that the major bleeding sinuses are occluded. However, it may not be possible to under-run all the bleeding points.

Parenteral oytocic agents (bolus doses of ergometrine or continuous infusion of syntocinon) may be used to cause contraction of the myometrium. This may not be effective in controlling bleeding from the lower segment as the myometrial constituent is significantly lower in this region. However, with good contraction of the upper segment, it may reduce the blood flowing to the lower segment and therefore reduce the haemorrhage. The bolus doses may be repeated if they are initially not very effective. Intramyometrial prostaglandin (hebamate) may be used to stimulate contraction. This is unlikely to be effective with severe haemorrhage, again, on the basis that there are fewer muscles in the lower segment.

The Brace suture would be considered one of the most effective means of controlling the haemorrhage at the time of surgery or even when the patient returns to the theatre. This suture is easy to apply for those who are familiar with it and does not require any expensive material. Various reports have demonstrated its efficacy in most patients. It reduces blood flow to the uterus and therefore controls the haemorrhage.

Where this cannot be applied, or has failed, other options would be internal iliac artery ligation, hysterectomy and embolization of the uterine artery. Ligation of the internal iliac artery is not a procedure with which most obstetricians are familiar. It is effective when used properly, but because the surgeon may not be familiar with the technique it may be too time-consuming. Uterine artery embolization is a new technique that has been tried and been shown to be effective. It requires a skilled radiologist, the correct equipment and easy access to the labour ward or radiology department. For a patient who is haemorrhaging this may be technically difficult; however, when available, it is quite effective. A hysterectomy is the last resort, however, there must be no delay in undertaking this procedure. Mortality from haemorrhage, especially that due to placenta praevia, is not uncommon because of a delay in performing a hysterectomy. This procedure is effective but requires considerable counselling after.

If the haemorrhage was noticed after the patient has left the theatre, the same principles will be applicable except that she may have to go back into theatre for a more effective control of the haemorrhage.

2. A woman who has just had a vaginal delivery is bleeding profusely from the vagina. Evaluate your management options.

Common mistakes

- Take a history and do a physical examination – there is no time to do this
- Discussing the details of all the procedures you performed
- Listing the things you do without evaluating
- Being illogical in your approach

A good answer will include some or all of these points

- Recognize that this is a cause of significant morbidity and mortality
- Secure an intravenous (i.v.) line. Collect blood for urgent cross-matching and blood grouping (most important step). Explain why the most important step
- Examine
  - Uterus – contracting? Stimulate contractions – most common cause – atony, especially if prolonged labour
  - Repeat oxytocic agents
  - i.v. syntocinon
  - Is the placenta complete?
  - Examine the genital tract and placenta and membranes
  - Uterine hypotonia – oxytocic agents, prostaglandins – intramyometrial
- Surgery – Brace suture, internal iliac ligation
- Uterine artery embolization
- Hysterectomy
- Packing the uterus – not very effective – false sense of security
- Involvement of haematologist and anaesthetist, senior obstetrician
- Other causes – inversion, ruptured uterus, retained placenta

Sample answer

Severe postpartum haemorrhage is an obstetric emergency, which may be associated with maternal mortality. The management must therefore be aggressive and multidisciplinary – involving the haematologist (as blood may be required), an anaesthetist (examination under anaesthesia (EUA) and exploration of the uterus or laparotomy may be required) and a senior obstetrician (who may be required to undertake the various surgical procedures).

One of the most important stages in the management of this patient is securing an intravenous (i.v.) line and also cross-matching blood. The i.v. access should be secured with a large-bore venflon. This will ensure that resuscitation would be possible if she collapses. It may be advisable to secure a second i.v. access as rapid replacement of fluid may be required to avoid maternal mortality. This is probably one of the most important steps in the management of this patient.

A quick examination of the abdomen will determine whether the uterus is contracting. If it is not, rubbing it may stimulate contractions and stem the bleeding. This is a simple measure that is effective where the cause of the bleeding is hypotonia of the uterus. If, despite this, the uterus fails to contract, i.v. oxytocic agents should be given – first as a bolus dose and then as a continuous infusion. If hypotonia is the cause, this may be enough to control the haemorrhage. It is important to determine whether the placenta was complete. It may be advisable to ask for it to be re-examined. If a missing lobe or cotyledon or membranes are identified then efforts must be made to remove them.

If, after all this, the patient continues to bleed, an examination of the genital tract should be undertaken. This will exclude trauma to the vulva, vagina and cervix as the cause of the haemorrhage. In the absence of trauma and if bleeding continues, an examination of the uterus under anaesthesia should be undertaken. This is to ensure that there are no retained products of conception. This is not uncommon, even when the placenta is thought to have been delivered complete.

For continuing uterine hypotonia and an empty uterus, intramyometrial prostaglandins may be administered. These are effective but may be associated with significant systemic side-effects. Although packing of the uterine cavity has been advocated by some to stem the bleeding, this has the disadvantage that it conceals any blood loss and by the time it has soaked through the gauze, it may be significant. It may be a temporary option but the pack cannot be left *in situ* indefinitely.

Where the above steps fail to stop the haemorrhage, laparatomy would be necessary. At this procedure, a Brace stitch could be inserted. This is cheap, easy to insert and very effective. It is easier than internal artery ligation and does not compromise fertility. Internal iliac artery ligation is difficult to perform and may require a gynaecological oncologist as most obstetricians might never have performed this technique. Fertility is also preserved with this step. An alternative is an abdominal hysterectomy. This will certainly stop the haemorrhage but fertility will be affected. It should therefore only be used as the last option. The advent of uterine artery embolization has provided an alternative to the management of massive post-partum haemorrhage. It is effective and safe but difficult to administer because of availability of radiologist and machine. These difficulties may make its availability for such an emergency difficult.

Other causes of such a haemorrhage that should be considered include uterine inversion, ruptured uterus, pulmonary embolus and retained placenta. Whatever the cause, the principles of general management are the same, although specific management may differ.

3. Justify the investigations you will perform on a woman six days after delivery presenting with a pyrexia of 38.6°C. She is breastfeeding and both breasts are normal.

Common mistakes

- Take a history and do a physical examination
- Treatment – details of antibiotics
- For exploration under general anaesthesia
- Laparotomy

A good answer will include some or all of these points

- Diagnosis is puerperial pyrexia
- Causes – urinary tract infection (UTI), breast infection, genital tract infection, chest infection, venous thrombo-embolism (VTE), pyrexia of unknown origin (PUO)
- Investigations – state type and give reason(s): full blood count (FBC); sputum; chest X-ray (CXR); midstream urine (MSU); Doppler scans, blood gases, electrocardiography (ECG), D-dimers; swabs – wound, vagina and endocervix; blood cultures

Sample answer

This patient has puerperial pyrexia, for which there are many causes. These include urinary tract and chest infections, wound infections, genital tract infections, pelvic collections, venous thrombo-embolism (VTE) and, in some cases, pyrexia of unknown origin (PUO). The investigations for the cause of this patient's pyrexia will therefore depend on the suspected cause.

A full blood count (FBC) will demonstrate leucocytosis in the case of bacterial infection. However, it is important to understand the normal physiological changes occurring in the blood after delivery. There is often a degree of leucocytosis and this must not be confused with that secondary to infection. A midstream specimen of urine (MSU) for urinalysis and also for microscopy, culture and sensitivity is mandatory. Urinary tract infection (UTI) is one of the most common cause of pueperial pyrexia. Urinalysis may indicate the presence of leucocytes, nitrites, proteins or blood, all of which may be suggestive of UTIs.

Other investigations will depend on the suspected cause of the pyrexia. Where an intra-uterine infection (endometritis) is suspected, then high vaginal and endocervical swabs for microscopy culture and sensitivity will be the most appropriate investigations. However, it is not uncommon to fail to isolate the organism responsible for the endometritis from these swabs. An ultrasound scan may reveal the presence of retained products of conception. However, the presence of retained products will not necessarily imply endometritis as the cause. It is not unusual after delivery to have blood clots within the uterus and ultrasound scan will invariably report these as retained products.

163

If the patient has chest symptoms, such as cough or positive signs on clinical examination, a sputum for culture and sensitivity and a chest X-ray (CXR) would be applicable. In some cases, there may be no obvious signs but tuberculosis must always be suspected, especially with the recent rising trends in pulmonary tuberculosis in the UK. In this case, therefore, a Mantoux test may be appropriate. Where this is a possibility, any sputum should be sent for acid-fast bacilli examination. If there is a suspicion of a deep vein thrombosis (DVT) or venous thrombo-embolism (VTE), investigations such as a venogram of the legs, Doppler scan of the leg vessels and an electrocardiograph (ECG) would be essential. A ventilation-perfusion scan will be necessary if there is suspicion of pulmonary embolism. The level of D-dimers in the maternal blood in the cases of VTE will be raised.

The patient's temperature is above 38°C, therefore a blood culture is necessary if the cause of the pyrexia is not yet identifiable. This must be for Gram-positive and Gram-negative organisms (that is, two cultures should be set up). Where the cause of the pyrexia is indeterminable, screening for tuberculosis must be undertaken. This will in addition to the investigations outlined above consist of early morning urine for microscopy culture and sensitivity. Although the breasts may appear normal, they must be examined carefully again and, if there are any features of mastitis, this must be treated accordingly. Other additional investigations will include wound swabs for suspected wound infections, especially following operative deliveries and pelvic ultrasound for localization of abscesses. This latter investigation will be very relevant if the patient has been suffering from a swinging pyrexia.

4. The recent confidential enquiries into maternal mortality revealed that psychiatric disorders have become an important cause of maternal mortality. What steps will you take to minimize this preventable cause of maternal mortality?

Common mistakes

- Listing all the types of psychiatric disorders in pregnancy
- Treatment of psychiatric illnesses
- Being too vague in your answer
- Deliver electively at 38–39 weeks' gestation

A good answer will include some or all of these points

- High-risk group
- Previous puerperal psychiatric disorders
- Known psychiatric illness
- Problem pregnancy
- Domestic violence
- Antenatal measures: education; plan care with psychiatrist; joint care – obstetrician, midwife, general practitioner (GP) and psychiatrist
- Postnatal: treatment of disorder – soon rather than later; support at home; warning signs; GP; mother and baby units

Sample answer

Psychiatric illness was the most common cause of indirect maternal mortality over the last triennium. Most of the mortalities occurred postpartum and after six weeks. A large number of them were suicides. An important factor thought to be responsible for this was failure to recognize this problem and deal with it properly. The best approach to reducing this cause of maternal mortality starts with recognition of the high-risk group, planning care both in the hospital and in the community during pregnancy and after.

Those at risk include women with known psychiatric illness as well as those with previous postnatal psychiatric diseases, such as depression. Women with known psychiatric disorders are also at an increased risk of psychiatric problems, especially after delivery. Other factors, which may increase the risk of psychiatric illness include complicated pregnancies, women suffering from domestic violence, poor social economic class, ethnic minorities, those with very little knowledge of English and single unsupported parents.

Antenatally, appropriate measures should be taken in the management of these high-risk women. Such measures should be taken by a combined effort from psychiatric nurses, general practitioners (GPs) and social workers where applicable. Such education will concentrate on the positive aspects of pregnancy and providing information about how to recognize early signs of postnatal psychiatric diseases.

After delivery, early treatment of the disorders should be instituted. Where this is identified, early involvement of a psychiatrist and community nurses is vital. Admission into dedicated mother and baby units should be offered early. Support should be offered at home and, again, early warning signs should be recognized and treated. It is better to institute treatment early rather than to delay it until severe depression sets in. Where there is poor support at home, this should be provided. It is important to recognize the fact that these illnesses may occur for the first time after the first six weeks of delivery and that suicides occur commonly within this time. Surveillance of at-risk women should be continued for at least one year after delivery. Institution of treatment should not be delayed even if the woman is breastfeeding. There are very few contraindications to breastfeeding and, even if the drug she would benefit from is contraindicated, it is preferable to switch the baby from the breast to the bottle in order to treat the disorder. A positive attitude towards the mother and other members of the family is vital. For those with a history of domestic violence, social workers should be involved.

16

Neonatology

1. What complications may the baby of a diabetic mother suffer from in the neonatal period?

2. Critically appraise your management of a neonate with hypothermia on the postnatal ward.

3. Justify your investigations of a baby with neonatal jaundice.

4. How will you counsel a mother whose baby refuses to feed on the first day after delivery?

1. What complications may the baby of a diabetic mother suffer from in the neonatal period?

Common mistakes

- Discussing antenatal complications
- Intrapartum complications
- Congenital malformations
- Risks of maternal infections and polyhydramnios

A good answer will include some or all of these points

- Most are related to macrosomia and intra-uterine hypoglycaemia
- Difficulties with siting venflon
- Metabolic – hypoglycaemia
- Respiratory – RDS, especially if preterm
- Haematological – polycythemia, NNJ, hyperviscosity, thrombosis
- Thermoregulation – hypothermia
- Others – biochemical (hypocalcaemia, hypomagnesaemia – tetany)

Sample answer

Diabetes mellitus is a common medical disorder of pregnancy, which may result in macrosomic babies. Occasionally, however, the baby may be growth restricted. The complications of babies of diabetic mothers include biochemical, respiratory, metabolic and haematological problems and those of macrosomia. Where there has been birth trauma, the effects may extend into the neonatal period.

The most common complications are hypoglycaemia and respiratory distress syndrome (RDS). Hypoglycaemia is seen in babies whose mother had poor diabetic control during pregnancy. In these babies, insulin levels are high as a result of the hyperglycaemia *in utero*. When the source of glucose is removed with separation from the mother, the high insulin levels continue to convert glucose in the neonate to glycogen with a resultant hypoglycaemia. Early feeding reduces this complication. The hypoglycaemic baby may become jittery, hypothermic and will feed poorly.

Biochemical complications that may occur in the neonate from a diabetic mother include hypomagnesaemia and hypocalcaemia – both of which may manifest as tetany. Temperature control may be a problem. Although the baby is macrosomic, the proportion of brown fat in the baby is small. Since babies do not undergo shivering thermogenesis, and depend entirely on brown fat for heat generation, they are more likely to suffer from hypothermia.

RDS is associated with a diminished production of phospholipids. Their production is inhibited by high glucose levels. This complication is more common in poorly controlled diabetic mothers. The diabetic baby is said to be a few weeks less mature than a non-diabetic baby. Consequently, RDS is more common in diabetic babies delivered after 38 weeks' gestation.

Haematological complications which may occur in the neonates are related to poly-cythaemia. These include neonatal jaundice, increased blood viscosity and thrombosis especially of the superior sagittal sinus.

2. Critically appraise your management of a neonate with hypothermia on the post-natal ward.

Common mistakes

- Refer to neonatologist
- Take a history and do a physical examination
- Describe the method of keeping the labour ward/delivery suite warm
- Education of staff on how to manage hypothermia
- Early recognition

A good answer will include some or all of these points

- Identify the at-risk fetus
  - At-risk fetus: preterm; intrauterine growth retardation (IUGR); baby of diabetic mother
- Prevention: kangaroo approach; thermo-neutral environment; early feeding; wrapping with warm clothes
- Treatment: provide warmth; transfer to neonatal unit; feed early; monitor closely

Sample answer

Neonatal temperature control is mainly by means of energy generation from brown fat. This is located over the scapula and the axilla. Since the production of heat from this fat is dependent on oxygen consumption, it is the fetal metabolic rate that determines temperature control in the neonatal period. It is therefore advisable to nurse the neonate in a thermo-neutral environment where the amount of energy required to maintain body temperature is minimal and therefore oxygen consumption and, by implication, metabolic rate is low.

Hypothermia is likely to occur in situations where there is inadequate brown fat to generate heat (as in intrauterine growth restricted (IUGR) fetuses, fetuses of diabetic mothers and premature babies).

The management of hypothermia must start with the identification of the babies at risk. These are those from the high-risk groups defined above. At the time of delivery, these babies need to be wrapped in warm clothing to minimize their heat loss from the surface area. This is more so as the ratio of body weight to surface area in the preterm neonate is disproportionate in favour of more heat loss. It is important to recognize that since the baby can lose heat easily, if the temperature is too high, it is unable to control it properly and could therefore have a febrile convulsion.

Neonates at risk of hypothermia should be nursed in an environment where the temperature is more than room temperature. The thermo-neutral environment is ideal for nursing. An open ward is not ideal for neonates. For preterm babies, therefore, nursing in an incubator is ideal. The IUGR neonate who does not require incubator nursing, however, should be nursed in a warm environment and early feeding initiated. Unfortunately, some of them have difficulties feeding and may have to be tube-fed. The disadvantage of wrapping neonates warmly is the danger of overheating, especially of preterm and IUGR neonates. Although incubators are readily available in developing countries, in some parts of the world they are uncommon. Adopting the kangaroo approach (body-to-body contact) between the mother and baby may provide an ideal thermo-neutral environment to maintain body heat. It is cheap and effective. However, there is an increased risk of infection, especially in preterm babies.

3. Justify your investigations of a baby with neonatal jaundice.

Common mistakes

- Treatment of neonatal jaundice
- Complications of neonatal jaundice
- Take a history and do a physical examination
- Do a cholangiogaphy
- Screen for chromosomal abnormalities

A good answer will include some or all of these points

- Introduction about how common neonatal jaundice is
- Causes of neonatal jaundice
- Haemotological investigations – FBC, blood groups, Coomb's test, G6PD status
- Biochemical – U&E, LFT
- Immunological
- Radiological – ultrasound
- Infection screen – MSU, swabs from umbilicus, throat, eyes
- Metabolic – thyroid function test

Sample answer

Jaundice is a common manifestation in the neonatal period. It is often physiological, although in some cases it is secondary to pathology. Investigations and management must therefore aim to identify the cause and offer the most appropriate treatment to prevent progression and subsequent development of kernicterus, especially where there is unconjugated hyper-bilirubinaemia.

The causes of neonatal jaundice include prematurity, physiological jaundice, obstruction of the biliary system, infections (either of the liver or generalized septicaemia), ABO incompatibility, Rhesus isoimmunization, haemolysis – as in cases of G6PD deficiency or hereditary sperocytosis and congenital malformations – such as choledodochal cysts and biliary atresia. In some cases the cause is unknown. Identification of the cause will depend on the history, findings on physical examination and, more importantly, the results of various investigations.

Investigations include a full blood count (FBC) for haemoglobin and differential count. In severe haemolysis, the haemoglobin drops, whereas in infections the white cell count (WCC) rises and the differential count may indicate whether it is a viral or bacterial infection. Reticulocytosis will indicate how the fetus is responding to haemolysis or anaemia. Blood for culture will identify an infective organism in cases of suspected septicaemia. A liver function test (LFT) will estimate the total and unconjugated bilirubin, the liver enzymes and serum albumin. The level of bilirubin often determines the type of treatment to be offered, whereas raised transaminases, for example, will suggest some hepato-cellular damage.

The baby's blood group, Rhesus typing, presence of atypical antibodies and its G6PD status are important and must be determined. Associated with this investigation is a Coomb's test. This allows for the identification of antibodies, which are responsible for the haemolysis in Rhesus isoimmunization. Stool and urine examinations are not very important in the investigation of neonatal jaundice. Infection screening must focus not only on the obvious bacterial infections but also on atypical organisms, including viruses. Blood must be collected for hepatitis, cytomegalovirus (CMG) and rubella screening. Urinalysis for the presence of proteins, nitrites, blood and culture will exclude infections. Very rarely, a liver biopsy should be performed to rule out obstruction. However, ultrasound of the liver and gallbladder will identify obstruction. Irrespective of the cause, treatment should be determined by the bilirubin levels, especially the unconjugated values.

4. How will you counsel a mother whose baby refuses to feed on the first day after delivery?

Common mistakes

- Assume that it is mechanical
- Investigate with ultrasound – what are you investigating?
- Offer X-rays – of what?
- Surgical treatment – Duhamel's operation for duodenal stenosis or congenital atresia of the duodenum
- Intravenous (i.v.) fluids the only means of treatment.

A good answer will include some or all of these points

- Discuss the symptom and possible causes
- Obtain information from the mother and notes
- Treat according to first principles
- Causes of refusal of feed
- Infections
- Hypoglycaemia
- Hypothermia
- Structural abnormalities

Sample answer

Refusal of feeds on the first day of life is an important symptom and one that could distress parents. A sensitive approach to investigating and treating this symptom is vital in order not to frighten the parents. The aetiology of this symptom varies from physiological, metabolic and infective to anatomical problems. In an attempt to manage this problem, its cause must be sought carefully.

Information from the parents is vital. It is essential to know whether the baby took and tolerated feeds before or had not really been fed. If the former is the case, a congenital mal-formation is unlikely, especially if there was no regurgitation or vomiting. An infective or physiological cause may therefore be considered. A quick review of the antenatal and birth record may reveal additional information. For example, there might have been poly-hydramnios or suspicion of bowel obstruction. It is unlikely to be the case here unless the baby had vomited its first feeds and this was not recognized.

The possible causes of this baby's problem, assuming that it was able to tolerate feeds before, could be hypoglycaemia, hypothermia or infections. Hypoglycaemia is more likely to occur in babies of diabetic mothers. This information should be available in the mother's records. If this is not possible, a simple blood glucose estimation (mother and baby) would indicate whether this is the case. Hypothermia is more common on an open ward, often associated with a draught and poor temperature control. Septicaemia, especially associated with meningitis, would be the most worrying cause for the parents. They must therefore be advised about the investigations and management. This must include an infection screening and initiation of intravenous (i.v.) antibiotics. Usually, this situation settles within a few days. The ultimate treatment of this baby if feeds continue to be refused is to offer i.v. nutrition or to tube feed. The advantage of tube feeding is that it bypasses the risk of introducing infections and also ensures that, if there is any upper gastrointestinal obstruction, the tube will identify it. All attempts must be made to avoid dehydration and the subsequent development of renal failure. The surface area of a baby is large compared to its body weight and failure to adequately rehydrate a baby which has not fed for a day may have important consequences. Finally, sedation should be excluded by information about medication from the mother. Some of these drugs, especially those that cross the placenta, may be responsible. Such babies require observation and possibly tube feeding until the effects of the drugs wear off.

Section Three

Short essay questions: gynaecology

1

Adolescent gynaecology

1. Justify your management of a newborn whom, on examination, is found to have ambiguous external genitalia.

2. A 25-year-old woman, whose pregnancy was uncomplicated, unexpectedly delivered a baby suspected to have Down's syndrome. The antenatal serum screening test had been normal (1:1500) and no ultrasound markers had been identified on ultrasound scan. Justify your subsequent management of this young woman.

3. A six-year-old girl has been referred to the gynaecology clinic with persistent vaginal discharge. Critically appraise your management of the patient.

4. A mother brings her eight-year-old daughter to you because she has been menstruating regularly for the past four months. Justify your management of the young girl.

5. Evaluate your management of a 10-year-old girl presenting with vaginal bleeding of one week's duration.

1. Justify your management of a newborn whom, on examination, is found to have ambiguous external genitalia.

Common mistakes

- Listing the causes of external ambiguous genitalia
- Discussing in detail the various chromosomal and genetic factors regulating the differentiation of the internal and external genitalia
- Undertaking a physical examination after taking a history – failing to address the problem as it is presented (a newborn and not anyone with external ambiguous genitalia)
- General discussion of the management of ambiguous genitalia – failing to justify (that is, give reasons for all the steps you take in the management of this neonate)
- Referring the patient to a psychosexual counsellor!!
- Involving a plastic surgeon in the management
- Listing investigations (again without justification) is not enough

A good answer will include some or all of these points

- The importance of assigning the correct sex at birth
- Communication with the parents about the uncertainty in the assignment
- Need to exclude congenital adrenal hyperplasia of the sodium-losing type – if missed may result in mortality
- Need for further investigations to exclude other causes
- Involvement of different teams – paediatricians, geneticists, if necessary, and clinical psychologist to support the parents
- Definitive management at birth and later
- Implications for ambiguous external genitalia
- It is important to advance reasons (that is, justify) every management step made

Sample answer

The finding of ambiguous external genitalia must be managed sensitively and tactfully, as assignment of the wrong sex to a child will have long-term implications both to the child and the family. Once the diagnosis is made, therefore, the parents must be informed of the uncertainty. An important step must be to exclude congenital adrenal hyperplasia of the salt-losing type, as failure to recognize this may be associated with mortality. This is excluded by serum measurement of urea and electrolytes (U&Es) and various adrenal hormones (e.g. urinary 17-oxosteroids and pregnanetriol or serum 17-hydroxyprogesterone).

A detailed drug history from the mother may identify exogenous virilizing causes, although this is uncommon. The involvement of a neonatologist will help with a more thorough

181

examination, aimed at locating the gonads if present in the inguinal region or as abdominal masses.

The karyotype must be determined to help assign the genetic sex. This can be from a buccal smear, where the presence of a Barr body will identify a 46XX neonate. However, a blood sample for karytyoping from peripheral lymphocytes will provide a definitive genetic sex. This is essential as it will be useful in defining the underlying cause and sex of rearing. For example, this could be a 46XX neonate with congenital adrenal hyperplasia (the most likely cause), whereas a 46XY neonate may be related to other factors.

Following the genetic studies, subsequent management will depend on the evaluation of the best possible sex of rearing for the child. Assessment must be with this in mind. Where congenital adrenal hyperplasia is the cause, cortisol replacement is all that is necessary, but the clitoris must be shortened at the age of two to three years. This is to reduce the psychological effects on the child.

2. A 25-year-old woman, whose pregnancy was uncomplicated, unexpectedly delivered a baby suspected to have Down's syndrome. The antenatal serum screening test had been normal (1:1500) and no ultrasound markers had been identified on ultrasound scan. Justify your subsequent management of this young woman.

Common mistakes

- Discussing the prenatal diagnosis of Down's syndrome
- Discussing the various test for prenatal diagnosis – advantages and disadvantages
- No need to critically appraise amniocentesis or chorionic villus sampling (CVS)
- It is irrelevant to say that this ought not to have happened
- Antenatal diagnosis of Down's syndrome
- Shortfalls of serum screening and ultrasound screening – unnecessary
- Criticism of the screening procedure

A good answer will include some or all of these points

- Recognize that parents and staff will be shocked at this diagnosis
- A truthful, careful and sensitive approach must be adopted to inform the parents
- They must be given time to assimilate the news
- The general practitioner (GP) and community midwife should be informed
- Paediatrician to be involved to inform the couple of the neonatal problems of Down's syndrome. Examination of the neonate to exclude malformations (especially those associated with Down syndrome, for example cardiac)
- Need to confirm the diagnosis – chromosomes – from a blood
- Involvement of a geneticist
- Explanation about why the diagnosis was missed
- Giving information to the couple about various support groups and the society
- Discussion about prenatal diagnosis in subsequent pregnancy, including the risk of recurrence

Sample answer

The unexpected diagnosis of Down's syndrome at birth is a shock not only to the parents but also to the staff. The approach, therefore, has to be sensitive, empathic and multidisciplinary. The first step must be to inform the parents of the diagnosis. By this stage, paediatricians would have been involved and they are most suited to inform the parents. Honesty must be paramount. The parents will no doubt be shocked and angry, and staff must be prepared to be support them to come to terms with the diagnosis.

Where a paediatrician is not already involved, one should be asked to examine the neonate, to confirm the diagnosis and then to exclude other congenital malformations that may be associated with Down's syndrome, especially cardiac abnormalities. No matter how certain the diagnosis is from this physical examination, the parents must be made to understand the importance of conforming the diagnosis by karyotyping. The presence of associated malformations will certainly have an effect on the quality of life of the newborn. It is also necessary for the paediatrician to counsel the couple on the immediate neonatal and long-term care of the baby. It may be appropriate at this stage to mention some possible complications associated with this problem. However, care must be taken not to give too much information to the parents at this early stage.

A blood sample is essential for chromosomal analysis to confirm the diagnosis of Down's syndrome. Involvement of the clinical geneticist will provide genetic support and counselling, whereas social workers, the patient's general practitioner (GP) and midwife will provide support in the community. At this stage it may not be necessary to involve the geneticist, but he or she needs to be informed. The geneticist may only see the couple if they wish to do so.

Once the couple have come to terms with the diagnosis, a plan needs to be made about the immediate care of the neonate. Some parents may be too shocked to take the baby home. Under such circumstances, arrangements should be made for the immediate care of the baby in the hospital. The obstetrician, neonatologist and geneticist must arrange to follow up the couple. The objective of this is, first, to explain how the diagnosis was not made antenatally and, second, to answer all questions that the couple may have. The option of having their karyotypes determined must be discussed. This will exclude translocations and therefore allow a more accurate estimation of the recurrence risk. If the couple decide to take the baby home, information must be provided on the possible complications that such babies may have and how to recognize the early symptoms (for example, recurrent chest infections). Pamphlets should be given to the parents – those prepared by the Down's Syndrome Association contain details about where to get help, the problems and how to cope with a Down's syndrome baby.

At a later date, the couple will be counselled about the risk of recurrence and prenatal diagnosis. In any subsequent pregnancy, antenatal diagnosis would be discussed and offered. Chorionic villus sampling (CVS) and amniocenteses are the two options to be discussed. Although most couples will opt to take the baby home, some may reject it and the option of late acceptance must be available, but simultaneously, plans must be made for adoption.

3. A six-year-old girl has been referred to the gynaecology clinic with persistent vaginal discharge. Critically appraise your management of the patient.

Common mistakes

- Listing the causes of vaginal discharge in this young girl
- Assuming it is due to sexual abuse and involving the police and social workers without justification
- Undertaking a vaginal and rectal examination
- Taking a high vaginal swab in the clinic
- Referring the girl to the Genito-Urinary Medicine (GUM) unit
- Treating with oestrogen creams and triple antibiotics, irrespective of the cause
- Failure to provide critical appraisal of management

A good answer will contain some or all of these points

- A good candidate will recognize that this is a distressing problem to the young girl and her parents
- Recognize the sensitivity involved and the implications
- Recognize that sexual abuse may be a cause and that suspicions of this must be handled with care because of the sensitivity and the implications of attaching such a label
- Take a good history to exclude associated symptoms of pruritus, bloody discharge, changes of clothing or soap. Any known allergies?
- Other investigations, such as examination under anaesthesia (EUA), swabs, stool examination, etc.
- Causes – atrophic vaginitis predisposing to infections, foreign body, threadworms, sexual abuse and, rarely, tumours
- Gentle inspection of the vulva and anus, looking for signs of trauma and noting atrophic changes. Taking swabs from the introitus and external urethra and rectum if necessary
- Gentle rectal examination may be necessary with little finger – identify foreign body in vagina (but best avoided in the clinic and undertaken under general anaesthesia)
- EUA – using a paediatric laryngoscope. Remove foreign body and gently cleanse vagina. Offer oral antibiotics if any infection or suspicion of infection
- Atrophic vaginitis – treat with sparing topical application of oestrogen cream to the vulva for about two weeks

Sample answer

Vaginal discharge in a young girl is distressing not only to her, but to her parents. The way it is managed is important as it may cause further distress to families, especially if a suspicion of sexual abuse is a possible cause of the discharge.

The first step in her management is to take an appropriate history from the girl and her parents. Although this may provide important clues to the cause of the discharge, information from this young girl may not be forthcoming. For example, a history suggestive of the insertion of foreign body or sexual abuse may not be obtained easily. However, if there is any associated itching then the discharge may be related to threadworms. On the other hand, a sudden change in bathing soap, underwear or other agents which may cause an allergic reaction must be excluded.

After this, a physical examination must be performed. In a six-year-old this is difficult as an internal examination may not only be difficult but may be very distressing. Such an examination needs to be performed by a doctor experienced in adolescent gynaecology so as to recognize tell-tale signs of sexual abuse. During the investigations, swabs for bacteriology and virology should be obtained to exclude infections. These may, however, not be very reliable in view of the fact that these will be mainly from the introitus. The presence of excoriations in the vulvo-perineal region should heighten the suspicion of sexual abuse. If this is the case, an expert must be notified to come and examine the child, and if possible, to take photographs. Unfortunately, this action will cause enormous distress to the family. The way it is handled must therefore be very tactful. It will not be necessary at this stage to involve the police and social workers unless the evidence is overwhelming.

Further investigations include an ultrasound scan and an abdominal X-ray. Abdominal X-rays will identify radio-opaque foreign bodies in the vagina, although if one is present as the cause of the discharge, it will need removal – probably under general anaesthesia (GA). Ultrasound scan may similarly identify the cause (for example, a foreign body) but, again, another procedure will be necessary for its removal. Examination under anaesthesia (EUA) will not only allow diagnosis, but the removal of any foreign bodies. This procedure, however, in the absence of radiological support may miss hidden foreign bodies.

Other treatment options will depend on the identifiable cause. Infections with threadworms will be treated accordingly. Where the treatment is a simple improvement in hygiene, education of the parents may be all that is needed. It is important not to be seen to be judgemental, and some parents may become resentful at the thought of being accused of negligence, to the distress of their daughter. Lastly, where sexual abuse is the cause, the appropriate gynaecologist/paediatrician must take over the care of this young girl.

4. A mother brings her eight-year-old daughter to you because she has been menstruating regularly for the past four months. Justify your management of the young girl.

Common mistakes

- Listing the causes of precocious puberty only
- Treating this girl as an adult
- Taking a history from the girl and performing a physical examination, such as vaginal and speculum examination – are these really relevant?
- Failing to recognize the need to involve paediatricians
- Failure to recognize the psychological implications and the other consequences, such as pregnancy
- Assuming that the cause is pathological and therefore concentrating on the diagnosis and treatment of the various pathological causes
- Remember that this question requires justification – give reasons for everything you do

A good answer will include some or all of these points

- This girl has precocious puberty
- Her management must be approached sensitively – it may not be embarrassing to the girl but to her parents
- The causes of precocious puberty include: constitutional – most cases are constitutional; iatrogenic – exogenous substances which may be responsible; other pathologies
- Need to investigate the causes of precocious puberty
- Recognize and mention the consequences of precocious puberty
- Bone development
- Risk of pregnancy and sexual abuse
- Psychological consequences on the child, especially when she compares herself with her peers
- Offer treatment – medical and otherwise
- Need for follow-up in the appropriate clinic

Sample answer

This girl most likely has precocious puberty, which may not only be embarrassing to her, especially among her peers, but also to her parents. Her management must, therefore, be approached with sufficient sensitivity and understanding. In most cases, it is usually accompanied by puberche, thelarche and adrenache, although their absence does not exclude it. Most cases are constitutional but various endocrinopathies may be responsible and these need to be excluded before management is instituted. The causes of precocious puberty include constitutional, hypothyroidism (usually of the autoimmune type), craniopharyngiomas, postinfective encephalitis, neurofibromatosis, congenital brain defects, McCune–Albright syndrome, tumours of the ovary or adrenal and exogenous oestrogens.

In the first instance, information will be obtained from the parents about the sequence of events that preceded the first period. Associated symptoms of hypothyroidism must be excluded. Other associated important factors that must be excluded include infective encephalitis, headaches, visual disturbances and fractures of the skull. These will point to possible aetiological factors for the precocious puberty. In constitutional cases, there may be a family history of precocious puberty. A careful drug history will exclude exogenous steroids as a cause.

Following the detailed history a thorough search for signs would be undertaken. The presence of these may suggest the cause of the precocious puberty. The presence of café au lait spots, for example, suggests neurofibromatosis. Other signs include an enlarged thyroid gland, hydrocephalus, visual field abnormalities, abdominal masses and an abnormal ratio of the various long bones. Investigations such as thyroid function test, FSH and LH, prolactin, testosterone, oestradiol, dehydro-epiandrosterone sulphate and ultrasound scan of the ovaries and adrenal glands would further help in the identification of the cause.

The definitive treatment will depend on the cause. However, implications for this condition must also be addressed. If the girl is ovulating, the possibility of pregnancy if she is sexually exposed must be considered. Sensitive counselling must be offered in this regard. The second consequence of precocious puberty is premature closure of the epiphyses. Although the girl may initially be tall for her age, her ultimate height will be shorter. Treatment must not only be aimed at the cause but also at preventing premature closure of the epiphyses. Where the cause is constitutional, the treatment of choice is gonadotrophin-releasing hormone analogues. These will inhibit the pituitary function and therefore suppress ovarian activity. Exogenous oestrogens should be avoided as these are responsible for the premature closure of the epiphyses. Other causes should be treated accordingly. For example, hypothyroidism should be treated with thyroid replacement, whereas adrenal and ovarian causes may be treated by surgery. Other forms of treatment include neurosurgery or radiotherapy. Danazol could be used, but for its side-effects. Cyproterone acetate has been used in some cases with reasonable success. The advantage of this is that the anterior pituitary is not completely suppressed. Although medroyprogesterone acetate has been tried it does not appear to be associated with much success.

Whatever treatment the girl is offered, it must be accompanied by adequate psychological support. This will depend on her age and her needs. In other words, psychotherapy must be tailored to the needs of the patient.

References

Duncan SLB. Disorders of puberty. In: Shaw RW, Soutter PW, Stanton S (eds). *Gynaecology*. London: Churchill, 1997; 188–199.
Swaenepoel C, Chaussain CL, Reger M. Long-term results of long-acting luteinising hormone-releasing hormone in the central precocious puberty. *Hormone Research* 1991; 36: 126–130.

5. Evaluate your management of a 10-year-old girl presenting with vaginal bleeding of one week's duration.

Common mistakes

- Assuming that she has cancer and ignoring all other causes of bleeding *per vaginum*
- Treating her as an adult
- Taking a detailed sexual history and excluding features of pregnancy
- Performing a physical examination – general, vaginal and speculum, taking swabs for cervical smear and microbiological investigations
- Failing to recognize that infections and sexual abuse may be a cause
- Assuming she has precocious puberty and investigating for all the causes of this condition
- Treating her for menstrual problems

A good answer will include some or all of these points

- Recognize that this is a young patient and therefore a sensitive approach is required
- The co-operation of her parents is essential and, where possible, paediatricians may be involved
- Need to take a careful history (from the girl and her parents) to exclude: trauma; sexual abuse; infections; foreign body
- Investigations to include: examination under general anaesthesia (EUA) if possible; ultrasound scan; high vaginal swabs/rectal swabs; hormonal investigations
- If any tumours – biopsy
- Treatment – depending on the identified cause

Sample answer

The management of this young girl requires understanding of the psychological consequences of various investigations and treatment of the bleeding, on both the girl and her parents. An important first step is to take a thorough history. This will provide possible clues to the aetiology of the bleeding, for example trauma, a foreign body and menarche. Chronological development of secondary sexual characteristics culminating in vaginal bleeding suggest menarchial bleeding. Other possible causes include infections, sexual abuse and malignancies. Although information about sexual abuse is difficult to obtain, efforts must be made in a sensitive and non-threatening way to gauge whether this could be the cause. Often, this can only be suspected after a pelvic examination.

Physical examination is essential to eliminate possible causes of the abnormal vaginal bleeding. In the first instance, characteristics of puberty should be identified if present. These will include breast development, height, pubic hair and other features of puberty. An abdominal examination may identify masses in the pelvic area, such as oestrogen-secreting ovarian tumours, which may be responsible for the vaginal bleeding. Where infection is the suspected cause, swabs must be obtained from the vagina and other suspected sites, such as the urethra and rectum. A restrictive pelvic examination starting with a gentle inspection of the vulval and perianal area may point to an infection or trauma, which may be sexually related. A gentle rectal examination with the little finger may identify a foreign body in the vagina. It may also identify a tumour in the vagina, which may be responsible for the bleeding.

Where there is no obvious cause identified, further investigations should be performed. These will include an examination under anaesthesia (EUA). A paediatric laryngoscope may be used to examine the vagina. Where there is a tumour, a biopsy should be taken. The most common type of tumour in this age group is sarcoma botyroides. This has a fleshy appearance and is of vaginal origin. Although the appearances of such a lesion are characteristic, it is necessary to confirm the diagnosis by a biopsy under general anaesthesia (GA). An ultrasound scan of the abdomen and the lower genital tract will not only identify any ovarian pathology but may be able to identify foreign bodies in the vagina. A pregnancy presenting as threatened miscarriage can also be excluded by ultrasound scan.

Following these simple and extremely important stages, subsequent management will depend on the suspected cause of the bleeding. Where atrophic changes are thought to be the cause, simple but sparing application of topical oestrogen will suffice. However, this should not be offered for more than two weeks. If it is an infection, such as threadworms, there will be associated pruritus and deworming may be all that is needed with appropriate education about hygiene. The diagnosis of a vaginal malignancy will require surgery, but this needs to be undertaken by an adequately skilled surgeon.

2

Menstrual disorders

1. A 37-year-old lady presented to you with regular and heavy periods. After thorough investigations, no abnormality was identified. Briefly debate the options (excluding hysterectomy) available for the treatment of this lady.

2. Evaluate the surgical methods of treating a 33-year-old woman with menorrhagia.

3. Critically appraise your management of a woman with cyclical secondary dysmenorrhoea.

4. A 31-year-old para 2+1 presents with secondary amenorrhoea. A pelvic examination and various investigations performed on her were normal. Evaluate your subsequent management.

5. How will you justify your management of a 37-year-old teacher with severe pre-menstrual syndrome?

1. A 37-year-old lady presented to you with regular and heavy periods. After thorough investigations, no abnormality was identified. Briefly debate the options (excluding hysterectomy) available for the treatment of this lady.

Common mistakes

- Discussing the management of uterine fibroids
- Assuming that she has an infection
- Listing the causes of bleeding in this woman
- Assuming that she has completed her family
- Offering her a hysterectomy as the best treatment – you have been told to exclude this option
- Discussing hysteroscopy, endometrial biopsy and ultrasound as part of your management

A good answer will include some or all of these points

- The options available to this patient with menorrhagia are: medical/hormonal: combined oral contraceptive pill; antifibrinolytic agents; prostaglandin synthetase inhibitors; progestogens; progestogen-only intrauterine devices; anti-oestrogens; danazol; GnRH analogues; surgical: laser ablation of the endometrium; resection of the endometrium; balloon/microwave ablations
- For each of these methods, discuss the merits and demerits
- Conclusion – the best options for this patient (first choice, etc.)

Sample answer

This patient has dysfunctional uterine bleeding and her treatment can either be medical or surgical. The suitability of either option will depend on several factors.

The combined oral contraceptive pill is the first medical therapeutic option. It is cheap, efficacious and provides the additional benefit of contraception. However, in view of the patient's age it may not be very suitable, especially if she is a smoker, overweight, or is at risk of venous thrombo-embolism (VTE). An additional disadvantage is the need to take the pill regularly. Even if she has no need for contraception, this will still be an appropriate therapeutic option.

Antifibrinolytic agents are the second medical option. The most effective is tranexamic acid. A randomized controlled trial (Bonnar and Sheppard, 1996) concluded that this was the most effective treatment for menorrhagia. Its main advantage is that of proven efficacy. It is also cheap and does not increase the risk of venous VTE. However, the patient needs to take this medication during menstruation and unless her periods are as regular as clockwork, she may find the occasional early period unacceptable. Although the non-steroidal anti-inflammatory agent (NSAID) mefenamic acid is not as effective as tranexamic acid, it is an acceptable option.

In addition, it reduces the pain that may accompany heavy periods. These and other prostaglandin synthetase inhibitors are not as effective as tranexamic acid and may be associated with gastric ulceration.

The progestogen-only (levonorgestrel) intrauterine contraceptive device (Mirena) is an option that has many advantages. It is administered once every five years. It is effective and provides additional contraception if necessary. It reduces menstrual blood loss by about 80 per cent within six months of insertion. Although expensive, it is more cost-effective than the other options in the long term. It may be associated with irregular vaginal bleeding, especially during the first six months, and in a woman who has multiple sexual partners may increase the risk of pelvic inflammatory disease. It may also cause headaches, acne, breast tenderness and functional ovarian cysts. It requires skill to insert and, if ineffective, will need to be removed.

The use of anti-oestrogens or gonadotrophin releasing hormone analogues (GnRH) in this patient will in most cases produce excellent results. These drugs are very effective when administered regularly. The nasal sprays have to be taken regularly, whereas the depot injections have to be administered monthly. Depot GnRH analogues are administered by qualified persons only and therefore compliance is not an issue. They are expensive and are associated with menopausal symptoms. If used for more than six months, they may cause osteopenia unless combined with AddBack therapy. For danazol, the patient needs to be motivated to take the medication daily. Danazol is associated with several complications, which will affect compliance and therefore efficacy.

Cyclical progestogens, in the form of norethisterone are the least effective medical option in this patient. In the Dublin randomized trial, norethisterone was found to be the least effective in controlling menorrhagia (reducing blood loss in less than 40 per cent of patients), although it is the most commonly prescribed. It is cheap but has side-effects, such as breakthrough bleeding, breast tenderness and mood swings. Again, it has to be taken daily and failure to do so may be associated with unwanted side-effects, such as breakthrough bleeding.

Surgical options include laser ablation/resection of the endometrium and balloon/ microwave (or other local methods) destruction of the endometrium. These techniques require skill and special equipment. Most are undertaken in hospitals, although many are treated as day-cases. Recognised complications include haemorrhage, perforation and fluid overload. Studies suggest that these ablative techniques are most effective during the first year after treatment and thereafter the incidence of hysterectomy rises (Dwyer et al. 1993).

In the management of this patient, a systematic approach will be adopted, starting with the option with the least side-effects yet most effective, and then progressing through the more costly and still effective alternatives. Tranexamic acid will be the first option if contraception is not an issue. If it is, and there are no contraindications, the combined oral contraceptive pill will be the first preference. The last but very effective option will be surgery.

References

Bonnar J, Sheppard BL. Treatment of menorrhagia during menstruation: randomised controlled trial of ethamsylate, mefenamic acid and tranexamic acid. *BMJ* 1996; 313: 579–82.

Dwyer N, Hutton J, Stirrat GM. Randomised controlled trial comparing endometrial resection with abdominal hysterectomy for the surgical treatment of menorrhagia. *BJOG*, 1993; 100: 237–43.

2. Evaluate the surgical methods of treating a 33-year-old woman with menorrhagia.

Common mistakes

- Listing the treating methods and discussing the details of how they are administered
- Discussing the medial therapeutic options of this patient
- Stating that she ought not to have surgery without first trying the medical options – **this** may well be the case, but the question is not asking you to critically appraise the decision to offer her surgical treatment
- Failing to evaluate the options listed
- Taking a history and doing a physical examination. Although this is not irrelevant, it is unlikely to earn you many marks
- The definition of menorrhagia is standard, therefore, irregular menstrual periods should not be considered in the management of this patient
- Assuming that she has polycystic ovary disease and listing the treatment for this condition
- Discussing treatment for infertility
- Considering a uterine malignancy as a differential diagnosis, although this is possible, it is very unlikely in this patient; remember, common things occur commonly

A good answer will include some or all of these points

- Non-medical methods include: laser endometrial ablation; endometrial resection; balloon/diathermy endometrial ablation; hysterectomy
- Laser – expensive equipment. Failure rate, skilled operator, risk of perforation
- Resection – similar problems as with laser. Equipment less expensive. Risk of complications not as high, failure rate is similar to that of laser
- Thermal endometrial ablation – balloon, etc. less expensive, day case procedure, cheaper, however, mainly at very specialized centres though becoming more widespread, effective
- Other forms of local destructive treatment – mention them if you know their names, otherwise indicate that you are aware of this rapidly evolving therapeutic option
- Hysterectomy – final, expensive, etc.
- Myomectomy – if fibroids

Sample answer

The treatment of this patient will depend on several factors, the most important of which is her desire to have children, or more children, and also on the cause of her menorrhagia. Causes that will require specific surgical treatment include uterine fibroids, adenomyosis and endometriosis.

If the patient has dysfunctional uterine bleeding (that is, her menorrhagia is idiopathic), surgical options include destructive procedures of the endometrium and a hysterectomy. The destructive procedures (such as laser ablation, endometrial resection, balloon or thermal ablation and other newer techniques of destruction of the endometrium) are effective, easy to perform and associated with a lower morbidity. However, most are only performed in hospitals (as day cases) by gynaecologists. Because of the short operative time and early postoperative recovery, they have a significant advantage in a patient who is at a significant risk of venous thrombo-embolism (VTE) from prolonged surgery. In good hands, 70–80 per cent of patients are very satisfied with the results. When it fails it must be considered as an expensive option as it has to be superseded by a hysterectomy or a repeat procedure. A local destructive procedure will only be considered in this patient if she has completed her family.

The second surgical option, hysterectomy, is appropriate for idiopathic menorrhagia and that secondary to uterine fibroids, pelvic inflammatory disease, adenomyosis and endometriosis. The advantage of this is that it is the definitive treatment of menorrhagia. It is cost-effective and completely eliminates the problem. However, it is expensive and may be associated with complications, including mortality. Although very effective, it can only be performed in hospital and is associated with a prolonged recovery when compared to that of an ablative/destructive procedure. Its main advantage is the effectiveness of the treatment.

If the cause of the menorrhagia in this patient is uterine fibroids, another other option for her treatment would be a myomectomy. This surgical procedure is associated with complications, such as bleeding, adhesion formation and, in some cases, progression to a hysterectomy. It is the best option if the patient has not completed her family. Myomectomy is expensive and has to be performed by an experienced surgeon. The possible drawback is the fact that not all the fibroids may be removed. The patient may therefore represent with menorrhagia and require a repeat procedure.

Lastly, if endometriosis is the cause of the patient's menorrhagia, laser destruction of the endometriosis and uterosacral nerve division (LUNA) may reduce the menorrhagia. The success of these procedures is poor, although when combined with medical treatment there is significant benefit. These procedures may also be associated with complications, such as damage to the bladder, bowel and ureters.

3. Critically appraise your management of a woman with cyclical secondary dysmenorrhoea.

Common mistakes

- Taking a history and undertaking a physical examination, although this is important, you do not need to spend too much time on this
- Defining different types of cyclical dysmenorrhoea – primary and secondary. The question has already stated that the patient has secondary dysmenorrhoea, so focus on this only
- Devoting most of the essay to the causes of secondary dysmenorrhoea
- Detailed discussion on the differential diagnoses – these should only be mentioned
- Why is it important to make a diagnosis – trying to justify the distinction in the management approach between primary and secondary dysmenorrhoea
- Not critically appraising your answer but simply outlining or discussing the management

A good answer will include some or all of these points

- Definition of secondary dysmenorrhea
- Common causes of cyclical secondary dysmenorrhoea – only briefly mentioning these: endometriosis; adenomyosis; chronic pelvic inflammatory disease; no identifiable cause (idiopathic)
- Diagnosing the cause of dysmenorrhoea: specific symptoms may help diagnosis – limitations of history-taking; physical examination – limited but may exclude other pathologies; diagnostic laparoscopy – will exclude the main causes – expensive and will not exclude all causes, for example adenomyosis; ultrasound scan – will exclude adenomyosis and fibroids
- Treatment – depends on the cause: adenomyosis – danazol, GnRH analogues, etc.; endometriosis – treat accordingly; pelvic inflammatory disease – often difficult to treat
- Supportive care

Sample answer

Cyclical secondary dysmenorrhoea in this patient could be due to endometriosis, chronic pelvic inflammatory disease, adenomyosis, an intrauterine contraceptive device, cervical stenosis or it may be idiopathic. Some of these conditions may be suspected from a well-directed history. The clinical symptoms of some of them are unique. For example, in the presence of endometriosis there may be an associated deep dyspareunia. However, while history may be useful in suspecting some causes, it is unlikely to provide a definitive diagnosis. In addition, some of the causes of secondary dysmenorrhoea listed above may present with similar symptoms.

A physical examination may identify some signs of the pathologies causing the patient's dysmenorrhoea. These include retroversion with or without fixation, bilateral adnexal tenderness, adnexal masses, and a bulky uterus. The value of a clinical examination in the diagnosis of the cause of her symptoms is limited. The presence of these signs does not necessarily diagnose the cause of the dysmenorrhoea. It will, however, exclude major pelvic pathologies. A stenosed cervix, especially in a patient who has had a cone biopsy, will be suggestive of cervical stenosis. In some patients, a bulky uterus with a doughy consistency will suggest adenomyosis. Although a physical examination may be helpful, it may not be very accurate.

Specific investigations will, therefore, have to be performed to make a definitive diagnosis or to exclude all the suspected causes of the dysmenorrhoea. A diagnostic laparoscopy will exclude endometriosis, pelvic inflammatory disease and suggest adenomyosis. Unfortunately, the absence of obvious endometriosis does not exclude endometriosis. Similarly, the diagnosis of chronic pelvic inflammatory disease may not be conclusive at laparoscopy. Laparoscopy is expensive, has to be performed in the hospital – usually under general anaesthesia (GA) (although it can also be performed under conscious sedation). This procedure may be complicated by bowel and bladder injuries, haemorrhage or air embolism. It will, however, be the most important investigation in the management of this patient.

Another investigation of importance is ultrasound scan of the pelvis. This investigation depends on the expertise of the operator and the quality of the machine being used. Ultrasound scan will exclude adenomyosis and uterine fibroids. Ovarian endometriomata may also be diagnosed, however, the absence of pathology on scan does not exclude it. Thus, whilst this investigation is expensive and may provide hints on the possible cause of the dysmenorrhoea, it will only diagnose a cause in some cases.

The value of taking swabs from the cervix to exclude pelvic inflammatory disease is debatable. Pelvic inflammatory disease as a cause of dysmenorrhoea is difficult to diagnose from swabs from the endocervix or vagina. Although this may be useful in the diagnosis of acute infections, it will be ineffective in the diagnosis of chronic pelvic inflammatory disease.

The treatment of this patient will depend on the cause of the dysmenorrhoea. For endometriosis, the treatment options include the combined oral contraceptive pill, progestogens, danazol and GnRH analogues. The combined oral contraceptive pill is effective in a premenopausal patient with no contraindications. It has to be taken continuously and has the advantage of being an effective contraceptive; however, it may cause breakthrough vaginal bleeding. Another alternative is a progestogen. Again, this needs to be taken daily and may be associated with acne, weight gain and irregular vaginal bleeding. If the woman is older and a smoker, the combined oral contraceptive pill will an unacceptable option. Danazol will be effective in the treatment of endometriosis, adenomyosis and dysmenorrhoea of unknown aetiology. It is, however, associated with many side-effects, which may affect compliance and therefore efficacy. The GnRH analogues are probably the most effective but are associated with menopausal side-effects, which may also affect tolerance. Where the cause of the dysmenorrhoea is pelvic inflammatory disease, attempting to treat the cause may be impossible. However, suppressing ovulation and providing anti-inflammatory agents may be effective.

The last option before surgery is supportive care. Simply explaining the nature of the patient's symptoms and the diagnosed cause will go a long way towards increasing the success rate. Where all the options discussed above have failed, hysterectomy must be considered. This is an expensive major procedure, associated with short- and long-term complications, but it is cost-effective in the treatment of secondary dysmenorrhoea. The patient must have completed her family before considering this option.

4. A 31-year-old para 2+1 presents with secondary amenorrhoea. A pelvic examination and various investigations performed on her were normal. Evaluate your subsequent management.

Common mistakes

- Enumerating all the causes of secondary amenorrhoea
- Listing all the investigations of secondary amenorrhoea
- Ignoring the facts given and doing a physical examination (it has already been stated that a physical examination and hormonal investigations were all normal)
- Inducing ovulation – assuming that the patient's other problem is infertility (after investigating the male partner)
- Advising about *in vitro* fertilization (IVF) and GIFT and assuming the problem is ovarian

A good answer will include some or all of these points

- The problem is most likely uterine or hormonal (polycystic ovary syndrome)
- History to exclude causes, such as Asherman syndrome, from an evacuation after a miscarriage or delivery, myomectomy and infections (for example, tuberculosis) and the intrauterine contraceptive device
- Investigations: hysteroscopy – value – identify cause and may be therapeutic, for example division of adhesions; hysterosalpingography – identify cause but not therapeutic; infection – tuberculosis – Mantoux test and chest X-ray (CXR); ultrasound scan – polycystic ovary syndrome and hormonal profile
- Treatment – division of adhesions, intrauterine contraceptive device, oestrogens (poor results)
- Tuberculosis of the genital tract – treat with systemic medication but gynaecological prognosis is poor
- If desires future pregnancies – counsel
- If polycystic ovary syndrome – treat accordingly

Sample answer

The most likely problem in this patient is uterine, although a mild hormonal cause must be considered. The uterine cause most likely to be responsible is Asherman syndrome. Polycystic ovary syndrome should, however, be considered in the investigations and treatment.

A history will provide a clue to the possible cause of uterine synaechiae. Previous dilatation and curettage or evacuation of retained products of conception following an incomplete miscarriage or secondary postpartum haemorrhage may be divulged by the patient. If any of these procedures was followed by the amenorrhoea, it is likely to be responsible. Other causes of

Asherman syndrome include tuberculosis of the pelvis, previous surgery (such as myomectomy) or the use of an intrauterine contraceptive device. A careful and directed history may therefore provide clues to the possible cause of the amenorrhoea. Excessive weight gain, hirsutism and acne will raise suspicions of polycystic ovary syndrome.

Investigations will be extremely useful in this patient and will certainly help in making the diagnosis. These include a hysteroscopy and a hysterosalpingography. A hysteroscopy will identify intrauterine adhesions and a hypoplastic endometrium. It may also provide an opportunity for adhesiolysis to be performed at the same time. At the time of the hysteroscopy, an intrauterine contraceptive device may also be inserted. This procedure can be performed on an outpatient basis under local anaesthesia or under general anaesthesia (GA) as a day case procedure. A hysterosalpingography may also be performed to diagnose Asherman syndrome. However, this is not therapeutic, is extremely uncomfortable and, where the patient is allergic to the medium used, may pose more problems. It may also precipitate an acute on chronic pelvic inflammatory disease.

If pelvic tuberculosis is suspected, an endometrial biopsy should be performed and sent for histology. In addition, a Mantoux or Heaf test may be performed.

The treatment will depend on the aetiology of the amenorrhea. If it is Asherman syndrome, the treatment is hysteroscopic division of the adhesions, insertion of an intrauterine device to prevent reformation and oestrogen stimulation of regeneration of the endometrium from glands. Unfortunately, this treatment is not very successful. If the patient does not want any more children, reassurance is all that is needed. If she desires pregnancy, appropriate counselling will be required. Unless she resumes normal menstruation, the chances are slim. In addition, the risks of miscarriage, premature labour, placenta accreta and percreta are high with pregnancy. Where the cause is polycystic ovary syndrome, appropriate hormone treatment will be provided. Cyclical progestogens will induce normal menstruation and, after six months, this may be discontinued and hopefully normal menstruation will resume. Induction of ovulation will be appropriate if the patient desires further pregnancies.

5. How will you justify your management of a 37-year-old teacher with severe pre-menstrual syndrome?

Common mistakes

- Offering treatment before confirming diagnosis
- Physical examination to confirm diagnosis
- Hormone profile to confirm diagnosis
- Ultrasound – an important investigation
- Premenstrual syndrome may be a differential diagnosis of large uterine fibroids, pelvic inflammatory disease and endometriosis – discussing these differentials and their management
- Avoid vague phrases, such as *'Various drugs can be tried'*!

A good answer will include some or all of these points

- Diagnosis needs to be confirmed: best from a symptoms chart/diary/calender; therapeutic trial with GnRH analogues
- Management – multidisciplinary team approach, including psychologist/psychiatrist
- General comment about treatment methods – high placebo effect
- Treatments of proven benefit: suppress ovulation – combined oral contraceptive pill; progestogens; oestrogens; danazol; GnRH analogues; surgery – bilateral oophorectomy; selective serotonin re-uptake inhibitors (SSRIs); anti-depressants, for example Prozac
- Unproven benefits: evening primrose oil; B6, pyridoxine
- Quality of life assessment of success

Sample answer

Premenstrual syndrome is common at the extremes of reproductive life. Confirming the diagnosis is paramount and this is best done from a symptom calendar or chart. A therapeutic trial with a gonadotrophin releasing (GnRH) analogue maybe more precise and effective in some cases, however. Once the diagnosis is confirmed, subsequent management should ideally be multidisciplinary – involving gynaecologists, psychologist or psychiatrists where it is deemed necessary.

There are various treatment options for premenstrual syndrome. It also has a high placebo effect. In fact, placebo effects have been reported in excess of 90 per cent in some studies. The treatment of choice will be influenced by the patient's desire for contraception or contraindications to the various options. In the absence of contraindications, the combined oral contraceptive pill will be the drug of first choice. It suppresses ovulation but may still be associated with symptoms of premenstrual syndrome. This is more so with the trisequens, which contain high progestogens in the second half of the packages. The combined oral contraceptive pill may completely relieve the symptoms, limit them to one or two days premenstrually or it may be ineffective.

The second therapeutic option will be progestogens only. Taken in form of tablets or pessaries during the second half of the menstrual cycle, these may improve symptoms in some patients. Monthly or three-monthly progestogen injections may also be effective. The exact physiological basis for the effectiveness of this option is unclear. It is probably the least likely of all the hormone therapies to be effective.

Danazol, with its anti-oestrogenic and anti-gonadotrophic activities, is an effective treatment. The main drawback is the associated side-effects, which include weight gain, headaches, muscle cramps, hirsutism and voice changes. These may affect complaince.

Gonadotrophin releasing hormone (GnRH) analogues are probably the most effective medical option for this patient. They suppress ovarian activity by downregulating the pituitary gland. In this patient, not only may the symptoms be alleviated but it may enable the determination of what proportion of the symptoms are of ovarian/endocrine origin, and therefore whether she would benefit from bilateral oophorectomy. Although it may be accompanied by menopausal symptoms, these could be overcome by including AddBack therapy to the treatment. Where this combination is effective, therapy could be prolonged beyond six months.

More recent therapeutic regimens include selective serotonin re-uptake inhibitors (SSRIs). This option is based on the report of altered serotonergic function in patients with premenstrual syndrome. In these women, it is thought that serotonin deficiency possibly makes them more sensitive to their endogenous ovarian steroids and boosting serotonin should therefore improve symptoms. The use of SSRIs, such as clomipramine and fluoxetine, has been shown to be effective in some patients. What is uncertain is precisely who will benefit from SSRIs. In this patient, this option may be tried and only after assessing her response will it then be possible to assess possible benefits from the treatment.

Oestradiol implants and transdermal patches may also be tried in this patient. These suppress the ovarian cycle and have been demonstrated to be benefit some patients. However, the risks of endometrial hyerplasia may require combining them with a progestogen, which may cause premenstrual symptoms and subsequent poor compliance. Combining the implants with the levonorgestrel intrauterine contraceptive device, which theoretically has fewer systemic side-effects may overcome this problem. This option should only be considered if her premenstrual syndrome is very severe and other options have failed.

An effective option is bilateral oophorectomy. This is effective but will require oestrogen hormone replacement therapy (which being unopposed) should not be associated with re-occurrence of the symptoms. The selection of patients for this radical procedure is important and GnRH analogues may be useful in this regard. If her symptoms are eliminated over a period of three months on this regimen then oophorectomy would be successful.

Anti-depressants may also be used. Prozac has been shown to be effective in the treatment of premenstrual syndrome. In prescribing this treatment for this patient, extreme sensitivity must be shown as the patient may mistake the treatment to be that for depression.

The use of treatment regimens such as evening primrose oil, vitamin B6 and pyridoxine may alleviate her symptoms, but the efficacy of these non-hormonal regimens is unpredictable. A combination of these with psychotherapy may, however, be associated with better results.

3

Gynaecology, endocrinology

1. A 19-year-old woman has been referred to the gynaecologist by her general practitioner with hirsutism. You have investigated her and found no obvious cause. Evaluate the treatment options for this young woman.

2. What advice will you give a 34-year-old, well-educated woman with polycystic ovary disease about the wider health implications of her condition?

3. Critically appraise the management of a 27-year-old woman presenting with inappropriate galactorrhoea and secondary amenorrhoea.

4. An 18-year-old girl who is *virgo intacta* attended the gynaecololgy clinic because she is yet to start menstruating. She has two sisters and three brothers. Justify the steps you will take to manage this patient.

1. A 19-year-old woman has been referred to the gynaecologist by her general practitioner with hirsutism. You have investigated her and found no obvious cause. Evaluate the treatment options for this young girl.

Common mistakes

- Discussing the pathogenesis of hirsutism
- Listing all the causes of hirsutism
- Detailing the symptoms of polycystic ovary disease and the physiological bases of hyper-androgenism in polycystic ovary disease
- Management of infertility and menstrual abnormalities
- Defining hirsutism and the use of Galloway and Ferriman classifications of hirsutism
- Advising the patient to lose weight – not told that she is obese
- Treating all the associated symptoms of polycystic ovary syndrome, for example menstrual abnormalities, acne, infertility, obesity, etc.
- Use of trade names of very unfamiliar drugs

A good answer will include some or all of these points

- This is an aesthetically/socially embarrassing problem
- May be familial/racial
- History to exclude these aspects
- Reassurance may be all that is needed, especially if familial
- Specific treatment
- Medical: cyproterone acetate – alone; cyproterone acetate in combination with oestrogen (Dianette) – also combined oral contraceptive pill; other anti-androgens – spironolactone (not as effective), flutamide
- Mechanical – cheap, patient is treated as normal, that is, does not have a disease (not medicalized): bleaching; shaving; depilatory; electrolysis; laser

Sample answer

Hirsutism can be aesthetically unacceptable and socially embarrassing. In the management of this patient, therefore, empathy and appropriate sensitivity is necessary. Usually, there is no known cause and it is either racial or familial. This can be excluded by family history. If this is the case, all that is necessary is reassurance. In this group, this is effective and obviates the need for lengthy treatments, repeated hospital visits and the stigma of pathology.

In some cases, however, despite reassurance, the patient will still require treatment. Various options are available, starting from very simple methods of hair removal, to medication. The motivation of the patient is important in the choice of treatment. It is often preferable to start with the simple and effective methods before introducing the complex and expensive regimens.

The first option for this patient will be shaving the excessive hair. If this is unacceptable, other mechanical treatments, such as plucking and waxing, could be considered. These are cheap and effective but require repeated application. The myth that shaving increases hirsutism needs to be dismissed in order to motivate this patient appropriately. Where she objects to this, or has previously tried these methods unsuccessfully, she should be offered bleaching and/or laser treatment. These methods are effective but are more expensive. Electrolysis is thought to be the only permanent way of removing hair and gives the best cosmetic result. This may be offered as an option if the others are unsuccessful or unacceptable. However, it is expensive and needs to be performed by an experienced operator to minimize the risks of scarring or infection.

Medical treatment options will be the last option for this young woman. The first will be a combination of cyproterone acetate (an anti-androgen) and an oestrogen in the form of Dianette. This offers the added advantage of effective contraception if required and also corrects any menstrual abnormalities. It is cheap and effective, but compliance may be a problem as it has to be taken regularly. In a young woman this may be an important consideration. It is important to emphasize that the effects of this treatment are not immediate and it may take up to four months for a significant difference to be noticed. More than 70 per cent of women treated with this regimen report a significant improvement in symptoms within 12 months. Side-effects, of which the patient must be warned, include depression, weight gain and breast tenderness.

If the patient does not require contraception, cyproterone acetate may be offered on its own. Again, motivation is required as it is taken daily. There are side-effects of this treatment, which may be unacceptable to the patient and therefore result in poor compliance. If this is not acceptable, spironolactone (an aldosterone antagonist with androgenic receptor-blocking activity) or flutamide (a non-steroidal anti-androgen) may be used. Flutamide may also be used in combination with a combined oral contraceptive pill to achieve results comparable to those of spironolactone or cyproterone acetate. Flutamide has several side-effects and may be poorly tolerated. A comparative trial of spironolactone and cyproterone acetate did not show any significant difference in response between the two groups, but spironolactone is not the drug of choice because of its side-effects and cost. In addition, when used it must be combined with effective contraception.

Other less-effective options that may be considered include ketoconazole, a synthetic imidazole derivative, which blocks gonadal and adrenal steroidogenesiss. Unfortunately, marked side-effects, such as nausea, asthenia and alopecia, necessitate close monitoring during treatment and may also result in poor compliance. Clinical response to this option is also relatively poor.

Ovarian suppression with low-dose contraceptive pills and gonadotrophin-releasing (GnRH) analogous are effective in some patients. The former will be suitable in this young woman, but the latter will have severe hypoestrogenic side-effects, which may be effective and more acceptable.

An important aspect of her management is the emphasis on the absence of pathology. Such reassurance and encouraging the patient to have a more positive image of herself may be all that is necessary.

2. What advice will you give a 34-year-old, well-educated woman with polycystic ovary disease about the wider health implications of her condition?

Common mistakes

Discussing:
- Infertility in polycystic ovary syndrome
- Irregular periods and how to manage them
- Acne and hirsutism, and how to manage them
- Ovulation induction in women with polycystic ovary syndrome
- The patient did not present with specific symptoms (so do not state that this will depend on her symptoms)
- Do not advise on contraception and other related problems

A good answer will include some or all of these points

- Insulin resistance, resulting in diabetes mellitus
  - Need to watch out for early symptoms of diabetes mellitus and make regular check-ups with general practitioner (GP), and check urine
- Ischaemic heart disease due to abnormal cholesterol metabolism
  - General health advice – adequate and regular exercise
  - Dietary – aim to reduce cholesterol levels
  - Early warning signs of heart disease/attacks
- Hypertension – increased risk
  - Regular blood pressure check
  - Persistent headaches need to be checked
- Endometrial carcinoma
  - Perimenopausal irregular vaginal bleeding
  - Postmenopausal bleeding
- Excessive weight gain
  - Dietary control

Sample answer

Polycystic ovary syndrome is one of the most common gynaecological endocrinological problem, which is increasingly recognized to have important health implications for the individual. These implications vary from the wider cardiovascular and metabolic problems to those of the genital tract.

The first issue is the increased risk of cardiovascular disorders. These include hypertension and ischaemic heart disease. Abnormal cholesterol metabolism is responsible for this increased risk. The advice for the patient will, therefore, relate to early warning signs of hypertension and ischaemic heart disease. These include, headaches, easy fatiguability, shortness of breath and precordial chest pain. It is important that the patient reduces cholesterol in her diet and visits her general practitioner (GP) regularly. The GP must be informed of these increased health risks and will therefore monitor the patient's blood pressure, cholesterol levels and examine her cardiovascular system.

The patient is also at an increased risk of developing insulin resistance. This is due to hyperandrogenism and insulin-like growth factors in polycystic ovary syndrome. She must therefore be educated on the early symptoms of diabetes mellitus, such as polyuria, polydypsia and polyphagia. In addition, she must attend her GP regularly for urine testing and occasional blood-glucose estimation.

An important complication of polycystic ovary syndrome is the development of endometrial cancer. In educating this patient, it is important to be extremely sensitive and cautious as she could become unnecessarily alarmed. Irregular periods are a recognized symptom of polycystic ovary syndrome and may also be a presentation for endometrial cancer. Polycystic ovary syndrome is one condition in which endometrial cancer may occur before menopause. It is therefore important for the patient to visit her GP regularly with any unusual vaginal bleeding and, where necessary, ultrasound scans should be performed and endometrial biopsies taken. Early referral for hysteroscopic assessment of endometrium would be highlly recommended to her GP.

Lastly, obesity is an important sequelae of this condition. If the patient is not obese, she needs to be counselled about her diet and exercise. These will not only reduce the risk of the other wider health issues, such as hypertension and endometrial cancer, but will reduce the risks of diabetes.

The advice this patient will be given will need to be reinforced by information she receives from her GP and from information leaflets about the wider health implications of this common endocrine condition.

3. Critically appraise the management of a 27-year-old woman presenting with inappropriate galactorrhoea and secondary amenorrhoea.

Common mistakes

- Assuming that she has a prolactinoma – no definite cause has been provided
- Discussing the treatment of infertility
- Referring the patient to an endocrinologist – indicating that this is the best option and therefore a gynaecologist should not manage her!!
- Concentrating on history and physical examination – unnecessary to provide all the details

A good answer will include some or all of these points

- There are many causes of galactorrhoea
- History to exclude some of these causes
- Physical examination to exclude disturbances in the visual field; thyroid gland enlargement
- Investigations to identify the cause of the galactorrhoea: hormone profile – thyroid stimulating hormone (TSH), follicular stimulating hormone (FSH), luteinizing hormone (LH), free T4; skull X-ray – will only identify gross pathology. Best option is magnetic resonance imaging (MRI) of the skull, especially the pituitary fossa; computerized tomography (CT) scan if necessary
- Treatment will depend on the cause and the wishes of the patient
- Primary concern amenorrhoea – treat appropriately
- Infertility co-existing – treat accordingly
- May need to be referred to neurosurgeons for surgery for prolactinomas
- Treatment for prolactinomas: bromocrytine; carbergoline; polycystic ovary syndrome; osteoporosis

Sample answer

Inappropriate galactorrhoea is defined as milk production outside lactation. In some cases there may not be an obvious cause, but often it may be due to hyperprolactinaemia. The combination of amenorrhoea and inappropriate galactorrhoea suggests that the patient may be hyerprolactinaemic. In her management, possible causes of galactorrhoea should be excluded before initiating treatment for the amenorrhoea.

Recognized causes of hyperprolactinaemia, such as drugs that inhibit dopamine production or action (for example, phenothiaxides, benzodiazepines, steroids, antihypertensive agents, etc.) may be established from directed questioning of the patient. In addition, symptoms of hypothyroidism, intracranial lesions (headaches, nausea, vomiting, visual field disturbances), chronic renal failure and polycystic ovary syndrome or stress may be excluded from the history. Although the history may provide very useful information, it is important to recognize that the most common causes of hyperprolactinaemia are pituitary prolatinomas and idiopathic hypersecretion, both of which are more likely to be asymptomatic. The two pathologies may, indeed, be unrelated and therefore symptoms of other causes of secondary amenorrhoea need to be excluded.

A physical examination may identify signs suggestive of the possible cause of either the inappropriate galactorrhoea or amenorrhoea, or both. These will include visual field disturbances, thyroid enlargement, confirmation of galactorrhoea, features of polycystic ovary syndrome (such as hirsutism) and genital tract abnormalities. A series of investigations is essential to diagnose the causes of these problems. A hormone profile (thyroid stimulating hormone (TSH), free thyroxine (FT), follicular stimulating hormone (FSH), luteinizing hormone (LH) and prolactin) will confirm hyperprolactinaemia, if present, or other causes, for example hypothyroidism, polycystic ovary syndrome, etc. Magnetic resonance imaging (MRI) of the skull, especially of the pituitary fossa, will be required to identify prolactinomas. This offers a better resolution to detect small microprolactinomas, but computerized tomography (CT) scanning is an equally good alternative and, in the absence of these, an X-ray of the skull would be performed. Although hormone assays may identify causes, normal values do not necessarily exclude them. Similarly, microprolactinomas may not be defined easily from the radiological investigations. X-rays are now considered crude screening methods for gross abnormality of the pituitary fossa or calcification in a craniopharyngioma.

The treatment of this patient will depend on the cause of either the amenorrhoea or the galactorrhoea, or both. Where the causes are unrelated it may not be possible to treat them concurrently, in which case the predominant concern must be treated first. Since most causes of galactorrhoea due to hyperprolactinaemia are idiopathic or of the microprolactinoma varieties, the treatment of choice will initially be for this variety. The treatment of choice will be a dopamine agonist, such as bromocryptine. This is effective in shrinking prolactinomas and reducing prolactin levels in the idiopathic group. Attempts must be made to remove known iatrogenic causes of hyperprolactinaemia, such as drugs, if possible. It is important to counsel the patient on her fertility whilst she is taking bromocryptine. This may not be acceptable to her because of side-effects, such as headaches. In this case, alternatives, such as carbegoline or quinagolines, may be used.

For the macroadenomas, transphenoidal microsurgical excision is the treatment of choice. One of the main consequences of hyperprolactinaemia is osteoporosis. This should be addressed by instituting oestrogen therapy. This may be combined with bromocriptine. The treatment of the patient's amenorrhoea may be the combined oral contraceptive pill, but it must be remembered that this can itself cause hyperprolactinaemia.

4. An 18-year-old girl who is *virgo intacta* attended the gynaecololgy clinic because she is yet to start menstruating. She has two sisters and three brothers. Justify the steps you will take to manage this patient.

Common mistakes

- Assuming that she has a chromosomal abnormality and discussing the management of intersexual disorders
- Discussing postpill amenorrhoea and its treatment
- Justifying why she has polycystic ovary syndrome and detailing how to manage this
- Investigating her for infertility and offering treatment for this
- Assuming that she has an adrenal problem and discussing its management
- Listing all the causes of primary amenorrhoea in this young girl

A good answer will include some or all of these points

- The most likely diagnosis is primary amenorrhoea – define this
- Management should include: history, personal and family
- Physical examination: secondary sexual characterictics; gonads; rectal examination
- Investigations: ultrasound scan; hormone profile; karyotyping, if indicated
- Treatment: reasurrance; specific cause

Sample answer

The most likely problem is this young girl is primary amenorrhoea, which is defined as failure to start menstruation by the age of 16 years. She is already 18 but whether this is pathological or constitutional, as most cases are, will depend on several factors. In her management, therefore, attempts must made to exclude pathological causes and then tailor treatment according to the identified cause.

First, it is important to establish the various milestones of puberty. These will include the age at thelarche (the first pubertal secondary sexual characteristic) and puberche. Where these appeared in the right order and at the right age, primary ovarian function must be considered to be normal. The age at which her sisters attained menarche should be established. If this was at about her age, all that is necessary is reassurance as the most likely cause is familiar or constitutional. However, if they attained menarche at an earlier age, pathological causes should be excluded. This must not be considered as an obvious indication that there is a cause as it can still be constitutional. Among important factors that must be excluded from the history are trauma to the skull, features of an intracranial lesion (such as headaches), visual field abnormalities, galactorrhoea and features of thyroid dysfunction. Drugs which may induce amenorrhoea should also be excluded, especially those that may interfere with pituitary function, for example steroids, antihypertensive agents, etc. Most of these may do so by inducing hyperprolactinaemia.

SHORT ESSAY QUESTIONS: GYNAECOLOGY

A physical examination may identify possible causes of the primary amenorrhoea. Initially, the patient's height should be measured. If she is of short stature for her age, it could be an indication of a chromosomal problem, such as Turner's syndrome. Body proportions and secondary sexual characteristics, such as the breasts, pubic and axillary hair, the carrying angle of the arm, location of the nipples and the hair line should also be observed. Palpation of the abdomen and inguinal rings should be undertaken to exclude gonads as in a case of testicular feminization syndrome. Since she is *vigo intacta*, a vaginal examination would be inadvisable. However, a rectal examination may be able to palpate the uterus, although this may not be necessary, especially with the ready availability of ultrasound facilities.

A series of investigations are essential in helping make a diagnosis and therefore tailoring treatment. A complete hormonal profile is required. This will include serum follicular stimulating hormone (FSH), luteinizing hormone (LH), thyroid stimulating hormone (TSH), free T4, prolactin, testosterone, sex hormone binding globulin and 17-beta-oestrdiol. In addition, an ultrasound scan of the pelvis will be performed. This will define the uterus and ovaries. It must, however, be recognized that sometimes these radiological investigations fail to reveal pathology. Where there is a suspicion of a chromosomal abnormality, karyotyping should be performed. The best sample for this is peripheral blood where lymphocytes may be harvested.

The treatment will depend on the cause. Where it is constitutional, reassurance is often adequate. However, if this is unacceptable, the combined oral contraceptive pill may be used to induce menstruation. It must be recognized that when the patient comes off the pill, she may suffer from amenorrhoea and or irregular periods. Where the cause is polycystic ovary syndrome, as defined by an abnormal hormone profile, appropriate treatment could be instituted. This may take the form of the combined oral contraceptive pill or cyclical progestogens. Effectively, the choice is determined by the presence of other symptoms requiring treatment.

If the primary amenorrhoea is secondary to drugs, these should either be discontinued or modified. However, if it is not possible to do this, hormonal therapy should be instituted provided the hormones do not interfere with the drugs. Other causes, such as hypothyroidism, will be treated accordingly. The more difficult problems to treat are those related to agenesis of the Müllerian system and intersexual disorders. For disorders secondary to agenesis of the müllerian system, appropriate counselling is required and, if the vagina is not formed, a neo-vagina is created either by surgery or by use of sustained pressure as described by Ingram (Folch et al. 2001). Counselling about fertility is important in the management of this patient. Where the cause is Turner syndrome, secondary sexual characteristics will be absent and she could be short. Here, the treatment of choice is oestrogen to stimulate the uterus and induce growth. Once this has been achieved, the patient will start menstruation. However, she may be infertile and require ovum donation. If the cause of the amenorrhoea is testicular feminizing syndrome, the gonads need to be removed and the patient offered hormone replacement therapy. Again, appropriate counselling will be required to address the issue of fertility.

Reference

Folch M, Pigem I, Konje JC. Müllerian agenesis: etiology, diagnosis and management. *Obstetrics and Gynecological Survey* 2000; 55: 644–9.

4

Termination of pregnancy and early pregnancy complications

1. Critically appraise the methods of contraception you may offer a young woman of 21 following a termination of pregnancy at 12 weeks' gestation.

2. Justify your management of a septic incomplete miscarriage in a 26-year-old nulligravida.

3. Miss O wishes to have a termination of pregnancy. She has read that this can be done either surgically or medically. How will you counsel her?

4. All women undergoing a termination of pregnancy should be screened for *Chlamydia trachomatis*. Debate this statement.

5. A 26-year-old woman presents with six weeks' amenorrhoea and a slight vaginal bleed. She had an ultrasound scan which did not show any free fluid in the peritoneal cavity but identified a complex right adnexal mass with a fetal heartbeat seen. These appearances were diagnostic of an ectopic pregnancy. Critically appraise your management of this patient.

1. Critically appraise the methods of contraception you may offer a young woman of 21 following a termination of pregnancy at 12 weeks' gestation.

Common mistakes

- Listing all the methods of contraception available and failing to make references to the patient
- Discussing sterilization as the only method
- Discussing every method of contraception
- Referring the woman to a family planning specialist for advice

A good answer will include some or all of these points

- Determine any contraindications for contraception that she may have
- Surgical methods
- Barrier methods
- Combined oral contraceptives
- Progestogen-only contraceptives
- Intrauterine contraceptive devices

Sample answer

The type of contraception offered to this patient will depend on her needs, her perceived ability to comply with the method and any contraindications. The range of options available includes barrier methods, the combined oral contraceptive pill, the progestogen-only contraceptive pill, intrauterine contraceptive devices and sterilization. Each of these methods must be considered within the context of its advantages, potential complications or disadvantages and the anticipated problems in this young woman, especially those of compliance and suitability.

The first method is the combined oral contraceptive pill. This is effective, but requires the patient to take the pills daily. Compliance is therefore an important factor in its effectiveness. Contraindications to the use of the combined oral contraceptive pill must initially be excluded. These include focal migraine headaches, thrombophilia and previous venous thrombo-embolism (VTE). The advantage of this method of contraception is its ability to regulate irregular cycles, ameliorate the problem of menorrhagia and reduce the incidence of pelvic inflammatory disease. This patient could start to take the oral contraceptive pill before her discharge from the hospital. If she is not well-motivated, however, this may not be the best method of contraception for her.

The second option is the barrier method of contraception. In this young woman this may be adequate, provided it is acceptable to her and her partner. The barrier method will provide immediate contraception, but the failure rate is high. The barrier method may be the patient's most suitable method of contraception if she is not in a regular relationship and therefore has no need for regular contraception. The added advantages of the barrier method are protection against sexually transmitted diseases (STDs), no need to comply with daily administration and no systemic side-effects. In this patient, it could also be started immediately. The low efficacy of this method of contraception may be related to its application or to method failure itself. It is a method that is suitable for any couple unless they have an allergy to the substances used in the device. This patient may depend on her partner for the success of this method and such a lack of complete control may present a disadvantage.

Although the intrauterine contraceptive device may be an option, it must be considered in the context of an increased risk of pelvic inflammatory disease in a young woman. However, if the patient is married or in a stable relationship and is unable to tolerate any other method of contraception, this may be her only option. The main advantage is that she does not have to remember to take anything. It only has to be fitted once. In addition to the increased risk of pelvic inflammatory disease if the patient has multiple sexual partners, there may also be an increased risk of menstrual abnormalities and an increased incidence of ectopic pregnancies (both independently of pelvic inflammatory disease which may also present with these disorders). If this is her chosen method, the intrauterine contraceptive device could be inserted before the patient is discharged from hospital. Inserting it at the time of termination, however, is associated with higher perforation and expulsion rates.

Although sterilization is an option, it is likely to be unsuitable, especially if the patient has not completed her family. If she has, this could be performed at the same time as the termination. It is an effective method, which does not require motivation on the part of the patient. She must, however, understand that it is not always reversible and that the risk of ectopic gestation if it fails is higher. For a patient of this young age, this option should not be considered unless she demands it.

The last option is the progestogen-only contraceptive pill. The pill must be taken at the same time every day. The failure rate is higher and it is also associated with irregular vaginal bleeding. However, it may be used in patients who have a contraindication for use of oestrogens. Again, it may be started before the patient is discharged from hospital. Other progestogens, for example Depo-Provera administered three-monthly or subdermal implants (Norplant or Implanon) confer significant advantages over the mini-pill. There is no need for daily administration. However, the side-effects are similar and the implants require special skills for their insertion and removal.

2. Justify your management of a septic incomplete miscarriage in a 26-year-old nulligravida.

Common mistakes

- Listing all the methods available
- Treating a hypothetical patient
- Discussing the treatment of miscarriages in general
- Discussing the diagnosis of a miscarriage

A good answer will include some or all of these points

- The risks of septic incomplete miscarriage
- Broad-spectrum antibiotics to cover Gram-negative, Gram-positive and anaerobic organisms
- Surgical evacuation
- Precautions for haemorrhage
- Counselling about the risk of haemorrhage and proceeding to a hysterectomy and Asherman's syndrome

Sample answer

The diagnosis of a septic incomplete miscarriage would have been made based on a history of retained products of conception and a foul-smelling vaginal discharge, lower abdominal pain and pyrexia. Once this diagnosis is confirmed, the potential complications and need to be meticulous and aggressive in the management must be recognized. There is no place for conservative management of a septic incomplete miscarriage. The main complications are generalized septicaemia, pelvic inflammatory disease with associated tubo-ovarian abscess, infertility and chronic pelvic pain.

The definitive management of this patient is to evacuate the infected retained products of conception. Before the evacuation, she must be given broad-spectrum antibiotics to cover Gram-positive and Gram-negative organisms and anaerobic bacteria. The most commonly used antibiotics are a combination of metronidazole and a cephalosporin (cephalexin). Before their administration swabs should be sent for microscopy, culture and sensitivity. These antibiotics must be administered intravenously and preferably for at least eight hours before surgical evacuation. This is to minimize the risk of generalized septicaemia following the evacuation. A full blood count (FBC) and group and save should also be performed because during the surgical procedure there is always the risk of severe haemorrhage that may require transfusion.

Because of the potential complications enumerated above the procedure is best performed under general anaesthesia (GA). Prior to this, the patient should be counselled about potential complications, including septicaemia, haemorrhage (which may require transfusion and occasionally a hysterectomy) and Asherman syndrome which may be due to overzealous scraping of the endometrium. This complication is more likely after an evacuation for a septic miscarriage than after an uncomplicated incomplete miscarriage. The surgical procedure should also be performed by an experienced clinician because of the danger of overzealous curetting. Ideally, it is performed by suction rather than by curettage. It is also important to cover the procedure with intravenous (i.v.) sytontocinon or syntometrine. This reduces the risk of haemorrhage and therefore the need for blood transfusion and, very occasionally, a hysterectomy.

3. Miss O wishes to have a termination of pregnancy. She has read that this can be done either surgically or medically. How will you counsel her?

Common mistakes

- Discussing only the following:
  - Complications of termination of pregnancy
  - Advantages of surgical termination
  - Use of oxytocic agents and ergometrine
  - Methods of cervical priming before surgical termination

A good answer will include some or all of these points

- Two main methods – surgical and medical
- Advantages of surgical, and complications
- Advantages of medical, and complications
- Limitations of both procedures
- Factors that may influence choice of method: gestational age; local expertise; no contra-indications for both procedures; need for follow up

Sample answer

There are currently two methods of terminating a pregnancy. The first, and most commonly performed method, is surgery. However, the second is becoming increasingly popular and evidence to support the efficacy of medical termination of pregnancy is overwhelming. There are, however, some principles that must be taken into consideration before offering either method to a patient. Counselling this patient must take all these factors into consideration.

Surgical termination of pregnancy may be performed in all units up to the gestational age of 12–13 weeks. Beyond 13 weeks most gynaecologists will be reluctant to perform a surgical termination. Although it is still possible to perform a surgical procedure in pregnancies up to the gestational age of 18–20 weeks, these are often performed in a very selected number of units and by experts in late terminations. Although general anaesthesia (GA) is commonly offered, this is not invariable. In this procedure, the cervix is dilated and products evacuated by use of a vacuum pump. Complications include perforation of the uterus, cervical trauma and haemorrhage. Before surgical evacuation, prostaglandins, such as gemeprost, may be used to soften the cervix and therefore reduce the risk of complications such as cervical trauma. Although less likely, the uterus may not be completely evacuated. Where there is a bicornuate or double uterus only one horn may be evacuated and, if the pregnancy is in the other horn, it may continue. For this operation, expertise is required.

The advantages of surgical over medical termination include no need to stay in hospital for long periods, a guarantee that the procedure will be performed, in most cases completely, and the less likely risk of a second evacuation. However, if the patient has an infection in the lower genital tract, this may spread easily into the upper genital tract.

The medical method of termination is effective, but case selection is vital. This is facilitated with a combination of misoprostol and mifepritone. Usually, the mifepristone is administered 48 hours before the misoprostol, which may be administered vaginally every three to four hours. This vaginal administration commonly starts off the contractions. Only pregnancies before the gestational age of eight to nine and after 12 weeks are commonly terminated medically. However, for terminations for fetal reasons, this method may be performed up to term. The disadvantage of this method of termination is that of time spent in hospital waiting for the process to be completed. This may take a few hours or sometimes a day or two. There is no guarantee that the patient will not proceed to surgery. The success rate of this method of termination is in the order of 80 per cent.

Whether this patient is offered medical or surgical termination, therefore, will depend on the gestational age, the presence of contraindications to prostaglandins, and expertise in either the termination of late pregnancy or surgical evacuation and medical termination. She should be happy to return for monitoring by ultrasound scan if she opts for the medical termination.

4. All women undergoing a termination of pregnancy should be screened for *Chlamydia trachomatis*. Debate this statement.

Common mistakes

- Discussing the screening for *C. trachomatis* in general
- Enumerating the complications of *C. trachomatis* infection and how to recognize them.
- Discussing all the World Health Organization (WHO) criteria for screening for *C. trachomatis*
- Discussing the procedure for termination of pregnancy
- Aseptic precautions to avoid the risk of ascending infections

A good answer will include some or all of these points

- *C. trachomatis* is the most common sexually transmitted disease (STD) in the UK and is associated with tubal infertility
- Common in single women
- Prevalence could be as high as 10–15 per cent of single women undergoing termination of pregnancy
- Most are asymptomatic
- Treatment is cheap and effective
- Spread by men who are asymptomatic
- Screening prior to termination of pregnancy, and offering prophylactic therapy at the time of termination to all women allows contact tracing
- Cost effective
- Recall or contact tracing – problems
- Implications of a positive test – may result in break-up of relationships

Sample answer

Chlamydia trachomatis is the most common sexually transmitted disease (STD) in the UK. It commonly affects the young and it is associated with pelvic inflammatory disease and tubal infertility in a large proportion of these patients. The prevalence of this infection in populations undergoing termination of pregnancy has been reported to vary between 10 per cent and 15 per cent. In some populations, especially in the inner cities, this may be as high as 25–30 per cent. During termination there is the added risk of ascending infection, which may result in tubo-ovarian disease and infertility. In randomized controlled trials where screening for this infection before termination has been performed, the incidence of operative morbidity has been reduced drastically. The question, therefore, is whether all women attending for a termination of pregnancy should be screened for this infection.

Universal screening is justified if the condition is sufficiently common and there is a recognized diagnostic technique. There also has to be a therapy for the condition and its sequelae must be well-recognized. The screening method must also be reliable and the risk of false positive or false negative tests must be low. In addition, the test must do no harm. In the case of *C. trachomatis*, it is sufficiently common, there are well-recognized sequelae if infection goes untreated and the test itself is sensitive and specific. If identified, the treatment is effective and causes minimal harm. Therefore, the case for screening is made.

Screening before termination allows infected patients to be identified, treated and, therefore, postoperative morbidity of ascending infections minimised. It also provides an opportunity for counselling about protection against other STDs and their sequelae. For the screen-positive patients, there is the added advantage of contact-tracing and treatment, especially as this infection is notoriously asymptomatic in males and sometimes in females. Whether screening should be available before termination is debatable. There is an argument for the procedure to be undertaken and antibiotic against *C. trachomatis* administered after having screened the patient but before the results are available. This may not be very cost-effective, as over 50 per cent of patients will receive expensive antibiotics without needing them. However, it has been argued that this reduces morbidity from surgery. The ideal set-up would be to screen patients on their first visit and ensure that results are available before termination. This way, those who are screen-positive will receive antibiotics and also be channelled to the appropriate genito-urinary medicine (GUM) clinic for contact-tracing. The main disadvantage of universal screening is cost. Advantages include reducing morbidity, prevention of tubal infertility (and therefore the cost of its subsequent treatment) and contact-tracing and treatment, especially those who are aymptomatic. Taking all these advantages into consideration it may be argued that this approach is cheap and cost-effective.

The other option would be to offer antibiotics against *C. trachomatis* to every woman attending for termination of pregnancy. Although this may overcome the problem and cost of screening, it would inevitably result in failure to trace contacts and, therefore, would not reduce the spread of the disease, even to the same individual by her male counterpart. Even if it is argued that both partners should be treated, an assumption is made that the partner is the source of the infection and so there will certainly be many cases missed. Although there may be some value in this approach, especially as the cost of treating the infection with tetracycline or its derivative is very cheap, it is not justifiable.

Although screening, treating and contact-tracing, followed by screening and treatment is ideal, it may also pose some problems. Contact-tracing, for example, is a very sensitive problem and one which may result in broken relationships, especially if the male partner is screen-negative. In addition, additional resources will be required to trace contacts and to provide adequate education and treatment. If the screening of all women is not to be advocated, what is the alternative? Selective screening at-risk groups will definitely identify a large proportion of affected women and their partners. However, the assumption that low-risk populations are not at risk must be discounted. Although the prevalence of this infection in the low-risk population is low, it must be recognized that only a small proportion of women attending for termination of pregnancy come from this low-risk population. It may, therefore, be argued that selective screening could be seen as discriminatory, and since the proportion from the low-risk group is small, it may be beneficial to screen everyone. One option would be to screen everyone, to give antibiotics to the high-risk group, but to delay treating the low-risk group until test results are available. Whatever the argument, screening for *C. trachomatis* has more benefits than disadvantages and therefore, on balance, it is best offered to all women attending for termination of pregnancy.

5. A 26-year-old woman presents with six weeks' amenorrhoea and a slight vaginal bleed. She had an ultrasound scan which did not show any free fluid in the peritoneal cavity but identified a complex right adnexal mass with a fetal heartbeat seen. These appearances were diagnostic of an ectopic pregnancy. Critically appraise your management of this patient.

Common mistakes

- Take a history and perform a physical examination
- Confirm the diagnosis of ectopic pregnancy
- Serial beta-human chorionic gonadotrophin (βhCG) estimation
- Perform a transvaginal ultrasound scan
- Offer conservative observational treatment

A good answer will include some or all of these points

- The diagnosis is clearly that of an ectopic pregnancy
- Counselling must be the first step
- Treatment options: surgery – laparoscopic; laparotomy salpectomy, salpingotomy or milking it out; injection of hyperosmolar solutions, prostaglandins or methotrexate; intramuscular (i.m.) injection of methotrexate – follow-up with βhCG and ultrasound scan whenever it is indicated – may later require surgery (laparotomy)
- Follow-up
- Contraception
- Recurrence risk

Sample answer

The diagnosis of an ectopic pregnancy in this patient has been confirmed by an ultrasound scan showing an adnexal mass with a fetal heartbeat seen. Her management must focus on treating the ectopic gestation and should include adequate counselling and discussion of the treatment options available to her.

The first important step in this patient's management is adequate counselling. The diagnosis must be explained to the her. She needs to have a diagnostic laparoscopy. This procedure will allow assessment of the size of the size of the pregnancy, the other Fallopian tube and may, in fact, allow treatment to be offered. It could be argued that diagnostic laparoscopy should only be undertaken if laparoscopic treatment or conservative medical treatment are options acceptable to the patient. If she elects to have a laparotomy, or if the expertise for laparoscopic surgery is unavailable, there is some justification in proceeding straight to a laparotomy. The advantage of this is that it bypasses prolonged anaesthesia and the added complications of laparoscopy, which include bowel injury, gas embolism and damage to major arteries resulting in massive haemorrhage.

If the patient has completed her family or has been sterilized, the option for her will be a salpingectomy. This can be performed laparoscopically or at laparotomy. The advantages of laparoscopic surgery include reduced hospital stay, reduced morbidity from large abdominal incisions and reduced risk of complications, such as wound infection. However, the patient must understand that not every case may be treated laparoscopically. If, for example, the ectopic pregnancy is cornual or is too large to be dealt with laparoscopically, a laparotomy must be performed. If she has not completed her family, attempts at conserving the Fallopian tubes will be advisable. The treatment of choice will be a salpingotomy. This involves incising the antemesenteric site of the Fallopian tube and removing the ectopic pregnancy. Any bleeding from the bed of the pregnancy may then be coagulated. There is no need to close the linear incision on the Fallopian tube. Although this has the advantage of preserving the Fallopian tube, the patient must be followed up with serial βHCG measurements to ensure that all the trophoblastic tissues have been removed.

Another conservative option for this patient is injection of the ectopic pregnancy with methotrexate or a hyperosmolar solution, such as prostaglandins or 50 per cent glucose. For this to be performed, however, the gestational sac diameter should be less than 2 cm. In this case, this is unlikely, as the fetal heartbeat was seen on ultrasound scan. If, indeed, a decision is made to offer this treatment, serial monitoring with βHCGs must be offered The patient must also understand that with this type of treatment there is a chance that she may have to undergo a further laparotomy if the gestational sac does not gradually resolve. If this patient elects for medical treatment of her ectopic gestation, she could be offered intramuscular (i.m.) methotrexate, but it is likely that the size of the gestational sac may negate this type of treatment. However, if it is offered, the patient must be prepared to undergo serial βHCG monitoring and, if necessary, repeat methotrexate or subsequent laparoscopic or laparotomy treatment for persisting disease.

The last option is a laparotomy if the ectopic pregnancy is not suitable for laparoscopic surgery. At surgery, she may either have a salpingectomy, a salpingotomy or milking of the ectopic pregnancy. Whichever option is offered will depend on her need for further pregnancies, the state of the Fallopian tube and the size of the ectopic gestation. Salpingectomy will be performed if she does not desire children or the Fallopian tube is significantly damaged. However, the other Fallopian tube must be assessed to ensure that salpingectomy is not performed on the better tube and a severely damaged one left behind. This treatment has the advantage of better exposure and an opportunity of dealing with other pelvic pathologies, such as ovarian cysts and adhesions. Although it may not be advisable to deal with adhesions at the time of surgery, this may be performed, depending on the type and location of the adhesions.

Whichever treatment option the patient is offered, she must be counselled about recurrence and advised on contraception. The intrauterine contraceptive device is contraindicated, whereas the recurrence risk is about 10 per cent. She must be advised about the need to report early in her next pregnancy and to use a barrier method of contraception if she is not in a regular relationship.

5

Benign uterine lesions and endometriosis

1. Evaluate the options available for the treatment of uterine fibroids in a 26-year-old primigravida.

2. A 33-year-old woman presents with 26-week size uterine fibroids. Critically appraise her management.

3. Evaluate the management of a 42 year old human immunodeficiency virus (HIV) positive nulliparous woman presenting with menorrhagia who, on examination, is found to have 18-week size uterine fibroids and a haemoglobin of 9.7 g/gl.

4. Justify your management of a 41-year-old woman presenting with right iliac fossa cyclical pain of two years' duration. She had a hysterectomy and left salpingoophorectomy for endometriosis three years ago.

5. Evaluate the management options of a 33-year-old nulligravida with endometriosis, in whom the main symptom is painful and heavy periods.

1. Evaluate the options available for the treatment of uterine fibroids in a 26-year-old primigravida.

Common mistakes

- Taking a history and performing a physical examination
- Assuming that the patient must have symptoms
- Listing the symptoms of uterine fibroids
- Simply listing the treatment options available for this patient
- Concentrating on the treatment of menstrual dysfunction only
- Listing the investigations that you will perform on a patient with uterine fibroids

A good answer will include some or all of these points

- Uterine fibroids are the most common gynaecological tumours
- Most are asymptomatic – and therefore do not require treatment
- Treatment will depend on symptoms, location of fibroids, parity of the patient and her desire for more children. Remember that she is only 26 years old
- Treatment options include: none; medical treatment – danazol, gonadotrophin-releasing hormone (GnRH) analogues; surgical options – myomectomy (open or laparoscopic), hysteroscopic myomecomy and hysterectomy; other modern approaches, such as embolization – only available in a few centres for research

Sample answer

Uterine fibroids occur in approximately 20–30 per cent of women by the time of menopause. In most of these, they are asymptomatic. The treatment options will depend on the symptoms of the fibroids, their location and size and the facilities available in the unit.

If the patient is asymptomatic, there will be no need to offer her any treatment other than reassurance. This option avoids the side-effects of surgery and medical treatment. As the fibroids are likely to grow bigger, definitive treatment should be a future option depending on symptoms.

If she has symptoms, definitive treatment will depend on the size and location of the fibroids, her desire to have (more) children and the facilities available in the unit. The first option will be surgery. This is more cost-effective in a young patient, as medical treatment will only delay further growth of the fibroids. The different surgical options are myomectomy, hysteroscopic resection and a hysterectomy. Myomectomy, which can be performed by laparotomy or laparoscopy in a few centres, will remove most of the big fibroids and leave the uterus intact. The risk of this procedure is that of progression to a hysterectomy if there is severe and life-threatening haemorrhage. In addition, it may be complicated by adhesions, which may further compromise fertility in a woman who desires more children. Although this is expensive (requiring an inpatient stay and general anaesthesia, GA) it is an effective treatment option. It must be recognized that myomectomy may not remove all the fibroids and those left behind may re-grow. For most patients, the operation will be laparotomy, but where the fibroids are small and are subserous, this may be performed through laparoscopy at some highly specialized centres.

Where the patient is unsuitable for surgery or is reluctant to have surgery, anti-oestrogens such as danazol or gonadotrophin-releasing hormone (GnRH) analogues such as goserelin will be the treatment of choice. These are associated with severe side-effects and can result in a reduction in the size of the fibroids of between 40 per cent and 60 per cent. Danazol has several side-effects and therefore compliance may be poor. GnRH analogues have severe side-effects which may be unacceptable. If the patient wants to have a family, treatment has to be completed before she embarks on a pregnancy. For this young woman, this may not be an effective treatment option. It may, however, be used preoperatively to minimize blood loss at myomectomy and to reduce the size of the fibroids. Unfortunately it may make the myomectomy difficult.

The last option is uterine artery embolization. Although this technique is in the early stages and the Royal College of Obstetricians and Gynaecologists (RCOG) only recommend it as a treatment option in units as part of research, preliminary results indicate that it is an effective treatment and one which will not compromise the fertility of the patient. However, there are reported fatalities with this option and its long-term effects have yet to be evaluated.

The treatment options for this patient will be determined by a variety of factors and the best option for her will be decided after careful assessment and counselling.

2. A 33-year-old woman presents with 26-week size uterine fibroids. Critically appraise her management.

Common mistakes

- Assuming the patient has completed her family
- Management depends on whether or not the fibroids are symptomatic!
- Offering laparoscopic myomectomy/hysteroscopic resection – morcellation
- Use of antifibrinolytic agents to treat fibroids
- Assuming that she has menstrual problems
- Prostaglandin synthethase inhibitors – ineffective

A good answer will include some or all of these points

- These fibroids are very large and are therefore likely to be symptomatic
- Symptoms include menorrhagia, pressure symptoms, infertility or subfertility (information to be gleaned from a brief history)
- Investigations – haemoglobin (Hb) – anaemia; intravenous urogram/ultrasound scan (IVU/USS) – to exclude urinary tract obstruction; midstream specimen of urine (MSU) – to exclude urinary tract infection (UTI)
- Treatment will depend on many factors, including parity, desire for children or more children, ease of surgery and associated complications
- Completed family and accepts option: total abdominal hysterectomy – curative, but associated with morbidity and mortality; general anaesthesia (GA) and the risks
- Conservative: myomectomy – unlikely to remove all fibroids; associated morbidity; may proceed to total abdominal hysterectomy; preoperative treatment with gonadotrophin-releasing hormone (GnRH) analogues – reduces vascularity and size. Makes shelving difficult. Side-effects of GnRH analogues
- Embolization – new method. Research toll only
- Wants more children – need to discuss implications of multiple myomectomy on pregnancy and childbirth

Sample answer

The fibroids in this woman are large and therefore unlikely to be asymptomatic. The option of no treatment is therefore unlikely to be acceptable. The symptoms with which she may have presented include menorrhagia, pressure on her bladder, ureter, bowel or blood vessels, infertility/subfertility or an abdominal mass. This information will be gleaned from a careful history. The effect of the fibroids on other adjacent organs may not be easily available from the history but revealed only after investigations. These must aim to exclude anaemia, urinary tract infections (UTIs) and obstruction. The presence of urinary tract obstruction will indicate a more urgent approach to treatment.

A full blood count (FBC) will exclude anaemia and polycythaemia, which may complicate fibroids and increase the risk of thrombo-embolism during surgery. The absence of anaemia does not exclude this condition, especially if the patient has been receiving iron supplementation. Urine microscopy will exclude UTIs, whereas urea and electrolytes (U&Es) will exclude kidney compromise. The latter may be secondary to ureteric obstruction, the presence of which will necessitate early intervention to avoid further renal compromise. A normal renal function test does not, however, exclude obstruction. This can easily be identified by ultrasound scan or magnetic resonance imaging (MRI) of the abdomen, specifically of the kidneys.

The definitive treatment will depend on the many factors, including parity, the patient's desire for more children, ease of surgery and associated complications. If this 33-year-old woman has completed her family, the treatment of choice will be abdominal hysterectomy. This will remove the fibroids with no risk of recurrence. She will need to have a midline incision with the associated risk of incisional hernia. Hysterectomy is associated with a significant morbidity – related to the surgery and general anaesthesia (GA), although there is no reason why the procedure cannot be undertaken under regional anaesthesia.

Where the patient has not completed her family, the treatment of choice will be myomectomy. In view of the size of the fibroids, this cannot be done laparoscopically. A laparotomy will be necessary. This procedure will only remove the obvious fibroids (visible and palpable ones). There is, therefore, the risk of smaller fibroids growing to a significant size to cause more symptoms. At the time of surgery, there is always the danger of proceeding to a hysterectomy if there is a life-threatening haemorrhage. Consent for a hysterectomy must therefore be obtained before a myomectomy. This procedure may be complicated by adhesions, which may futher compromise fertility. The use of medical regimens, such as danazole or gonadotrophin-releasing hormone (GnRH) analogues, prior to myomectomy have been reported to minimize blood loss, but they may be associated with difficulties with shelving the fibroids and thus an increase in the risk of progression to hysterectomy. A successful myomectomy should not have implications for vaginal childbirth in the future, however, where the uterus has been extensively dissected, an elective Caesarean section may be necessary.

If this woman is unsuitable for surgery, an interim measure may be the option of medical treatment with GnRH analogues or danazol. These agents will reduce the size of the fibroids by up to 60 per cent, but once treatment is discontinued the fibroids re-grow. In addition, this treatment is likely to be discontinued after six months in view of the side-effects of anti-oestrogens on the musculoskeletal, genital, cardiovascular, metabolic and haematological systems. Although Add-Back therapy may obviate some of these symptoms. Unfortunately these treatment regimens cannot be continued indefinitely.

The last option for this patient is uterine artery embolization. This option will be advantageous if the patient is a surgical risk. The procedure is still in the early stage of evaluation, but early reports indicate that it is effective. The Royal College of Obstetricians and Gynaecologists (RCOG) recommends that this option is available only in tertiary centres where research on its suitability in treating fibroids is being assessed.

3. Evaluate the management of a 42-year-old human immunodeficiency virus (HIV) positive nulliparous woman presenting with menorrhagia who, on examination, is found to have an 18-week size uterine fibroids and a haemoglobin of 9.7 g/gl.

Common mistakes

- Management of human immunodeficiency virus (HIV)/counselling prepregnancy
- List treatment options – without evaluating
- Debate treatment/management options: no need to mention magnetic resonance imaging (MRI)/intravenous urogram (IVU); ineffective medical treatments, such as mefenamic acid, tranexamic acid, mirena coil, resection, vaginal hysterectomy
- Unhelpful: history and duration of symptoms/intermenstrual bleeding, duration of HIV, etc.; critically appraise – what is the question asking?

A good answer will include some or all of these points

- The dilemma posed by this clinical problem
- Risk to staff and to patient if she is immunocompromised
- Therefore, need to attempt conservative measures first
- Associated features of complications which will require urgent treatment, for example ureteric obstruction
- Treatment will depend on the fertility needs of the patient
- Start treatment with haematinic agent for anaemia
- Medical options – first if no need for urgent treatment
- Danazol – cheap, effective, poor compliance because of side-effects and need for daily administration
- Gonadotrophin-releasing hormone (GnRH) analogues – expensive but effective. Compliance not a problem. Side-effects of menopausal symptoms. May be used as adjuvant treatment prior to surgery – benefits of reduction in size of fibroids and blood loss at surgery
- Improve anaemia and general health before surgery: embolization – option but mainly recommended to be used for research (Royal College of Obstetricians and Gynaecologists, RCOG); surgery – myomectomy – advantages and disadvantages, total abdominal hysterectomy – advantages and disadvantages; must ensure universal precautions to minimize risk of transferring HIV to staff and protect patient from opportunistic infections by broad-spectrum antibiotics; collaborate with genito-urinary medicine (GUM) department specialists

Sample answer

This patient's clinical problem poses an important dilemma for the clinician. She presents a significant risk to staff and, if she is immunocompromised, she will have an increased risk of acquired infections, especially in hospital following invasive management. In her treatment, therefore, these considerations must be carefully evaluated before any definitive therapy is offered.

The definitive treatment will depend on the complications, which require urgent treatment, and the patient's fertility needs. As her haemoglobin is low, the first and most important stage in her management will be the provision of haematinic agents to effectively correct her anaemia.

In view of the human immunodeficiency virus (HIV), the anaemia and the size of the fibroids, medical options will be the best approach in the first instance. These could be in the form of danazol or gonadotrophin-releasing hormone (GnRH) analogues. Danazol, an anti-oestrogen, is not as effective as GnRH analogues. It is associated with severe side-effects, which may affect compliance and therefore efficacy. On the other hand, GnRH analogues will down-regulate the pituitary gland and therefore induce amenorrhoea. This treatment is expensive but, if effective, provides the best cost-effective treatment for this condition. Therefore, this will be the first line of management for this patient. That said, she may discontinue this treatment because of menopausal symptoms. If this is the case, AddBack therapy could be added. GnRH analogues are not advised for longer than six months unless combined with AddBack therapy as taking them may induce osteopenia. It could reduce the size of the fibroid by as much as 60 per cent. This will benefit further surgery if it is considered. As the woman is 42, it is possible to maintain her on this regimen and avoid surgery. Unfortunately, once the GnRH therapy is discontinued, the fibroids re-grow.

If medical management fails, surgery will be the option of choice. The definitive surgery will depend on the patient's fertility needs. If she has completed her family, hysterectomy will be the operation of choice. Before, this, however, her anaemia must be corrected. This could be through a combination of GnRH analogues to reduce the size of the fibroids, vascularity, and also to create a state of amenorrhoea therefore allowing her haemoglobin to rise. The advantage of hysterectomy is that it is straightforward with a reduced risk of transmitting the disease to staff compared to the risk involved with myomectomy. It is the operation of choice as it will remove the fibroids and avoid reccurrence of the anaemia. Myomectomy will be the operation of choice if the patient desires children. However, apart from the increase risk of transmitting HIV to staff, there is always the risk of proceeding to a hysterectomy.

In this patient, uterine artery embolization is probably one of the best options. It is associated with minimal risk of transmitting HIV to staff and reduces the risk of cross-hospital infection to the patient. Unfortunately, this procedure does not have long-term follow-up to assess its efficacy. It is also only available in tertiary centres where research is continuing. In this patient, this treatment will be offered as the first option if medical options fail. Whatever treatment, the genito-urinary medicine (GUM) team must be involved in her care.

4. Justify your management of a 41-year-old woman presenting with right iliac fossa cyclical pain of two years' duration. She had a hysterectomy and left salpingo-oophorectomy for endometriosis three years ago.

Common mistakes

- Taking a history and physical examination to exclude pelvic inflammatory disease
- Managing the patient as if she had chronic pelvic pain syndrome
- Treating her for bowel problems
- Ignoring the information about previous endometriosis
- Assuming that a pelvic examination and other investigations have been made and the diagnosis confirmed
- Asking about the history of sexually transmitted diseases (STDs) and discussing their differentials
- Failing to consider differential diagnoses
- Not justifying

A good answer will include some or all of these points

- Most likely recurrent endometriosis, however, other differentials need to be considered
- Confirmation of diagnosis: is the pain cyclical? examination – why? To detect masses, tenderness and induration – all clinical signs of endometriosis; ultrasound – why? diagnostic laparoscopy – ? therapeutic trial of gonadotrophin-releasing hormone (GnRH analogues)
- Consider the differential diagnoses
- Treatment: medical – analgesics, reassurance, drugs for endometriosis; endometrioma (ovarian) – surgery; hormone replacement therapy (HRT) if oophorectomy

Sample answer

The most likely diagnosis in this patient is recurrent endometriosis. However, other differential diagnoses, such as ovarian pathology, bowel disorders and adhesions must be considered. The diagnosis of the cause of the cyclical pain in this patient needs to be confirmed. In the first instance, more information about the nature of the pain is required. For endometriosis, a cyclical pain is typical although not exclusive. Other associated symptoms of endometriosis that have to be excluded include cyclical urinary symptoms, bleeding from other possible endometriotic sites and, of course, symptoms which will exclude abdominal pathologies, such as irritable bowel syndrome.

A physical examination to identify signs of endometriosis or other pathologies will be undertaken next. The presence of an adnexal mass, adnexal tenderness or induration will be highly suggestive of endometriosis. Following this examination, investigations have to be undertaken to confirm the diagnosis and exclude other possible causes of pain. The two relevant investigations for this patient are ultrasound scan and diagnostic laparoscopy. An ultrasound scan will identify an ovarian endometrioma or other ovarian pathologies, which are not endometriotic, for example, a haemorrhagic ovarian cyst. The renal tract should also be assessed as there may be a ureteric obstruction secondary to endometriosis over the ureters.

A diagnostic laparoscopy will have to be undertaken to locate any recurrent endometriosis and ovarian endometriomata. The main concern with such a procedure in this patient is the risk of bowel injury. This is more likely in a patient who has had surgery for endometriosis. The laparoscopy will also exclude other ovarian pathologies, such as benign ovarian cysts, which may have other complications. Unfortunately, a diagnostic laparoscopy may not provide the diagnosis in this patient if she has adhesions, which may render the ovary inaccessible. Consideration must therefore be given to a therapeutic trial for endometriosis in the form of gonadotrophin-releasing hormone (GnRH) analogues for two or three months. If her symptoms improve during this time, the most likely cause of the cyclical pain is endometriosis. If it fails to rid the patient of her symptoms, the diagnosis is unlikely to be endometriosis.

Once the diagnosis is confirmed, the treatment of choice will be surgery. Where the patient is unsuitable for surgery, GnRH analogues should be offered for six months. These may be offered in the first instance without Addback therapy, although there is no evidence that such a combination at the outset reduces efficacy in endometriosis. The surgical options will be oophorectomy and adhesiolysis (if adhesions are present). Before surgery the patient must be counselled appropriately on the complications associated with adhesions and the importance of hormone replacement therapy (HRT), which in her case will be long-term. Symptomatic treatment may be useful if the patient is unsuitable for hormonal or surgical treatment. It is important to consider symptomatic relief as this may be adequate in some cases. Potent analgesics may be sufficient, in which case other forms of therapy would be unnecessary. However, it is very likely that the patient's general practitioner (GP) will have tried this option unsuccessfully before referring her to the hospital.

5. Evaluate the management options of a 33-year-old nulligravida with endometriosis, in whom the main symptom is painful and heavy periods.

Common mistakes

- Discussing the symptoms of endometriosis and how to make a diagnosis
- The value of diagnostic laparoscopy in making a diagnosis
- The need for *in vitro* fertilization (IVF) and GIFT
- Total abdominal hysterectomy for her menorrhagia
- Presentation with an abdominal mass – discussing the diagnosis and treatment
- Assuming that the endometriosis is mild/severe or moderate!

A good answer will include some or all of these points

- Severity is important in tailoring treatment for this patient
- Options – for symptom relief: medical treatment; surgical treatment
- Symptom relief – best option – tranexamic acid and androgens: decrease menstrual loss (most effective treatment) and therefore may be combined with analgesics
- Medical treatment with the combined oral contraceptive pill – provided no risk factors. Effective, cheap and provides contraception. However, side-effects
- Gonadotrophin-releasing hormone (GnRH analogues – best value. Sprays/monthly depot doses – compliance not an issue with depot injections. Side-effects. Expensive
- Danazol – side-effects, compliance may be poor
- The levonorgestrel intrauterine system (Mirena)
- Surgery – laparoscopy – laser, diathermy, oophorectomy, uterosacral nerve division/ excision
- If heavy periods secondary to endometriosis, total abdominal hysterectomy
- Treatment may achieve pregnancy

Sample answer

The management of this patient will depend to a large extent on the severity of her symptoms. She has two treatment options – surgery and medical therapy. The choice of treatment will be determined by the wishes of the patient, contraindications to some of the options, availability and acceptability.

For symptom relief alone, the best option will be the antifibrinolytic agent tranexamic acid, given as 1 g four times a day during menstruation. It is effective in decreasing menstrual loss (Bonnar and Sheppard, 1996). Although it may reduce blood loss, tranexamic acid is unlikely to reduce the severity of pelvic pain secondary to endometriosis. Combining it with a potent analgesic may therefore be more effective in symptom control. The only drawback of this option is the need to continue with the therapy for an indefinite period as it is symptomatic therapy rather than treatment for endometriosis. It may, therefore, not be the most cost-effective therapeutic regimen for this patient.

A combination of tranexamic acid and an androgen, such as danazol or gestrionone, may overcome the need to continue treatment indefinitely. The androgen acts at the level of the pituitary gland, hypothalamus and ovary to counteract the effect of oestrogens on the endometriosis. It may therefore lead to a significant regression of the endometriotic lesions and eventually to a significant improvement in clinical symptoms. The side-effects of danazol may result in poor compliance, but the choice of the less-androgenic alternative, gestrinone (Dimetrios), may be associated with fewer side-effects and therefore better compliance. This combination is effective and negates the need for surgery. Given for six months, adequate response may be achieved in up to 70 per cent of patients. However, like other forms of treatment for endometriosis, the reccurrence risk of the symptoms is approximately 40 per cent.

The combined oral contraceptive pill taken continuously (without the pill-free interval) is an effective, cheap alternative for this patient. It has the added advantage of offering contraception if it is necessary. There have to be no contraindications for this treatment. These include thrombophilias, focal migraines and previous venous thrombo-embolism (VTE). For this regimen, the patient has to be well-motivated, as compliance is an important factor to its success. Side-effects, such as breakthrough bleeding, may affect its efficacy.

Gonadotrophin-releasing hormone (GnRH) analogues are the most cost-effective medical treatment for this patient. These will downregulate the pituitary gland and thus cause the endometriosis and associated biochemical changes in the peritoneum to regress. Treatment is usually for six months. Beyond this time limit, it is associated with oestrogen deficiency effects, such as osteopenia. To counteract this, AddBack therapy in the form of oestrogens or Livial maybe included and treatment prolonged. More recently, this combination is being offered from the outset and there is no evidence to suggest that it reduces the efficacy of GnRH analogues. Menopausal symptoms may affect compliance with preparations requiring frequent administration, however, with depot preparations, compliance tends not be an issue.

The surgical option (for this patient) is laparoscopic laser/diathermy of the endometriosis, division or total excision of the uterosacral ligaments or oophorectomy. Laparoscopic destruction of the endometriotic lesions is not typically considered a very effective treatment. This is because, it is unlikely that all the lesions will be destroyed, especially as the clinical absence of endometriotic lesions does not exclude disease. Additionally, lesions on surfaces that do not lend themselves to destructive therapy are unlikely to be destroyed. A combination of these surgical and medical therapeutic options is likely to achieve the best results. Surgery is expensive, associated with complications and is not very effective in isolation. Bilateral oophorectomy is the most effective treatment. In this 33-year-old woman, this should be considered as the last option. It should be offered with or without a hysterectomy. If she has completed her family, a hysterectomy should be considered. Although at the outset, it is the most expensive option, it certainly produces the best results. The patient must, however, be counselled on the need for prolonged hormone replacement therapy (HRT). Since this will take the form of continuous oestrogen, the risk of recurrence of the endometriosis is minimal. However, if the patient has not completed her family, oophorectomy alone may be performed, provided she understands that future pregnancies will require ovum donation. Although it has been suggested that superovulation followed by ova retrieval and storage could be considered in such patients, this must only be considered as a last resort and following appropriate counselling, as *in vitro* fertilization (IVF) has a low success rate.

An alternative that must not be forgotten in this patient is pregnancy. If there is no reason for her to delay pregnancy, she could be encouraged on the basis that pregnancy will significantly improve her symptoms. This must be done with extreme caution as difficulties in conceiving due to the endometriosis may cause extreme anxiety and generate more problems.

Reference

Bonnar J and Sheppard BC. Treatment of menorrhagia during menstruation: randomised controlled trial of ethamsylate, mefenamic acid, and tranexemic acid. *BMJ* 1996; 313: 579–82.

6

Benign ovarian lesions

1. A 38-year-old woman presents to the gynaecology clinic with a swelling in the lower abdomen. You suspect that she has an ovarian cyst. Justify the steps you will take in her management.

2. A 27-year-old woman presents with intermittent lower abdominal pain. She also noticed that she has been putting on weight and her clothes have been getting tighter. On examination, you find an abdominal mass consistent with a 36 weeks' gestation. The origin of the mass is uncertain but you suspect that it is ovarian. Outline the steps you will take to manage this patient giving reasons for each stage.

3. You saw a young girl of 17 years presenting as an emergency with intermittent lower abdominal pain of three days' duration. The pain is now constant and is mainly on the right side and radiating to her back. Her last menstrual period of a 28-day regular cycle was one week ago. Critically appraise your management of this patient.

1. A 38-year-old woman presents to the gynaecology clinic with a swelling in the lower abdomen. You suspect that she has an ovarian cyst. Justify the steps you will take in her management.

Common mistakes

- Restating the information given in the question
- Discussing the management of malignant ovarian tumours
- Omitting to obtain more information from a history
- Treatment depends on parity – without first defining the type of ovarian tumour she has
- Assuming that she has an ovarian malignancy and treating her as such
- Refer to a tertiary centre with gynaecological oncologist because such patients should not be managed in the District Hospital!!
- Diagnostic laparoscopy as an investigation – you need to explain when it will be useful
- Justify means that you offer a reason for every statement you write down

A good answer will include some or all of these points

- Need to obtain more information from the history
- Identification of various clinical features of ovarian tumours, with emphasis on excluding malignant features
- Undertaking various investigations to confirm the diagnosis: ultrasound scan; role of magnetic resonance imaging (MRI) in the identification of malignancies and secondaries in the liver and abdominal lymph nodes; CA125; urea and electrolytes (U&Es) – if suspicion of urinary tract obstruction; laparoscopy?
- Treatment – depends on the diagnosis: laparotomy and oopherectomy or cystectomy; laparoscopic oophorectomy/cystectomy; more extensive if malignant – total abdominal hysterectomy, bilateral salpingoophorectomy, omentectomy with or without removal of nodes followed by adjuvant chemotherapy
- Ovarian endometrioma – treatment (medical or surgery)

Sample answer

In the management of this patient, obtaining more information about her presenting complaints is essential. The swelling may be associated with abdominal pain. If the pain is intermittent, then torsion may be a complication of the cyst. The pain may also be constant and increasing in intensity. This will point to the possibility of haemorrhage into an ovarian cyst. Where a cyst has ruptured, the pain tends to be excruciating and of very sudden onset. However, where the pain started intermittently and later became constant, the likely cause will be torsion. Associated symptoms may depend on the size of the ovarian cyst. These will usually be gastro-intestinal and include dyspepsia, constipation and bloatedness of the abdomen.

Following this, a clinical examination should be undertaken to identify signs of ovarian pathology. These include the origin and size of the mass, associated ascites, fixity, pleural effusion and cachexia. A pelvic examination will confirm the presence of a pelvic mass, although this may be completely abdominal and thus difficult to feel vaginally. Bilaterality of the tumour, its consistency and fixity to the pelvis may indicate a possible malignancy.

Necessary investigations include a serum CA125. This may be raised in ovarian epithelial cancers, endometriosis, other epithelial cell tumours and infections. A high value is therefore not necessarily indicative of malignancy. It is, however, important to establish a baseline in case serial monitoring is necessary. An ultrasound scan will define the origin of the cyst more precisely, although this is not always the case. Other features which may be identified on ultrasound scan include bilaterality of the tumour, the characteristics of the cysts, such as the presence of solid areas, irregular walls with excreciencies, papillary growths, bright material within the cyst and the size of the cyst. These features may distinguish a benign from a suspected malignant ovarian cyst. If the ultrasound scan is inconclusive, magnetic resonance imaging (MRI) or computerized tomography (CT) may be necessary. In addition to defining the ovarian cyst and other features suggestive of malignancy, this will exclude secondaries in the liver and enlarged lymph nodes. A very large ovarian cyst may cause ureteric obstruction. This may be identified (by ultrasound or MRI of the kidneys) as hydronephrosis and/or dilation of the ureters. In some cases, ultrasound scan may not be conclusive, especially if the cyst is small; a diagnostic laparoscopy may therefore be better at defining the nature and origin of the pelvic pathology. In addition, definitive treatment may be offered at the time of the laparoscopy.

The treatment will depend on the type of cyst, its size and associated complications. Ovarian endomeriomata are best treated by oophorectomy, ovarian cystectomy or a combination of ovariotomy and medical therapy. Where the cyst is torted, it must be treated as an emergency. At the time of surgery, whether or not the ovary is saved (that is, a cystectomy is performed) will depend on the viability of the ovary after it is untwisted. Oophorectomy will be performed if the ovary is not viable. In these situations the Fallopian tube tends to become necrotic with the ovary, and often a salpingoophorectomy is the treatment of choice. For an uncomplicated benign cyst, a cystectomy will be performed either laparoscopically or via laparotomy. Where a malignancy is suspected, the patient should be referred to an oncologist for the most appropriate management, which will consist of a total abdominal hysterectomy, bilateral salpingoophorectomy and node dissection followed by chemotherapy. Whatever the pathology of the cyst in this patient, her management will only be completed after histological examination of the cyst or ovary.

2. A 27-year-old woman presents with intermittent lower abdominal pain. She also noticed that she has been putting on weight and her clothes have been getting tighter. On examination, you find an abdominal mass consistent with a 36 weeks' gestation. The origin of the mass is uncertain but you suspect that it is ovarian. Outline the steps you will take to manage this patient giving reasons for each stage.

Common mistakes

- Her management depends on her age, parity and desire for further pregnancy
- Management to be determined by an oncologist
- She has ovarian cancer and therefore should not be managed by an general gynaecologist
- Counselling about family history of breast and colon cancer
- Screening for ovarian cancer – listing all the methods for screening for ovarian cancer

A good answer will include some or all of these points

- History to exclude features of malignancy, for example anorexia, loss of appetite, dyspepsia
- Examination to exclude the presence of ascities
- Investigations: blood, urea and electrolytes (U&Es), liver function test (LFT), CA125; ultrasound; magnetic resonance imaging (MRI)
- Treatment
- Discussion with oncologist
- Surgery – incision, details of surgery
- Follow-up

Sample answer

The abdominal mass in this patient is likely to be an ovarian mucinous cystadenoma. However, this diagnosis will have to be confirmed as soon as possible before definitive treatment may be offered. Initially, additional symptoms have to be obtained from the patient. These include loss of appetite, the duration of the abdominal swelling and pressure symptoms, such as swelling of the feet and vulva, varicose veins, haemorrhoids, and gastro-intestinal symptoms, such as dyspepsia and constipation.

A clinical examination is needed to characterize associated features of the abdominal mass. These include the nature of the cyst – solid, irregular, associated ascites or secondaries in the chest and abdomen, oedema of the lower limbs and vulva. Following this, ancillary investigations should then be undertaken. Urea and electrolytes (U&Es) would indicate renal involvement in the form of ureteric obstruction. In addition, if the cyst is malignant, the patient will require adjuvant chemotherapy and, for this, renal function needs to be normal. A liver function test (LFT) will be performed for similar reasons – to assess the involvement of the liver with secondaries and whether chemotherapy could be offered. An estimation of carcinoma antigen CA125 is essential. This is raised in epithelial cancers, endometriosis and pelvic inflammatory disease. An ultrasound scan will define the nature of the cyst, associated ascites, liver secondaries and renal tract obstruction. However, this, may not be conclusive. In this case, magnetic resonance imaging (MRI) would be undertaken. This has the added advantage of screening for lymphadenopathy of the paraortic nodes.

The definitive treatment of this patient is surgery. Although a malignancy is unlikely, it must be considered before surgery is untaken. Discussions with the patient must therefore include the nature of the abdominal incision – which in this case will be vertical. In addition, a gynaecological oncologist should be notified and available if needed. At surgery, the contra-lateral ovary would be inspected for tumours. Any ascites should be sampled, its colour noted and then sent for histology, and if none is present, a saline wash out of the pelvis and paraortic gutters would be performed and sent for histology. The ovarian tumour should then be characterized, essentially identifying features suggestive of malignancy. These include an intact capsule, secondaries on the liver surface or omentum, enlarged abdominal nodes and further characteristics of the ovary – whether cystic or partly solid and cystic. If there are no features of malignancy, treatment will simply be removal of the ovary, omental biopsy and where nodes are palpable, biopsy. If a malignancy is suspected, an abdominal hysterectomy, bilateral salpingoophorectomy and omentectomy will be performed. The definitive treatment will only be completed after histology.

3. You saw a young girl of 17 years presenting as an emergency with intermittent lower abdominal pain of three days' duration. The pain is now constant and is mainly on the right side and radiating to her back. Her last menstrual period of a 28-day regular cycle was one week ago. Critically appraise your management of this patient.

Common mistakes

- Screening for ovarian cancer and await results before management
- Ultrasound scan must be performed before surgery
- Uterine fibroids are the likely cause
- An ectopic pregnancy is the first differential until proved otherwise

A good answer will include some or all of these points

- The most likely diagnosis is torsion of an ovarian cyst
- Dermoid cyst – the most likely type of cyst in this young girl
- It is an emergency, hence no place for conservative management
- Diagnostic laparoscopy if out of hours and no facilities for emergency ultrasound scan
- Surgery – laparoscopic or lapratomy
- Ovarian cystectomy or oophorectomy
- Fixation of the contralateral ovary
- Counselling after treatment

Sample answer

The most likely diagnosis in this young girl is torsion of the ovary. This diagnosis will have to be confirmed at either laparoscopy or laparotomy. Associated symptoms include nausea and vomiting and, depending on the size of the cyst, abdominal bloatedness and constipation. A previously diagnosed ovarian cyst may also be obtained from the history. A physical examination may identify an abdominal or pelvic mass, tenderness with rebound or guarding. The presence of a mass may also be confirmed on pelvic examination.

Essential investigations include a full blood count (FBC). A raised white cell count (WCC) is recognized to be associated with a torted ovarian cyst. In addition to this, blood should be grouped and saved. A differential diagnosis in this patient is haemorrhage into an ovarian cyst. The cyst may also have ruptured and severe haemorrhage may require transfusion. An ultrasound scan will confirm the presence of an ovarian cyst but this is unlikely to suggest torsion. The disadvantage of waiting for this before proceeding with surgery is that this facility may not be available out of hours. However, if it is available, it will provide details about the cyst, the size, and what type it may be. If this facility is unavailable, and the ovarian cyst is not more than 12-week gestation in size, a diagnostic laparoscopy may be performed. This procedure has the advantage of defining the type of ovarian pathology and the complication. Where the expertise exists, an ovarian cystectomy or oophorectomy could be performed laparoscopically.

The definitive treatment for this patient will be an ovarian cystectomy or oophorectomy. This is easily performed through a laparotomy. If the torsion has resulted in gangrene of the ovary (and usually this is with the Fallopian tube), a salpingoophorectomy will be the treatment of choice. If the ovary is still viable after untwisting, a cystectomy will be performed. The ovary on the opposite side has to be inspected to ensure that there is no a cyst on it. If there is a cyst, it has to be removed otherwise it could undergo a similar complication. The remnant ovary on the affected side and the unaffected ovary should then be fixed to avoid a recurrence of the torsion.

7

Vulval and vaginal disorders

1. Justify your management of a 19-year-old woman presenting with a painful swollen right labium majorum.

2. Mrs TP is 24 years old. She presented to the gynaecology outpatient with primary amenorrhoea. Following investigations, a diagnosis of Müllerian agenesis was made. Critically appraise how you will manage this patient.

3. What steps will take in the management of a 76-year-old woman with a diagnosis of carcinoma of the vagina.

1. Justify your management of a 19-year-old woman presenting with a painful swollen right labium majorum.

Common mistakes

- Take a history and do a physical examination, although this is an important part of management it needs to be a targeted history and physical examination. Just stating that you will take a history and do a physical examination is not enough
- Refer her to a genito-urinary medicine (GUM) clinic, although the swelling may be secondary to a sexually transmitted disease (STD), referring her to the GUM clinic without making a diagnosis is assuming that all swellings in the vulva are caused by STDs
- Exclude vulval cancer, although this is a possibility it is highly unlikely in this 19-year-old
- Listing all the gynaecological investigations for a vaginal discharge is not appropriate. Although you may need to undertake some of them, they must be related to the symptoms and signs you elicit
- Failing to justify your management – remember that *justify* means offering an explanation for everything you do for the patient

A good answer will include some or all of these points

- More information is required to help make a diagnosis – the history is a focused one
- Physical examination to define the location of the swelling, again, this is focused and should demonstrate that you are thinking of the causes of this swelling and the associated signs which you may demonstrate
- Investigations – these must be specific to this patient
- Treatment – this will depend on the cause of the swelling
- Differential diagnoses: Bartholin's cyst/abscess; trauma – haematoma; STD

Sample answer

The definitive management of this young woman will depend on the cause of the vulval swelling. In the first instance, therefore, more information is required to help focus on its possible cause. A Bartholin's abscess is the most likely diagnosis; however, other differential diagnosis, such as trauma with a haematoma, a hernia and a lipoma have to be considered. An associated vaginal discharge and the patient's sexual history are of particular relevance to making a diagnosis. A Bartholin's abscess will present with a swelling that is gradually getting worse and is red and tender. A history of trauma to the vulva will suggest a haematoma and associated with this may be urinary retention or a swelling in the vagina if the haematoma extends into the paravaginal area. Another possible cause is an inguino-labial hernia, which has become strangulated or obstructed. This is, however, uncommon in this age group. In this case, there may be a longstanding history of a swelling that was reducible initially. The patient may also give a history of the swelling getting worse with coughing and possible associated complications, such as constipation. Lipomas of the vulva are uncommon and they tend to occur in the older age group. These tend to be painless and located in the anterior portion of the vulva.

A physical examination will reveal signs of the possible cause of the swelling. A Bartholin's cyst or abscess is located on the posterior medial aspect of the labium majorum. It will be tense, fluctuant and tender, and it may be inflamed. Associated with this may be a vaginal discharge. If there is a gonococcal infection, a purulent urethral discharge may be identified. Evidence of trauma will confirm the diagnoses of a vulval haematoma, whereas a soft non-tender swelling located on the anterior vulva may be diagnostic of a lipoma. A bimanual examination is important as it will reveal associated features, such as bilateral adnexal tenderness associated with pelvic inflammatory disease or a paravaginal swelling in the case of trauma causing a haematoma. Thorough examination of the inguinal ring and a negative cough impulse will exclude an inguinal hernia.

Once the diagnosis has been made, the most appropriate treatment would be offered. If a Bartholin's abscess or cyst is the cause of the swelling, the treatment of choice is marsupialization and antibiotic therapy. Antibiotic therapy must cover Gram-negative and Gram-positive organisms and also be effective against *Neisseria gonorrhoea*. A sample of the pus drained from the abscess should be sent for microbiology and needs to be transported in a medium suitable for the culture of *N. gonorrhoea*. If a haematoma is the cause, it has to be drained. A lipoma will be excised, whereas a hernia will be referred to a general surgeon for repair. If the bowel is strangulated, there may have to be resection during surgery. There are other causes of a vulval swelling but these are rare and the treatment will depends to a large extent on the cause. In this young woman, if a Bartholin's abscess is the diagnosis, sexually transmitted diseases (STDs) must be considered and excluded as they may co-exist.

2. Mrs TP is 24 years old. She presented to the gynaecology outpatient with primary amenorrhoea. Following investigations, a diagnosis of Müllerian agenesis was made. Critically appraise how you will manage this patient.

Common mistakes

- Take a history and physical examination
- Discussing the causes of primary amenorrhoea
- Investigations of primary amenorrhoea
- Investigations to confirm Müllerian agenesis – the diagnosis has already been made. No need therefore to confirm

A good answer will include some or all of these points

- The extent of the agenesis
- Education/counselling of the patient
- Treatment options
- Neovagina
- Pregnancy
- Conclusion

Sample answer

Müllerian agenesis is a common cause of primary amenorrhoea. Patients presenting with primary amenorrhoea do not usually expect to be told that they have an agenesis of the lower genital tract. Typical Müllerian agenesis consists of an absent uterus and vagina. In this patient, therefore, it is important to establish how severe the agenesis is. An important early step is to inform the patient of the diagnosis, its implications and the subsequent management plan.

The complete syndrome includes an absent vagina and uterus. In the incomplete variety, there may be partial fusion of the upper portion of the Müllerian system. There may therefore be a rudimentary uterus, usually with no vagina. Communication about the diagnosis needs to be very tactful and sensitive. Most patients will initially respond by denial and then anger, but will eventually come to terms with it. If available, psychological support from staff with appropriate skills in counselling should be offered. Subsequently, counselling must enlighten the patient of the implications of the condition (she will remain amenorrhoeic and will not be able to have children).

The next step will be to discuss the options available to the patient and to determine her needs. It is unlikely that she is sexually active. In fact, she may have experienced apareunia and offering an explanation for this may be very reassuring. The main treatment option is to create a new vagina. This is probably the only treatment that she could be offered.

A neovagina may be created surgically or by non-surgical means. If it is to be created surgically, the patient would have to be referred to someone with an experience in the creation of a neovagina. This is often successful initially but is commonly followed by adhesions and therefore the results may not be as good. A neovagina can also be created by use of vaginal dilators and an Ingram's bicycle seat. This requires the patient to apply dilators of increasing size and length for 30 minutes every day for about three to six months. If the patient is well-motivated, and can tolerate this, the results are often very good. Some patients, however, do experience a pulling sensation in the vagina after completing the therapy. The disadvantage of this option is that after creation of the neovagina, it must be maintained by frequent dilatation. Often, this is done by sexual intercourse.

The long-term consequence of the diagnosis, relating to the patient's inability to become pregnant, must be discussed. She needs to be informed that although she cannot become pregnant, she could have children from her own eggs through surrogacy. However, adoption is another option that should be discussed. A diagnosis of Müllerian agenesis requires a team approach to its management. In some cases, a clinical psychologist or a psychotherapist may be necessary.

3. What steps will take in the management of a 76-year-old woman with a diagnosis of carcinoma of the vagina.

Common mistakes

- Take a history and perform a physical examination
- Discussing the aetiology of vaginal carcinoma
- Symptoms of vaginal carcinoma
- Details of the screening for vaginal intraepithelial neoplasia (VAIN)
- Management of VAIN

A good answer will include some or all of these points

- Carcinoma of the vagina is rare
- Need for a thorough examination under general anaesthesia (GA)
- More elaborate assessment depending on the suspected extent of the disease
- Need for a full thickness biopsy
- Surgery – vaginectomy, radical hysterectomy
- Radiotherapy
- Combination or both (surgery and/or radiotherapy)
- Follow-up

Sample answer

Carcinoma of the vagina is uncommon and best managed by a gynaecological oncologist, to whom the patient should be referred. It typically presents with postmenopausal bleeding. Once the diagnosis is made, attempts must be made to define the extent of the disease. This is best done by examination under anaesthesia (EUA). During this procedure, a colposcopy may also be performed to identify co-existing VAIN and also to define the location of the lesion. EUA is incomplete without a combined rectal and vaginal examination.

If, during EUA, an anterior or posterior spread is suspected, a cystoscopy and/or a proctosigmoidosccopy, respectively, should be performed. A generous full thickness biopsy should also be taken for an adequate histological evaluation. Further investigations would be undertaken to exclude distant metastases. A chest X-ray (CXR) will exclude secondaries in the lungs, whereas an intravenous urogram (IVU) will exclude parametrial spread affecting the ureters. However, an IVU may be avoided if an ultrasound scan of the renal system is performed. Lymphangiography has been recommended by some experts to help map out any nodal involvement but this is not universally available.

The treatment of choice for this patient is surgery. This will depend on the stage of the disease and her suitability for surgery. If she has stage I disease, the treatment of choice will be a radical hysterectomy, radical vaginectomy and lymphadenectomy. For more advanced diseases, an exenteration is the treatment of choice. This will depend on the extension of the disease. For an anterior spread, this will take the form of an anterior exenteration and re-implantation of the ureters in the bowel or creating an ileal conduit. For a posterior spread, a posterior exenteration with the creation of a colostomy will be the surgery of choice. If the spread is both anterior and posterior, a total exenteration will be the treatment of choice. These radical options will only be offered if the patient is fit. Where she is unable to withstand such extensive surgery, radiotherapy should be offered as the treatment of choice. In fact, it is regarded as the treatment of choice in some patients by some oncologists. It is associated with less morbidity and mortality, especially for older patients. This is offered as combined internal and external radiotherapy. Whatever the treatment, regular follow-up is essential to identify recurrences.

8

Infertility

1. A couple investigated for infertility were categorized as 'unexplained infertility'. Summarize the options available to them.

2. Critically assess the methods of assessing tubal function in the investigation of infertility.

3. Evaluate your options for ovulation induction in a 25-year-old patient with polycystic ovary syndrome.

4. What steps will take to minimize the risk of ovarian hyperstimulation syndrome and how will you recognize it?

5. A couple attending the infertility clinic have been investigated and the husband's semen analysis was described as oligozoospermic. Evaluate the options available to the couple.

1. A couple investigated for infertility were categorized as 'unexplained infertility'. Summarize the options available to them.

Common mistakes

- Discussing the causes of infertility – there is no need to list the causes of infertility as the question explicitly demands summarizing options for a particular type of infertility – the unexplained type
- Do not discuss the contributions of every factor involved in infertility
- Take a history and doing a physical examination is irrelevant. The couple have already been investigated and categorized as unexplained!!
- Details of infertility treatment in general, for example ovulation induction regimens in women with anovulation, *in vitro* fertilization with embryo transfer (IVF-ET), etc. These are irrelevant to this question

A good answer will include some or all of these points

- What is the definition of unexplained infertility and its prevalence
- Factors that may influence outcome (chances of a successful outcome) – secondary infertility has a better prognosis than primary
- Counselling – the first important stage: supportive; success rate; influence of natural conception rates superimposed as infertility
- Assisted reproductive techniques – IVF-ET, gamete intra-Fallopian transfer (GIFT), artificial insemination by husband (AIH), artificial insemination by donor (AID); expensive; complications; psychological problems with failure
- Surrogacy

Sample answer

Unexplained infertility is defined as infertility in which all investigations have failed to identify a cause. This definition depends to a large extent on the extent and complexity of the facilities that are available for the investigations. These are more likely to be more extensive in tertiary centres than in primary or secondary units. Prevalence is thought to vary from 10 per cent to 39 per cent of all infertile couples (Templeton and Penney, 1982).

It is well-recognized that the outcome of unexplained infertility depends on various factors. These include the age of the female patient, the duration and type of infertility. If the woman is over the age of 35, the success of expectant management is poor. Hull *et al.* (1985) showed that the chances of spontaneous conception are closely related to the duration of infertility and whether it is primary or secondary in nature.

The first option for any couple with this diagnosis, therefore, is counselling and reassurance. The eventual pregnancy rate after three years' expectant management is between 60 per cent and 70 per cent (Hull *et al.*, 1985). In this option, sympathetic explanations of the diagnosis and the success rate of expectant management are offered to the couple. The most likely couple to succeed with this option is the young one. This option is frustrating at the best of times, not only to the couple but also to the physician. For older women the success rate is lower simply because age has an important effect on spontaneous conception rates.

The next option for the couple is assisted reproduction techniques for infertility. Although there is no evidence to indicate that detailed investigations and treatment have a better success rate, it may provide a psychological boost to the couple – the perception that something is being done to overcome the problem. The drawback to this option is that pregnancies occurring during this time could be wrongly attributed to the investigations and empirical treatment rather than to natural conception. Options include artificial insemination with the husband's semen (AIH). This is inexpensive and likely to be acceptable to the couple. *In vitro* fertilization and embryo transfer (IVF-ET) may also be offered. Here, superovulation is induced and, after harvesting the eggs, fertilization is facilitated *in vitro* and the fertilized embryo transferred into the uterus. The advantage of this technique is that fertilization is guaranteed and extra embryos may be stored for further attempts. However, this is a very expensive option and one whose failure may be associated with many psychological problems. A third intervention option is gamete intra-Fallopian transfer (GIFT). Again, this is an invasive option. Some couples may be offered ovulation induction but allowing 'natural conception' to take place. This option ensures that ovulation (and possibly multiple ovulation) has occurred. It is expensive and may be complicated by ovarian hyperstimulation syndrome, with associated severe morbidity and sometimes mortality.

The last option for the couple is adoption. Adopting may sometimes remove the anxiety associated with attempting to conceive and result in a natural conception. Whatever the case, there is the need to be more pro-active in the older than the younger couple. Those with primary infertility have a lower success rate with expectant management than those with secondary infertility. Where the duration of infertility is less than three years, expectant management is associated with an eight per cent success rate.

Reference

Hull MG, Glazener CM, Kelly NJ *et al.* Population study of causes, treatment and outcome of infertility. *BMJ* 1985; 291: 1693–7.
Templeton AA, Penny GC. The incidence, characteristics and prognosis of patients whose infertility is unexplained. *Fertil Steril* 1982; 37: 175–82.

2. Critically assess the methods of assessing tubal function in the investigation of infertility.

Common mistakes

- Causes of tubal infertility – the question specifically asks about assessing tubal function
- Although tubal function can be in the male partner, it is unusual for the gynaecologist to assess him
- Listing all the causes of infertility
- History, physical examination and investigations
- Treatment of causes of tubal infertility

A good answer will include some or all of these points

- Tubal function consists of anatomical (external and internal) and physiological components
- Methods of assessment: hysterosalpingography – radiological, painful, traumatic to the cervix, outlines the uterus and Fallopian tubes. Tends to test for tubal patency and peritubal adhesions. Advantages – able to identify uterine and tubal synaechiae. May diagnose tuberculosis and cervical incompetence. Does not identify endometriosis and adhesions. May produce false negatives because of tubal spasm. Patient may have a vasovagal attack; laparoscopy and hydrotubation – requires anaesthesia. Assesses tubal patency and the exterior of tube. Enables the diagnosis of endometriosis and other pelvic pathology. Fails to identify level of obstruction and intrauterine status; ultrasound scan – saline hysterosalpinography. Enables ovarian cysts to be diagnosed. May be useful in the diagnosis of Asherman syndrome. Requires skilled personnel and equipment. Contrast ultrasound (Echovist) similar to saline ultrasonography; falloposcopy; salpingoscopy – useful to assess the internal anatomy of the tubes. Requires general anaesthesia (GA) and a very skilled operator and equipment. Unlikely to be available to all patients
- Conclusion – most methods of tubal function assessment are complimentary – laparoscopy and hysterosalpingography

Sample answer

Tubal factors are responsible for approximate 15 per cent of cases of infertility. Although they may be present in isolation, they sometimes co-exist with other factors, which may be extrauterine or intrauterine. In the course of assessing tubal function, therefore, it will certainly be advantageous if other associated factors could be excluded. Tubal function is normal if anatomic (gross and histological) and physiological aspects are normal as these constituents are essential for fertilization and transport through the tube. There are various approaches to assessing tubal function. These include hysterosalpingography, laparoscopy and dye test, falloposcopy, salpingoscopy and hygroscopic sonograpphy with contrast medium (HyCoSy) or saline.

Hysterosalpingography is an outpatient procedure usually performed without general anaesthesia (GA). It involves the administration of a contrast medium (for example, Urograffin) through the cervical and uterine canals into the Fallopian tubes. This allows visualization of the course of the tubes, localization of any blockage and peritubal adhesions. It has the added advantage of being able to diagnose cervical weakness (incompetence) and intrauterine adhesions. In addition, pathognomonic appearances may aid in the diagnosis of pelvic tuberculosis affecting the Fallopian tubes. The major disadvantages of this procedure include flare-up of subclinical chronic pelvic inflammatory disease, vasovagal attacks and trauma to the cervix. In addition, false positive tubal blockages may be reported because of tubal spasm. Unfortunately, this procedure does not allow for the examination of the rest of the pelvis and therefore the exclusion of other factors associated with infertility, such as endometriosis.

Diagnostic laparoscopy and dye testing is the most common method of assessing tubal patency. Although it can be performed under sedation and local anaesthesia, it is most commonly performed under GA in the UK. The advantages include its ability to identify abnormal fimbriae and associated pelvic pathologies, such as adhesions and endometriosis. In addition, some of these pathologies may be treated (for example, adhesiolysis) during the procedure. Unfortunately, it does not define the site of tubal obstruction and cannot exclude uterine pathology, such as synechiae. Skilled clinicians need to perform the procedure, which is more expensive than hysterosalpingography. Where *in vitro* fertilization may be a treatment option for the infertility, it allows for the assessment of the ovaries *vis-à-vis* oocyte retrieval. Although the above two diagnostic procedures are most common, others, such as falloposcopy (examination of the internal surface of the fallopian tubes through the uterine canal) and salpingoscopy (examination of the internal surfaces of the Fallopian tubes through the external ostium of the tubes at laparoscopy), are available for the assessment of tubal function, these procedures are quite specialized and therefore are only available in few units. They require skill and expensive equipment. The advantage of both procedures is their ability to identify intratubal pathologies, which neither of the other two methods will identify. These include thinning of the epithelium and adhesions (synechiae). Again, they are commonly performed under GA, although they can be performed under sedation and local anaesthesia. These additional assessments may help in the counselling of patients on their suitability for tubal surgery or gamete intra-Fallopian transfer (GIFT).

Recently, there has been a move towards contrast or saline hysterosonography using ultrasound for tubal patency assessment. These procedures have the same advantages as those of hysterosalpingography, but tubal function has to be assessed dynamically during the procedure. The main advantage over the latter is the use of ultrasound, which may allow the exclusion of ovarian pathology and intramural fibroids (a possible factor infertility which laparoscopy may identify).

There are unfortunately no robust methods of assessing the physiological functions of the Fallopian tubes, and the various techniques assess mainly the anatomical components of tubal function. Inevitably, a tube that allows fertilization and successful transfer into the uterine cavity is physiologically normal.

3. Evaluate your options for ovulation induction in a 25-year-old patient with poly-cystic ovary syndrome.

Common mistakes

- Induction of ovulation and treatment for infertility
- Discussing options for infertility treatment
- Concentrating on drug therapy only
- Treatment of male infertility
- Details of IUF/ET or GIFT etc.

A good answer will include some or all of these points

- Induction of ovulation – methods: weight loss; medical or surgical options
- Anti-oestrogens – clomifene citrate or cyclofenil, gonadotrophins (Metrodin)
- Gonadotrophin-releasing hormone (GnRH) analogues and gonadotrophins
- Metformin
- Surgical
- Ovarian diathermy/laser
- Wedge resection of the ovary

Sample answer

Polycystic ovary syndrome is one of the most common gynaecological endocrinological disorders. Infertility is one of the symptoms with which these patients present and it is commonly due to anovulation. Ovulation induction in polycystic ovary syndrome may be achieved through medical or surgical options. However, as some of these patients are over-weight, simple measures such as weight loss may be effective in inducing ovulation. This has the added advantage that it does not require any medication, is free of side-effects and is inexpensive. In addition, if successful, conception rates are higher following induction of ovulation as a result of weight loss than that of other methods.

Of the medical methods of inducing ovulation, clomifene citrate is the most commonly used. This is an anti-oestogen, usually administered in the early menstrual phase. It is inexpensive and induces ovulation successfully in about 30–40 per cent of patients with polycystic ovary syndrome, although that rate may be as high as 80 per cent in properly selected patients. The six months' cumulative conception rate, where ovulation has been suc-cessfully induced, is similar to that of normal fertility (60 per cent) with most occurring in the first six ovulatory cycles. It has the added advantage that the multiple pregnancy rate is only five to 10 per cent and significant ovarian hyperstimulation syndrome is rare compared to that after ovulation induction with gonadotrophins. Unfortunately, because of the anti-oestrogenic effects, clomifene citrate may induce ovulation but not result in successful pregnancy. Often, therefore, patients may have to take multiple courses before pregnancy can be achieved.

Where clomifene citrate has been unsuccessful in inducing ovulation and pregnancy, cyclofenil could be the next option. It is also an anti-oestrogen but it has less anti-oestrogenic effects on the cervical mucus. It may theoretically be associated with higher pregnancy rates than clomifene citrate. However, cyclofenil is more expensive and associated with more side-effects when compared to those of clomifene citrate.

Human menopausal gonadotrophins (HMG) and pure follicle-stimulating hormone (FSH) (pergonal, normagon or metrodin), extracted from the urine of postmenopausal women, are effective but more expensive methods of ovulation induction in patients with polycystic ovary syndrome, preferably when anti-oestrogen agents have failed. They are available as FSH and luteinizing hormone (LH) (for example, pergonal and normagon) of pure FSH (for example, metrodin). Recombinant FSH is now available, with the advantage of being free of extraneous proteins to which some patients may develop allergic reactions or antibodies. This is an effective but more expensive method of ovulation induction than the previous two options. They also have to be administered parenterally (usually daily and starting in the menstrual phase). Ideally, the patient should have follicular tracking and serial oestradiol monitoring to time the administration of human chorionic gondadotrophins (HCG), in order to minimize the risk of multiple pregnancies and ovarian hyperstimulation syndrome. A combination of these is certainly more expensive than the previous oral regimens. As these patients are more sensitive to HMG, treatment is usually initiated on lower doses (75 IU) and monitored every five days. The 12 months' cumulative pregnancy rate following this regimen in polycystic ovary syndrome patients is much higher than in those with hypo-pituitary dysfunction. The risk of ovarian hyperstimulation syndrome is one to two per cent, whereas there is a 25 per cent incidence of pregnancies of higher orders. Unfortunately, the miscarriage risk associated with this method of induction of ovulation is between 32 per cent and 40 per cent.

For this patient, the surgical methods of ovulation induction include laparoscopic laser or diathermy drilling of the ovaries. Although successful, the main disadvantages of the surgical options are the short-lasting effects of treatment. The procedure itself is expensive and involves a laparoscopy and hospital care even if this only during the time of treatment. There are associated complications of the procedure and the ever-present risk of adhesion formation. In skilled hands, this may be best performed at the time of laparoscopic assessment of tubal function. The original method of ovulation induction in patients with polycystic ovary syndrome was wedge resection of the ovary. Although this has generally been superseded by modern techniques, it may still be considered in some developing countries. Very recently, metformin has been being used to induce ovulation in overweight diabetic women. This must be an option in this patient if she is obese. The pregnancy rate after induction of ovulation by weight loss is higher than in that after other methods of ovulation induction.

4. What steps will you take to minimize the risk of ovarian hyperstimulation syndrome and how will you recognize it?

Common mistakes

- Classification and details of ovarian hyperstimulation syndrome
- Treatment and management of the causes of ovarian hyperstimulation syndrome
- Mentioning irrelevant points, for example, ovarian hyperstimulation syndrome does not occur with gondadotrophin-releasing hormone (GnRH) analogues (this is not true and if you are uncertain do not mention it). Ovarian hyperstimulation syndrome occurs in natural cycles!
- Vaginal examination is contraindicated in ovarian hyperstimulation syndrome
- Scanning before induction of ovulation to determine suitability for induction. Listing investigations for ovarian hyperstimulation syndrome
- Inaccurate facts, for example, features of ovarian hyperstimulation syndrome include hirsutism, irregular periods and vaginal bleeding
- Use of clomid for more than six months inadvisable because of ovarian hyperstimulation syndrome
- Only occurs in polycystic ovary syndrome patients in whom injudicious use of gonadotrophins has occurred

A good answer will include some or all of these points

- Define the features of ovarian hyperstimulation syndrome (enlarged ovaries, abdominal distension, nausea, vomiting, diarrhoea, and in severe forms, ascites, pleural effusions, hypovolaemia, hypotension and polycythaemia)
- Ovarian hyperstimulation syndrome results from superovulation. Potentially fatal
- Predisposing factors: large number of follicles (especially induced by gonadotrophins and beta-human chorionic gonadotrophins, βHCG); βHCG administration; younger patients; pregnancy – four times higher incidence in conception cycles. Pregnancy increases ×3 in ovarian hyperstimulation syndrome cycles; low body mass index (weight) (BMI <19); polycystic ovary syndrome
- Minimizing the risk
  - Serial follicular tracking to ensure no HCG administration for more follicles
  - Oestradiol levels >6000 pmol, do not administer βHCG
  - Advice against sexual intercourse if oestradiol levels high or large number of follicles
  - Progestogens rather than βHCG to support pregnancy
  - Ovarian drilling /diathermy for polycystic ovary syndrome
  - Clomid rather than gonadotrophins
  - Human menopausal gonadotrophins (HMG) + gonadotrophin-releasing hormone (GnRH) agonists increase the prevalence of ovarian hyperstimulation syndrome
- Recognition

- Symptoms – mild, moderate or severe (abdominal pain, vomiting, chest pain enlarged abdomen)
- Ultrasound – follicles, ascites
- Biochemistry – deranged urea and electrolytes (U&Es), hypovolaemia, low urine output, pleural effusion – chest X-ray (CXR)

Sample answer

Ovarian hyperstimulation syndrome is a complication of induction of superovulation. Its incidence varies from approximately 10 per cent to 20 per cent, depending on severity. This includes mild, through moderate, to severe varieties. Ovarian hyperstimulation syndrome consists of ovarian enlargement, abdominal distension, ascites, nausea, vomiting and diarrhoea, and in severe forms, pleural effusion, hypovolaemia, hypotension and poly-cythaemia. If improperly managed, it could be fatal.

To minimize the risk of hyperstimulation, the factors predisposing to ovarian hyper-stimulation syndrome must be identified. In the the younger patient, polycystic ovary syndrome, low body mass index (BMI <19), beta-human chorionic gonadotrophin (βHCG) administration, high serum oestradiol levels during ovulation induction, a larger number of follicles (>18–20 mm in diameter) during ovulation and pregnancy. Pregnancy is three times more likely in ovarian hyperstimulation syndrome cycles.

Minimizing the risk of ovarian hyperstimulation syndrome, therefore, must involve reducing the predisposing factors. First, ovulation induction is best undertaken by drugs that are least likely to induce the condition. For example, the use of anti-oestrogen agents, such as clomifene citrate instead of gonadotrophins. However, this may not necessarily be the case, as these drugs may be ineffective. Alternatives to gonadotrophins, such as ovarian drilling, must also be considered. Where gonadotrophins are employed, the ovulation induction process must be monitored closely. This will include follicular tracking with ultrasound to ensure that there are not too many follicles ready to rupture. This can be complemented with serum oestradiol estimations. If the number of follicles above 12 mm in diameter is more than 15, or serum oestradiol levels are above 2000 pg/ml, then βHCG should be withheld. This will delay, or prevent, release of the ova from the follicles. In some cases, it has been suggested that delay-ing rather than omitting the βHCG may also minimize the risk of ovarian hyperstimulation syndrome.

Where ovulation induction is for a natural conception, advising against sexual intercourse will minimize the risk of ovarian hyperstimulation syndrome. This will prevent pregnancy and therefore reduce the chances of ovarian hyperstimulation syndrome developing. If pregnancy does occur, the use of progestogens rather than HCG to support the early phase of pregnancy will significantly minimize the risk of ovarian hyperstimulation syndrome.

Ovulation induction with gonadotrophin-releasing hormone (GnRH) agonists with HCG or HMG is associated with a lower risk of ovarian hyperstimulation syndrome compared to the use of HMG and HCG. Used in a pulsatile fashion, this has been shown to result in successful pregnancy without the risk of developing the condition. GnRH agonists with HCG or HMG may be used in patients who have raised oestradiol levels during induction of ovula-tion with gonadotrophins. Imoedemhe et al. (1991) used eight-hourly intranasal buserelin in patients with >4000 pg/ml oestradiol levels and achieved a 22 per cent pregnancy rate with no case of ovarian hyperstimulation syndrome. Alternatively, follicular aspiration may be used. Pregnancies after *in vitro* fertilization (IVF) are rarely complicated by ovarian hyper-stimulation syndrome. This is because of aspiration of the follicles. Therefore, where there are many follicles above the threshold diameter, repeated aspiration will minimize the risk of ovarian hyperstimulation syndrome.

Although other methods of minimizing the risk of ovarian hyperstimulation syndrome have been employed, such as intravenous (i.v.) administration of albumin and also cortico-steroids, these are not commonly used. The most effective method of minimizing this compli-cation of superovulation is to monitor the patient closely and to offer interventions that will minimize it. It is also important to identify early symptoms and signs of ovarian hyper-stimulation syndrome and to take the steps necessary to prevent progression. Early symptoms include abdominal pain, vomiting chest pain and an enlarged abdomen. Ultrasound monitor-ing of follicles during superovulation with gonadotrophins and ready investigation for bio-chemical derangements suggestive of early ovarian hyperstimulation syndrome are essential. Close monitoring of the patient's urine output may also indicate the early onset of ovarian hyperstimulation syndrome. Once these are identified, avoiding βHCG will minimize the severity of the condition.

References

Imoedemhe DAG, Chan RCW, Signe AB, Papaco ELA, Olaza AB. A new approach to the management of patients at risk of ovarian hyperstimulation in an *in vitro* fertilization programme. *Human Reproduction* 1991; 6: 1088–1091.

Rizk B. Ovarian hyperstimulation syndrome. In: Studd J (Ed.). *Progress in Obstetrics and Gynaecology*. London: Churchill Livingstone, 1994; Vol. 12; 311–349.

5. A couple attending the infertility clinic have been investigated and the husband's semen analysis was described as oligozoospermic. Evaluate the options available to the couple.

Common mistakes

- Taking a history and doing a physical examination – this would have been done before the investigations
- Details of investigations for infertility are irrelevant
- Use of very simplistic language, such as *'Place sperms in the woman'* for artificial insemination
- Offer a procedure and then state that it is most unlikely to succeed – if so, why offer it in the first place? If you were the patient would you accept it?
- You have been asked to evaluate the options and not to outline how to investigate the infertile couple

A good answer will include some or all of these points

- Assumption – repeat semen analysis remains abnormal and female investigations are normal
- Options – three main ones:
  - Identify cause of oligozoospemia and correct if treatable. This is the most cost-effective option and there is no need for invasive procedures, which may be associated with higher pregnancy rates. May need referral to a urologist. Modification of lifestyle to remove risk factors
  - Assisted conception techniques: artificial insemination by husband (AIH/IUI) – sperm preparation and concentration. Only extra requirement is sperm preparation. Success rate may be improved by induction of ovulation. Use of husband's sperm, therefore biological father – more acceptable; artificial insemination by donor (AID) – least likely to be accepted at the outset (as first suggestion); AIH and AID cheaper than *in vitro* fertilization (IVF) or gamete intra-Fallopian transfer (GIFT)
  - Advanced assisted conception techniques: IVF – expensive and low success rate. May still need donor sperm; GIFT – cheapest of the three. May still need donor sperm; intracytoplasmic sperm injection (ICSI) – if sperms cannot fertilize or are morphologically abnormal; expensive and associated with the complications of superovulation and ovarian hyperstimulation syndrome
- Adoption: child not biological offspring of parents

Sample answer

It is to be assumed that the semen analysis was performed at least twice in this couple and that the results were basically similar. There is therefore no need to repeat the semen analysis. In the first instance, the cause of the oligozoospermia should be identified if possible. If treatable, this will be the most suitable option to be offered. In most cases, however, the cause is difficult to identify and treatment is neither a logical nor a satisfactory option. If there is no known cause, the husband should be referred to a urologist for further evaluation and management if necessary. Sometimes a simple modification of lifestyle, such as working habits, smoking, drugs, etc., may be all that is necessary to improve the quality of the semen. Before referral, therefore, information about lifestyle factors that could influence semen analysis should be elicited and appropriate counselling offered.

The second option is artificial insemination with the husband's sperms (AIH). In this case, the sperms have to be prepared so that only normal ones are present and, in addition, the concentration is significantly improved. This may go in tandem with ovulation induction in order to improve the success rare. For this option, the only requirements are facilities for sperm preparation and introduction into the cervical canal. The main advantage is involvement of both partners and the offspring will be genetically from both parents. However, artificial insemination by donor (AID) may be another alternative. In this case, the biological father is a donor. Psychologically, this may be more difficult for the couple to accept.

Advanced assisted conception techniques may be offered in three different ways. The first is *in vitro* fertilization (IVF) or gamete intra-Fallopian transfer (GIFT), where ovulation induction is undertaken followed by fertilization with the husband's sperms (specially prepared) if they are morphologically normal) or by intracytoplasmic sperm injection (ICSI) using spermatids aspirated from the testis. This option is expensive and some couples may not be able to afford it, especially where it is only available privately. ICSI is likely to be an option only in highly specialized tertiary centres or private units. Complications with these advanced techniques may negate their availability.

The last option for the couple is adoption. This is complex, time-consuming and also very lengthy. All of this may make it a very frustrating option for the couple. In addition, the couple are not the biological parents of the adopted child and may be apprehensive about this. Oligozoospermia is a complication that must be handled with sensitivity and adequate empathy. The treatment options are many but, the couple have to be very comfortable with the one they eventually choose.

9

Family planning

1. A 31-year-old woman has attended the clinic requesting reversal of sterilization. What principles will underpin your management?

2. Briefly outline the non-contraceptive uses of the combined oral contraceptive pill.

3. Critically appraise the non-contraceptive uses of norethisterone in gynaecology.

4. What advice will you offer a perimenopausal woman about contraception and hormone replacement therapy (HRT)?

1. A 31-year-old woman has attended the clinic requesting reversal of sterilization. What principles will underpin your management?

Common mistakes

- Illogical in management – not following a logical order
- Describing the details of reversal of sterilization – microsurgical or macrosurgical techniques; describing these in detail, etc.
- Listing the reasons why a reversal should be performed
- Justifying why the procedure is necessary
- Highlighting the cost of reversal

A good answer will include some or all of these points

- The request needs to be justified (this is not a scientific concept)
- Information about the type of sterilization (from history or from gynaecology notes if patient cannot remember. If notes are not available, request them – diathermy poor success rate, clips or rings – good success rate
- Ovulating or not – investigate
- Semen analysis – normal?
- Assess Fallopian tubes at laparoscopy – what will be the length of Fallopian tube left after reversal?
- If residual Fallopian tube is less than 4 cm success rate is poor
- Type of reversal – microsopic or macroscopic
- Complications
- Alternatives to reversal of sterilization if unaccepted

Sample answer

A request for reversal of sterilization is not uncommon, especially as approximately 10 per cent of women in the UK regret the decision to undergo sterilization. In the first instance, this request needs to be assessed to determine whether is it justified. For most units, there are strict criteria that have to be fulfilled before a reversal can be allowed.

Following justification of the procedure, additional information is required about the type of sterilization the patient had. A laparoscopic sterilization with clips offers the best success rate after a reversal followed by sterilization by rings. An open sterilization, where portions of the Fallopian tubes were excised, or diathermy sterilization have poor success rates following reversals. In fact, if the patient had diathermy sterilization then the success rate is very poor and it might not be advisable to offer this patient a reversal.

Factors which could potentially affect the success rate of a reversal must be excluded. These include ovulation and good-quality semen. If any of these is abnormal, attempts have to be made to identify the cause and to correct them before the reversal. Assessment of ovulation is best done by serial luteal phase progesterone assays, whereas a semen analysis will identify any abnormal male factor.

If the decision is to offer a reversal, the next principle will be to determine how much residual Fallopian tube will be left after the process. This may be assessed at the time of the reversal or as a separate procedure. The advantage of making such an assessment as a separate procedure is the opportunity it provides for the assessment of the pelvis for co-existing factors, such as endometriosis or pelvic adhesions, which could affect fertility if not rectified. Some surgeons believe that such a separate procedure exposes the patient to an unnecessary risk of repeated general anaesthesia (GA). However, there are others who believe that this separate assessment is important as it provides an opportunity for a prognostic assessment before surgery. If the residual Fallopian tube is judged to be considerably less than 4 cm, it may not be worth undertaking the procedure.

Where the patient is suitable for reversal, the success of the procedure will depend on the type of reversal and the expertise of the operator. Microscopic reversal has a higher success rate than macroscopic reversal. In addition, when performed by a skilled operator the procedure has a better success rate. In good hands, and by use of microsurgical techniques, the success rate is in order of 70–80 per cent. Any complications (especially infections) arising after the procedure will influence success. Attempts must therefore be made to maintain meticulous asepsis and also to offer prophylactic antibiotics to minimize this risk. The success rate will also be influenced by the interval between the reversal and pregnancy. It is highest within the first 12 months of surgery. Counselling before reversal must, therefore, emphasize this point as there is no benefit in undertaking the procedure if the patient has no certainty of trying for a baby for at least 12 months.

2. Briefly outline the non-contraceptive uses of the combined oral contraceptive pill.

Common mistakes

- Listing the indications for the combined oral contraceptive pill
- Advantages and disadvantages of the combined oral contraceptive pill
- Different types of the combined oral contraceptive pill
- Complications of the combined oral contraceptive pill

A good answer will include some or all of these points

- Most common combination of oestrogens and progstogens
- Control of menstrual problems
- Regulation of menstruation
- Treatment of amenorrhoea
- Premenstrual syndrome
- Stimulation of the uterus in Asherman syndrome
- Control of menopausal symptoms
- Control of dysmenorrhoea
- Treatment of endometriosis
- Hirsutism and acne in polycystic ovary syndrome

Sample answer

The combined oral contraceptive pill is a popular method of contraception. By virtue of its oestrogen and progestogen constituents, it has many other non-contraceptive applications in gynaecology.

The most common application of combined oral contraceptive pill is in the control of menstrual problems. It may be used in the treatment of menorrhagia, irregular vaginal bleeding and dysmenorrhoea. In the treatment of these menstrual dysfunctions, it is administered in a similar way to its use as a contraceptive. In most of these situations, it provides a dual role – of contraception and of menstrual dysfunction control. In perimenarchal girls with heavy and painful periods, it is are effective. However, caution must be exercised when prescribing for this group of patients as the oestrogen component may affect the ultimate height of the young patient.

Another application is in the treatment of endometriosis. This is offered continuously without the pill-free interval. The duration of treatment is commonly six months. The major drawback is breakthrough bleeding. Its use in the treatment of adenomyosis has not been shown to be as effective as that in endometriosis.

The combined oral contraceptive pill may be used in premenstrual syndrome, although there is no strong evidence to support the effectiveness of this treatment. In some patients, however, this treatment may make the symptoms worse. Other non-contraceptive uses of the combined oral contraceptive pill include the control of menopausal symptoms and treatment of amenorrhoea where the cause is secondary to oestrogen deficiency. In polycystic ovary syndrome, where there is oligo-amenorrhoea or irregular vaginal bleeding, the less androgenic combined oral contraceptive pill may be used to regulate the menstrual cycle. Some patients with polycystic ovary syndrome and hirsutism may also be treated with the less androgenic combined oral contraceptive pill or one containing cyproterone acetate (Diannette).

Other uncommon uses of the combined combined oral contraceptive pill include the treatment of patients with Asherman syndrome. In this condition, high doses of oestrogens are given to induce proliferation of the epithelium of the deep glands following separation of the adhesions. Although oestrogens are more effective, the combined oral contraceptive pill may also be used.

3. Critically appraise the non-contraceptive uses of norethisterone in gynaecology.

Common mistakes

- Complications of norethisterone
- Describing how to prescribe norethisterone and the relevant doses
- Listing the various methods of administering norethisterone
- Contraindications of norethisterone therapy

A good answer will include some or all of these points

- Norethisterone – androgenic progestogen
- Indications
  - Control of irregular bleeding
  - Treatment of menorrhagia
  - Progesterone challenge test
  - Treatment of heavy bleeding
  - Treatment of hyperplasia of the endometrium
  - Used in conjuction with oestrogens
  - Breast cancer

Sample answer

Norethsterone is a C-19 progestogen, which is available in a variety of combined oral contraceptive pills. It is also commonly available as a single hormone which can be used in different gynaecological conditions. As a single agent, it has various uses in gynaecology. These vary from benign conditions to its use as adjuvant therapy for gynaecological malignancies.

The most common use of norethisterone is in the treatment of menorrhagia. Not only is this the most commonly used agent in primary care but it is also used widely in secondary and sometimes tertiary care. As a form of treatment for menorrhagia, there is overwhelming evidence to indicate that it is ineffective. It is associated with breakthrough bleeding and other side-effects, such as weight gain, breast tenderness and premenstrual-like symptoms. It is not a cost-effective treatment for this common gynaecological condition.

Norethisterone is most effective when used to treat irregular menstrual cycles, especially those due to luteal phase dysfunction or of anovulatory nature. In this treatment, norethisterone may be administered cyclically. Common cyclical regimens include days five to 25 and days 19 to 25. It stabilizes the endometrium and induces a controlled withdrawal bleed within about five days of stopping treatment. The major advantage of this treatment is that it is not associated with the oestrogenic side-effects of the combined oral contraceptive pill. However, it does not provide effective contraception if it is required. Because of its mild androgenicity, it may induce mild virilization of a female fetus *in utero*. Occasionally, however, the treatment is not provided in the most appropriate regimen and therefore it may not be successful. The side-effects are similar to those outlined above under the treatment of menorrhagia.

Norethisterone may be used to challenge the endometrium in a patient with amenorrhoea (progesterone challenge test). Its advantage in this therapeutic investigation is the ease with which it is administered and minimal side-effects. However, because of its androgenecity, it may not be as effective as a less androgenic progestogen, such as dihydrogesterone. Again, the side-effects are similar to those detailed above. Because of the shorter period of administration, these side-effects tend to be mild. A negative test, therefore, does not necessarily indicate failure of the endometrium to be stimulated by endogenous oestrogens.

In women presenting with heavy continuous bleeding, norethisterone administered in high doses and continuously may help in controlling the bleeding. This is an effective and inexpensive treatment, although because of the high dosages involved, side-effects such as nausea may not be well tolerated.

Other uncommon uses of norethisterone include the treatment of endometrial hyperplasia where the patient is unsuitable for surgery or refuses surgery. The advantage is inhibition of proliferative activity of the endometrium but this may not prevent progression to malignancy in all cases. It may provide a false sense of security in the patient being treated. Norethisterone may also be used in cases of metastatic endometrial carcinoma. This is not as effective as medroxyprogesterone acetate. It may also be used to treat breast cancer.

4. What advice will you offer a perimenopausal women about contraception and hormone replacement therapy (HRT)?

Common mistakes

- Details of hormone replacement therapy (HRT) in a perimenopausal woman
- Advantages of HRT
- Diagnosis of menopause
- Contraindications to HRT
- HRT and contraception
- Contraception in a perimenopausal woman

A good answer will include some or all of these points

- HRT is offered when indicated – to alleviate symptoms
- Contraception important as pregnancy can occur – hormone levels do not exclude the risk of pregnancy
- Age <50 – contraception for two years
- Age >50 contraception for one year
- On HRT before menopause – stop and wait for six months, then check hormone levels/remains amenorrhoeic
- Intrauterine contraceptive device (IUCD), surgical sterilization, combined oral contraceptive pill

Sample answer

The perimenpausal period is often regarded as that including the years before the onset of menopause. During this time, periods are usually irregular and or are commonly anovulatory. However, ovulation may occur and pregnancy is possible. Contraceptive advice during this period is therefore extremely important. It is also important to recognize the fact that during this period, fertility is significantly reduced. Therefore, the contraceptive needs of the woman are distinctly different from those of women in the early reproductive years. An important factor that must always be considered is the potential for associated medical conditions which may be contraindications for hormonal contraception and the increasing prevalence of systemic diseases in the older woman.

The type of contraception a woman may be offered will depend on the presence of any contraindications, her preferred choice, whether she has a current form of contraception and existing conditions which may be contraindications to different forms of contraception.

Assuming that there are no contraindications, and the woman's partner has not been sterilized, the options will include the combined oral contraceptive pill, the minipill, the intrauterine contraceptive device (IUCD), Depo-Provera and sterilization.

The IUCD, is more effective in this age group compared to the younger age groups. However, this must be acceptable to the patient. The complication of irregular vaginal bleeding, especially during the early months after insertion may result in early discontinuation. For most women, adequate counselling will result in a high continuation rate. Since the duration of this form of contraception depends of the type of device, the choice of device could be such that, once inserted, it potentially covers the rest of the reproductive life of the woman. The major disadvantage in such women is irregular vaginal bleeding, which may be a complication of the IUCD but may generate significant anxiety and may need investigating.

The combined oral contraceptive is another option. The low-dose oestrogen combined oral contraceptive pill will be more suitable in this age group. However, since this is associated with an increased risk of venous thrombo-embolism (VTE), the risk factors for this complication, such as smoking, obesity, hypertension, family history and thrombophilia, must be excluded. Again, this is more effective in this age group. It may provide the added benefit of counter-acting perimenopausal symptoms, which may require hormone replacement therapy (HRT). The minipill is an effective form of contraception, however, the complication of irregular vaginal bleeding may cause unnecessary anxiety derived from the need to exclude hyperplasia or endometrial carcinoma. However, the minipill may offer some relative protection against oestrogen-induced endometrial hyperplasia.

Sterilization is an ideal method for any age group. In the perimenopausal woman, this is even more ideal and it is unlikely that she will return requesting for reversal. During counselling, however, the frequent occurrence of irregular periods in this age group must be emphasized as some women may blame the irregularity of their periods on the sterilization.

Contraceptive advice is extremely important in the woman who is on cyclical HRT or is about to start HRT and is perimenopausal. She should continue with an adequate form of contraception for up to two years after the presumed age of menopause. Because this is difficult to ascertain, it may be advisable for the woman to stop the HRT and contraception for six months and see whether her periods resume or measure hormone levels and ascertain that ovulation does not occur. Stopping contraception in these women could be extremely difficult. In those who are less than 50 years of age, it is advisable to continue contraception for two years after the age of 50 before stopping, and for those after the age of 50, continuation should be for one year.

10

Pelvic infections, pelvic pain, chronic vaginal discharge

1. What principles will you follow in the management of a patient who has been suffering from chronic pelvic pain for the past three years?

2. A 30-year-old woman presented with lower abdominal pain, low-grade pyrexia and a history of chronic vaginal discharge. On examination, she was found to have a lower abdominal mass, which was tender but there was no ascites. An ultrasound scan showed a multiloculated cystic mass in the pouch of Douglas but no free ascites. A CA125 was slightly raised. You suspect she has a large tubo-ovarian abscess. Critically appraise your management of the patient.

3. Justify your management of a 27-year-old woman presenting with chronic vaginal discharge.

4. Critically appraise the measures you will undertake to reduce the prevalence of *Chlamydia trachomatis* genital infections.

1. What principles will you follow in the management of a patient who has been suffering from chronic pelvic pain for the past three years?

Common mistakes

- Take a history and do a physical examination
- Cause of pain is psychological – it is not possible to make this assumption on the basis of the information provided. However, it is recognized that this is a possible but not very likely scenario
- Treat with psychotherapy – this cannot be the only method of treating this patient. It has to be combined with another treatment modality
- Offer treatment for infertility after investigating the patient and her partner. This is completely irrelevant. You are not expected to even broach the subject of fertility
- Exclude human immunodeficiency virus (HIV) – on what basis? HIV does not cause pelvic pain
- Assume she has endometriosis and treat – this diagnosis should only be one of the differential diagnoses rather than the sole cause

A good answer will include some or all of these points

- This is a common symptom that could be due to many causes – the most important principle in the treatment is to identify a cause if possible; recognizing that the cause may not be identifiable in some cases
- A good history will be required to identify some of the common causes – this needs to be focused and directed
- Physical examination may be useful but often not
- Investigations – most important – diagnostic laparoscopy
- Treatment – depends on the cause
- Medical: combined oral contraceptive pill; progestogens; gonadotrophin-releasing hormone (GnRH) analogues; danazol; analgesics
- Surgery: bilateral salpingoophorectomy; total abdominal hysterectomy + bilateral salpingoophorectomy; laparotic uterosacral nerve division (LUNA), etc.
- Psychotherapy

Sample answer

Chronic pelvic pain is a common symptom. It may be due to a variety of gynaecological and non-gynaecological causes. In the management of this patient, fundamental principles that have to be followed include establishing the cause of the pain and directing treatment to this cause. This can only be achieved through a thorough history, physical examination and appropriate investigations.

The relationship of this patient's symptoms to her menstrual cycle must be established. In addition, other associated symptoms, such as vaginal discharge, infertility and deep dyspareunia need to be excluded. A physical examination to identify associated signs, such as vaginal discharge, cervical excitation tenderness and adnexal masses, is the next important step in her management.

Investigations that have to be performed include endocervical and high vaginal swabs. It is unlikely that these will provide any additional information to the diagnosis. However, for completeness, these have to be performed to exclude associated infections. The most important diagnostic investigation is a laparoscopy. This will exclude endometriosis and chronic pelvic inflammatory disease. It is unlikely to exclude irritable bowel syndrome and other non-gynaecological causes of the chronic pelvic pain.

The treatment of choice will depend on the identified cause. If it is endometriosis, treatment options will include the combined oral contraceptive pill, progestogen-only, danazol or gonadotrophin-releasing hormone (GnRH) analogues. The most effective treatment will be either danazol or GnRH analogues. However, the complications of these drugs must be considered during counselling before treatment.

If chronic pelvic inflammatory disease is the diagnosis, treatment has to be tailored to this. There are no randomized controlled trials of the efficacy of antibiotics in the treatment of chronic pelvic inflammatory disease but in this patient an antibiotic covering *Chlamydia trachomatis*, Gram-negative and Gram-positive organisms, and anaerobes may be offered. Subsequent supportive treatment will be tailored to the patient's symptoms. These will include psychotherapy, surgery and steroids.

Surgical options include total abdominal hysterectomy and bilateral salpingoophorectomy, bilateral salpingoophorectomy alone and laparoscopic uterosacral nerve division (LUNA). In those with pelvic pain of no definite cause, a total abdominal hysterectomy will only eliminate menstrual problems, whereas oophorectomy will alleviate cyclical symptoms related to the ovarian cycle. There is need to counsel the patient about possible failings of these radical treatment options.

2. A 30-year-old woman presented with lower abdominal pain, low-grade pyrexia and a history of chronic vaginal discharge. On examination, she was found to have a lower abdominal mass, which was tender but there was no ascites. An ultrasound scan showed a multiloculated cystic mass in the pouch of Douglas but no free ascites. A CA125 was slightly raised. You suspect she has a large tubo-ovarian abscess. Critically appraise your management of the patient.

Common mistakes

- Take a history and do a physical examination
- Diagnostic laparoscopy to confirm the diagnosis
- Take a sexual history
- Investigate for infertility
- Hormone profile

A good answer will include some or all of these points

- The most likely cause of this patient's symptoms is a sexually transmitted disease (STD)
- The organism responsible must be identified
- Definitive treatment – surgery
- Antibiotics before surgery
- Adequate counselling prior to surgery
- Options at surgery: drainage of the abscess; removal of the Fallopian tubes if necessary; complete antibiotic therapy
- Appropriate counselling after surgery re: fertility and ectopic pregnancy
- Refer to genito-urinary medicine (GUM) clinic if necessary for contact-tracing
- Laparoscopic surgery

Sample answer

The cause of this patient's tubo-ovarian abscess is likely to be sexually transmitted. This may be difficult to identify unless samples can be obtained for microscopy culture and sensitivity. However, a sexual history and associated symptoms, such as vaginal discharge and dysuria, are important. Since *Chlamydia trachomatis* is the most common sexually transmitted disease (STD) associated with pelvic inflammation, attempts must be made to confirm or exclude this diagnosis. A blood sample should therefore be obtained from the patient for chlamydia antigen testing. The presence of IgG antibodies against chlamydia will not suggest recent infection, however, the presence of IgM antibodies will indicate recent infection.

The mainstay of treatment is antibiotics and surgery. In the first instance, she will be offered broad-spectrum parenteral antibiotics. These should cover Gram-negative, Gram-positive and anaerobic organisms, and *C. trachomatis*. The most popular combination will be a cephalosporin, metronidazole and a tetracycline derivative. These will be modified, depending on the sensitivity of the organisms identified from the cultures and sensitivity test.

Laparotomy is essential to drain the abscess. Although the abscess could be managed with ultrasound-guided aspiration, the best approach is laparotomy. At laparotomy, the definitive treatment will depend on the findings. The most likely scenario is a severely damaged Fallopian tube with the ovary stuck to the tube. In such cases, the best option may be to remove the Fallopian tube; swabs must also be obtained for microscopy, culture and sensitivity. After surgery, the course of antibiotics should be completed. Laparoscopic drainage of the abscess is an alternative to laparotomy. Although the morbidity associated with this procedure is lower than that after laparotomy, it requires expertise and special instruments. In addition, the risk of visceral injury may be considerable in view of the adhesions, which tend to co-exist as a result of the infection. This procedure should therefore be limited to very skilled clinicians.

An important aspect of the management is counselling after surgery. The counselling needs to emphasize the fertility problems associated with such complications. She needs to be told that pregnancy is unlikely in view of the consequences of the infection on her fertility, and that she may need *in vitro* fertilization (IVF) in future. If the cause of her infection is chlamydia or another STD, contact-tracing should be initiated and the patient referred to the genito-urinary medicine (GUM) clinic where she will be screened for other STDs and the appropriate steps taken.

3. Justify your management of a 27-year-old women presenting with chronic vaginal discharge.

Common mistakes

- Stating that she has a sexually transmitted disease (STD) and therefore focusing the rest of your essay on managing this
- Screening for human immunodeficiency virus (HIV) – this is unlikely to be applicable unless you can demonstrate that she is at risk. In contemporary practice in the UK, this is not justified. It may be the case in the near future
- History of alcohol and drug abuse – what is the relevance of this to the question
- Diagnostic laparoscopy – why? Ensure that you justify all your answer – why are you subjecting the patient to any investigation or treatment

A good answer will include some or all of these points

- Consequences – devastating /psychologically morale sapping
- History – exclude associated symptoms, for example pruritus, and predisposing factors, such as: STDs or other infections, for example threadworms; allergy – soaps, underwear, powders, etc.; drug-induced; systemic diseases; previous treatment of any discharge; contraceptives – oral contraceptive pill, intrauterine contraceptive device (IUCD); associated symptoms, such as irritation, pruritus, bloody discharge; colour of discharge; last cervical smear
- Examination: systemic; localized pelvic – vulva, vagina; colour of discharge; bimanual
- Investigations: swabs – wet film, rectal threadworms, Gram stain, *Chlamydia trachomatis* specific test
- Treatment: hygiene/remove allergen if known; specific treatment – *Trachomatis vaginalis*/bacterial vaginosis – metronidazole; other specific treatments – cryotherapy; contact-tracing if STD; reassurance – oral contraceptive pill and leucorrhoea

Sample answer

Chronic vaginal discharge is a devastating symptom and one that can also be extremely difficult to treat. In this young woman, a systematic approach to diagnose the cause of the discharge, followed by tailored therapy, is essential.

The first stage in her management is to identify other associated symptoms with the discharge. These include pruritus, superficial dyspareunia and predisposing factors of the discharge, such as sexually transmitted diseases (STDs), allergy, drug-induced or systemic diseases. The use of the contraceptive pill or an intrauterine contraceptive device (IUCD) may provide a clue to the cause of the discharge. The nature of the discharge, its colour, associated bleeding and dysuria are important. The time of the patient's last cervical smear must be ascertained.

A general examination will identify systemic diseases, which may cause chronic vaginal discharge. During a pelvic examination, swabs should be taken from the high vagina, the endocervix, urethra and rectum. Careful attention must be paid to the character of the discharge, the appearance of the vagina, tenderness in the adnexa and adnexal masses. The swabs obtained should be sent for the following investigations: *Chlamydia trachomatis*, *Neisseria gonorrhoea*, *Candida albicans* and for bacterial vaginosis. Threadworms should be excluded if there is associated pruritus. If potassium hydroxide is applied to a wet preparation from the high vaginal swab, a fishy smell or the presence of clue cells on the slide will confirm *Gardnerella vaginalis* infection.

The treatment will depend on the causes identified. Simple measures, such as hygiene, to remove possible causes and allergens should be offered if applicable. For specific infections (such as *C. albicans*, *Trachomatis vaginalis*, *G. vaginalis*, chlamydia and *N. gonorrhoea*) the most appropriate treatment should be instituted. *T. vaginalis* infection or bacterial vaginosis should be treated with metronidazole, Chlamydia with a tetracycline derivative or azithromycin and *N. gonorrhoea* with a cephalosporin. For some patients, there may be an obvious cervical erosion which is responsible for the discharge. This may be treated with cryo-cautery or diathermy. Where the identified cause is an STD, attempts must be made to trace all contacts and offer appropriate treatment. The patient should be screened for other STDs. The genito-urinary medicine (GUM) clinic should be involved in this aspect of her treatment.

In most cases, no cause for the discharge will be identified. It could, therefore, be explained as leucorrhoea, which is normal in some patients. In such cases, adequate counselling and education may be adequate. The use of betadine douches has been shown to be helpful in some women. Simple sanitation methods, such as changing of pads and avoiding the use of tampons, may also be all that is required.

4. Critically appraise the measures you will undertake to reduce the prevalence of *Chlamydia trachomatis* genital infections.

Common mistakes

- Discussing treatment for *Chlamydia trachomatis* in general
- Listing the various methods of diagnosing *C. trachomatis*
- Being too general
- Failing to critically appraise

A good answer will include some or all of these points

- *C. trachomatis* infection is one of the most common sexually transmitted diseases (STDs) and causes tubal infertility and chronic pelvic inflammatory disease
- Reducing the prevalence must start with identifying the at-risk groups
- At-risk groups: those aged <25 years having at least two partners within 12 months; women from low socio-economic class who smoke and are single; infections with other STDs; those undergoing termination of pregnancy; partners of those who have been infected; previous or ectopic pregnancy
- Reduction of prevalence: reduce the infection rate – public health education. Mass media, classroom, schools and television. Expensive and no guarantee that it will reach target population; universal screening or targeted screening? Advantages and disadvantages? screening all at-risk groups when the opportunity arises – termination of pregnancy, family planning – especially emergency contraception. Insertion of intra-uterine contraceptive device (IUCD); prophylactic antibiotics to all at-risk groups? Dangers – expensive but increases the risk of causing a drug-resistant strains
- Limitation of spread from infected patients: appropriate treatment; contact-tracing; leaflets; infertility clinics/ectopic pregnancy; diagnosis procedure – how reliable?

Sample answer

Chlamydia trachomatis infection is a common sexually transmitted disease (STD) in the UK. It is the most common cause of tubal infertility and pelvic inflammatory disease. To reduce the prevalence of this infection, at-risk groups must be identified and targeted measures taken to reduce the risk of transmission. In addition, once the diagnosis is made, institution of the most appropriate treatment and contact tracing will help to minimize the prevalence of the condition. There must be a concerted effort by general practitioners (GPs), other clinicians and the media to educate the public at large, and those at risk in particular, of the risks, early symptoms and sequelae of this infection and the benefits of barrier contraception. This could be offered through the mass media, the classrooms and schools. Such programmes may be directed specifically at at-risk groups or at the general population. They are expensive and may be seen as encouraging promiscuity if not managed properly.

Those most at risk are women under the age of 25, who have had more than two sexual partners, those from a low socio-economic class, those with other STDs, those undergoing termination of pregnancy or those who have had an ectopic pregnancy. In these at-risk groups, screening for the infection is important. It will identify those with the infection, offer treatment and also allow for contact-tracing and treatment. Targeting this at-risk population is thought to be more cost-effective than universal screening, but it will invariably result in some cases being missed within the low-risk population.

The second approach, therefore, is to screen all sexually active women for *C. trachomatis*. This approach ensures that all those at risk are screened. However, such universal screening is not cost-effective, especially in areas where the population is low risk. A disadvantage of such targeted screening is that of labelling a defined population as high-risk. This may discourage others from seeking services that will immediately label them as high-risk.

Instead of targeted screening, prophylaxis has been proposed as a means of reducing the prevalence of *C. trachomatis* in the high-risk population. In this approach, antibiotics sensitive to *C. trachomatis* are offered to all women undergoing termination of pregnancy, or having an intrauterine contraceptive device (IUCD) inserted. Such an approach will ensure that all cases are treated but the major disadvantage is that, without screening, those who are chlamydia-positive will not be identified and therefore their sexual contacts will also not be identified and treated. Such an approach runs the risk of minimizing the infection temporarily, but repeated infection and its consequences are more likely.

Once the infection has been identified, institution of appropriate treatment not only to the patient but to her contact(s) will significantly minimize the prevalence of this infection. Education of those with the infection and/or those at risk about the symptoms and the consequences of the disease is important in prevention. It is essential that screening should employ modern and reliable techniques. Such screening should be available in various clinics, such as infertility units, and other areas attended by at-risk groups. Where patients present with features suggestive of pelvic inflammatory disease, chlamydia screening should be considered. Such an approach will reduce the prevalence, and therefore the spread, of the disease.

11

Menopause

1. A 45-year old business executive has been suffering from menopausal symptoms. She wishes to go on hormone replacement therapy (HRT). How will you counsel her?

2. Criticize the use of pipelle/vibra aspirators in outpatient endometrial biopsy in the evaluation of postmenopausal women with irregular vaginal bleeding.

3. Critically appraise your management of a 72-year-old patient presenting with post-menopausal bleeding.

4. The use of outpatient hysteroscopy has negated the role of ultrasound in the management of women with postmenopausal bleeding. Do you agree with this statement?

1. A 45-year old business executive has been suffering from menopausal symptoms. She wishes to go on hormone replacement therapy (HRT). How will you counsel her?

Common mistakes

- Discussion of hormone replacement therapy (HRT) in general
- Advantages
- Types
- How to administer
- Complications
- Contraindications
- Cardiovascular disease is the most common cause of female mortality
- Telling patient about low and high density lipoproteins and apolipoprotein a
- Check follicle stimulating hormone (FSH) and FSH and luteinizing hormone (LH)
- Determine her gravidity and parity – why?

A good answer will include some or all of these points

- HRT has significant advantages
- What specific symptoms does she have?
- Contraindications – does she have any? – relative or absolute? Identifying some may require a physical examination and screening, for example blood pressure
- Is the uterus intact or not
- Is she still menstruating or not
- These will help determine the type of HRT and, therefore, the route of administration (contraception is important).
- Side-effects – breast cancer (after 10 years' use)
- Need for monitoring
- Check contraceptive needs and tailor HRT accordingly
- Selective oestrogen receptor modulators (SERMS)

Sample answer

Hormone replacement therapy (HRT) has several advantages but before commencing any patient on HRT it must first be ascertained that she does requires HRT and that there are no contraindications. Counselling must therefore aim to identify all these factors and also offer her the most appropriate options available.

First, it must be established whether the patient does need HRT. This will be determined by her symptoms. In addition, it is important to establish whether or not she has had a hysterectomy as this will influence the type of HRT offered. If she has not had a hysterectomy, it is important to know whether or not she is still menstruating. Having established her symptoms and physical status, the next step is to ensure that she does not have any contraindications to HRT.

Contraindications are absolute and relative. Absolute contraindications include active cancer of the uterus and breast, active venous thrombo-embolism (VTE) and active liver disease. Relative contraindications include previous VTE, previous breast cancer and hypertension.

The choice of HRT for this patient also depends on her needs. If she has an intact uterus and no absolute contraindications, she will need combined HRT to minimize the risk of endometrial cancer. If she has had a hysterectomy, she could have oestrogens only. These may be administered in the form of tablets, patches or implants. The disadvantage of implants is mainly that of tachyphylaxis. Before commencing HRT the patient should be examined to ensure that her blood pressure is normal and that there are no breast masses. Counselling about the side-effects of HRT, such as breast tenderness, premenstrual symptoms, depression, weight gain and breast cancer after more than 10 years' therapy, must also be offered. The ultimate choice of HRT will depend on any contraindications. Lastly, the patient's contraceptive needs must be considered before HRT is offered. It may be that she still requires contraception, in which case this may be combined with HRT. Where there are contraindications, other forms of HRT, such as SERMS, progestogens and phyto-oestrognes should be considered.

2. Criticize the use of pipelle/vibra aspirators in outpatient endometrial biopsy in the evaluation of postmenopausal women with irregular vaginal bleeding.

Common mistakes

- Discussing the use of pipelle or vibra aspirators – indications and how to apply them
- Describing the management of postmenopausal bleeding – ultrasound scan, etc.
- Listing the advantages of hysteroscopy and the management of postmenopausal bleeding
- Detailing the causes of postmenopausal bleeding

A good answer will include some or all of these points

- Use of these devices to investigate postmenopausal bleeding
- Advantages of these procedures
- Major drawbacks
- Need to combined them with hysteroscopy and ultrasound

Sample answer

Postmenopausal bleeding is a common gynaecological problem. The aim of investigating patients presenting with this complaint is to exclude endometrial carcinoma. This is best achieved from histological examination. An endometrial sample is therefore essential for this examination. This can be obtained either as an outpatient procedure with or without local analgesia or under general anaesthesia (GA). The availability of the pipelle or vibra aspirators has been responsible for the ease with which these biopsies can be taken on an outpatient basis. They do, however, have disadvantages, which must be recognized when using them in clinical practice.

In most cases, there is no need for anaesthesia and the devices are commonly used during routine pelvic examination at gynaecological consultations. They are also commonly used with outpatient hysteroscopy for biopsies. The advantages of these devices are therefore the avoidance of GA and cervical dilatation (which may be very painful). Tissues are obtained after consultation and patients do not have to go on long waiting lists for hysteroscopy, where this is offered on outpatient basis. Despite these advantages, application of the devices is blind. Directed biopsies are therefore not obtained. There is a tendency for tissues to be taken mainly from the body of the uterus and pathology limited to the cornual regions of the uterus may thus be missed. The accuracy of these devices in identifying endometrial cancer is thought to be approximately 75–80 per cent. Another disadvantage is their inability to exclude other causes of postmenopausal bleeding, such as endometrial polyps. Failure to obtain tissue does not reliably exclude all the cause of postmenopausal bleeding. Combining the use of these devices with ultrasound or saline sonography is thought to be more effective. In women with fibrotic lesions, such as those taking tamoxifen, the use of these devices to sample the endometrium is ineffective.

The success of obtaining endometrial biopsies depends of the ability of these devices to pass through the cervix. In patients with a very stenosed cervix this may be difficult and persisting with the attempt to pass them may be associated with vaso-vagal attacks. In addition, there is the added complication of infections and perforation of the uterus. Ideally, therefore, these devices should be used in conjunction with ultrasound or outpatient hysteroscopy to allow for a more effective means of diagnosis. The use of ultrasound and or hysteroscopy will exclude other causes of postmenopausal bleeding and will direct the clinician to a specific focus from which the endometrial biopsy should be taken. In the absence of a thickened endometrium, the use of these devices may not be necessary.

Overall, these devices are now routinely available in all gynaecological outpatient departments in the UK. Their use will therefore continue. Clinicians must be aware of their shortfalls and recognize that where they have produced tissue which excludes a malignancy, and yet the symptoms persist, further investigations must be performed. As long as these drawbacks are appreciated, the use of the pipelle or the vibra aspirator to investigate postmenopausal women with abnormal bleeding will remain an acceptable practice.

3. Critically appraise your management of a 72-year-old patient presenting with post-menopausal bleeding.

Common mistakes

- Take a history and perform a physical examination – not being critical
- Listing all the steps in the management of the patient
- Assuming that she has endometrial cancer and discussing the management of endometrial cancer
- Discussing the uses of endometrial biopsies and outpatient hysteroscopy

A good answer will include some or all of these points

- The primary aim is to exclude endometrial cancer and then to identify other causes, which could be treated
- Discuss the importance of a good history; elaborate on the limitations of this
- Physical examination – benefits and limitations
- Investigations: outpatient endometrial biopsy – pipelle/vibra aspirator; hysteroscopy; ultrasound scan
- Treatment – no need to go into the details of the pathologies that could cause post-menopausal bleeding

Sample answer

In this 72-year-old patient, the most important diagnosis that must be excluded is endometrial cancer. An appropriate method of excluding this is histological examination of a biopsy of the endometrium. Prior to doing this, however, it is necessary to identify possible factors for endometrial cancer or other causes of her postmenopausal bleeding. If she is nulliparous or of low parity, suffers from diabetes mellitus or hypertension, or has been on oestrogen-only hormone replacement therapy (HRT), her risk of endometrial cancer is certainly greater. In addition, a history of polycystic ovary syndrome or infertility associated with irregular periods during her reproductive years may also increase the risks of her developing endometrial cancer. If she is taking tamoxifen for breast cancer, the risk of endometrial malignancy is considerably higher. Although a good history may shed some light on the possible causes of the postmenopausal bleeing, it should be recognized that in most cases, there are no risk factors in the patient's history. However, there may be other factors, such as medical disorders and drug therapy, which may influence the type of treatment that the patient may receive.

Following the history, a physical examination has to be performed. The most important part of this examination will be the abdomen and the pelvis. However, other systemic features, such as hypertension, cardiac and respiratory signs, must be excluded. The presence of all these may influence treatment, for example the patient's suitability for surgery. Essential findings on abdominal examination will include an abdomino-pelvic mass. The presence of such a mass may suggest endometrial carcinoma, although classically, patients with endometrial carcinoma do not have an abdominally palpable uterus. However, the presence of ovarian masses may suggest the possibility of a functioning ovarian tumour. A pelvic examination may identify atrophic vaginitis and cervicitis, and a bulky uterus or adnexal masses. In most women with postmenopausal bleeding, these examinations are negative but do not exclude pathology. So, although a pelvic examination may identify possible causes of postmenopausal bleeding, it has significant limitations, as endometrial pathology cannot be excluded by these means.

To exclude endometrial pathology, therefore, an endometrial biopsy is needed. This can be done at the time of the pelvic examination in the clinic by use of a pipelle or a vibra aspirator. However, the success of this procedure will depend on the ease with which these instruments can be inserted through the cervix. In addition, a negative biopsy does not completely exclude pathology as it does not identify polyps and is only reliable in approximately 70–80 per cent of cases. Hysteroscopy performed at the time of the biopsy may improve the accuracy of this biopsy. It will also diagnose polyps. The only disadvantage is that this is unlikely to be performed at the outpatient visit. There are patients who may not tolerate these rather invasive procedures properly, hence they may have to be abandoned. An alternative to an endometrial biopsy or hysteroscopy is an ultrasound scan to assess endometrial thickness. This will identify the thickness of the endometrium and adnexal pathology, which the other diagnostic methods will not do. If the endometrium is more than 4 mm thick, the patient could be offered a biopsy.

Having made the diagnosis, treatment will depend on the cause. If the patient has atrophic vaginitis or cervicitis, oestrogen creams administered sparingly will be adequate. It must be recognized that their prolonged administration can led to endometrial cancer. If the patient has polyps, these could be removed at hysteroscopy. For endometrial cancer, the treatment of choice will be an abdominal hysterectomy, bilateral salpingoophorectomy and node dissection, if appropriate. Adjuvant chemotherapy or radiotherapy will be offered if indicated. For an oestrogen-dependent pathology the most appropriate treatment will be total abdominal hysterectomy and bilateral salpingoophorectomy and omemtectomy, followed by adjuvant chemotherapy if necessary.

4. The use of outpatient hysteroscopy has negated the role of ultrasound in the management of women with postmenopausal bleeding. Do you agree with this statement?

Common mistakes

- The management of postmenopausal bleeding
- Day case versus inpatient hysteroscopy
- Avoid stating that hysteroscopy provides a histological diagnosis
- Both procedures are diagnostic so do not state that one is and the other is not. Both procedures are also used for screening
- The question is not asking which is used first – hysteroscopy or ultrasound

A good answer will include some or all of these points

- There is no need to answer yes or no
- Both procedures are diagnostic
- Outpatient hysteroscopy: what at the benefits? – allows visualization of the uterine cavity – directed biopsies may be taken at the same time – polyps may be removed, therefore may be therapeutic; disadvantages – training – equipment – may not be feasible in all patients – stenosed cervix – may be associated with vaso-vagal attacks – risk of fluid overload – may not be acceptable to some patients – risks of perforation and infections
- Ultrasound: equipment; training; assess adnexal and endometrial cavity; not therapeutic; need to perform a separate biopsy to make a diagnosis; transvaginal scan may be more acceptable; evidence that it is effective in screening for postmenopausal bleeding; does not negate the need for hysteroscopy
- Conclusion – both procedures are complementary and not mutually exclusive. There is a role for both in the management of postmenopausal bleeding

Sample answer

These two procedures are important in the management of irregular vaginal bleeding, especially in postmenopausal women. In general, they complement each other.

Outpatient hysteroscopy allows visualization of the endometrium. Directed biopsies may, therefore, be taken from well-defined sites. Endometrial polyps cannot only be diagnosed but may also be removed during the hysteroscopy. The disadvantages of outpatient hysteroscopy include the need to train staff to perform the procedure and the cost of setting up units for this procedure. It may not be possible in some patients because of cervical stenosis. Vaso-vagal attacks may result from grasping the cervix in some cases and, where fluid is the distension medium, overload with resulting circulatory failure may occur, especially in those who are frail and who have cardiovascular compromise. Some patients may find it intrusive and there is always the risk of perforation of the uterus. Although uncommon, infections may occur as a complication of this procedure. In addition to these disadvantages, outpatient hysteroscopy does not allow the diagnosis of adnexal pathologies, which may be responsible for the post-menopausal bleeding (for example, oestrogen-producing ovarian tumours).

Ultrasound, on the other hand, has the advantage of identifying adnexal pathologies and uterine pathologies, such as polyps. As endometrial thickness needs to be more than 4–5 mm for an endometrial biopsy to be performed, many women are spared the discomfort of unnecessary attempts at biopsy. Ultrasound scan, especially by the transabdominal route, may be more acceptable to some patients than hysteroscopy. There are, however, several disadvantages to the use of ultrasound in the management of patients with postmenopausal bleeding. Ultrasound, unlike hysteroscopy, does not offer an opportunity to treat some of the causes of postmenopausal bleeding. It must be accompanied by endometrial biopsy to be valuable in the diagnosis of endometrial carcinoma. The transabdominal approach requires a full bladder, which some patients may find unacceptable. The transvaginal approach, on the other hand, though better at defining endometrial and pelvic pathology is considered by some as intrusive. Ultrasound machines are expensive and skilled manpower is necessary for the procedure to be reliable. Even in excellent hands, the reliability of this investigation depends on the individual undertaking the procedure and the route of scanning (transabdominal or transvaginal).

Outpatient hysteroscopy and endometrial biopsy, and ultrasound and endometrial biopsy, although very useful in the management of postmenopausal bleeding, are not interchangeable. Indeed, they complement each other and therefore the argument that one can negate the use of the other is unlikely to be tenable. It may be concluded that these procedures are complementary.

12

Genital prolapse and urinary incontinence

1. A very obese, hypertensive, known asthmatic woman presents with urinary incontinence. Urogynaecological investigations have confirmed that she has significant urodynamic (genuine) stress incontinence. Critically appraise the options for her management.

2. A 65-year-old woman has returned to the urogynaecology clinic with recurrent urinary incontinence four years after as successful colposuspension. Justify your subsequent management.

3. A 26-year-old woman with one child presents with genital prolapse. Critically appraise your management of this patient.

4. Evaluate your management options of a 67-year-old woman with vault prolapse.

5. Mrs AB had a colposuspension operation 12 months ago. She comes to see you again complaining of stress urinary incontinence, urgency and urge urinary incontinence. Justify the steps you will take in her management.

6. Critically appraise your management of a 57-year-old fit patient with a low compliance bladder.

1. A very obese, hypertensive, known asthmatic woman presents with urinary inconti-
    nence. Urogynaecological investigations have confirmed that she has significant
    urodynamic (genuine) stress incontinence. Critically appraise the options for her
    management.

Common mistakes

- Simply listing the diagnosis and management of urodynamic (genuine) stress incontinence – these must be related to the unique characteristics of the patient presented in
  this question
- Describing how the diagnosis of urodynamic (genuine) stress incontinence is made –
  this is unnecessary as the diagnosis has already been made
- Performing a urogynaecological investigation – same comment as above
- Concentrating on the treatment of her hypertension and asthma – these are already
  known problems, so you must assume that they are being treated. Even so, you should
  ask the appropriate specialists for advice
- Offering her surgery for genital prolapse without evidence of having diagnosed prolapse
  – making such an assumption without first confirming its presence is incorrect
- Assuming that she has mixed incontinence – she has urodynamic (genuine) stress
  incontinence and not mixed incontinence
- Treating for urinary tract infections (UTIs) only

A good answer will include some or all of these points

- This patient has significant medical problems that may affect her treatment
- Need to exclude genital prolapse co-existing with the urodynamic (genuine) stress
  incontinence
- Significant urodynamic (genuine) stress incontinence implies there is a need for some
  form of treatment rather than being conservative
- Options: physiotherapy – advantages and disadvantages; surgery – colposuspension –
  advantages and disadvantages – success rate, complications, including morbidity –
  Stamey operation – advantages and disadvantages – tension free vaginal tape (TVT) –
  advantages and disadvantages – anterior repair if prolapse – advantages and disadvantages
- Need to involve physicians and anaesthetist in her care

Sample answer

This patient has significant medical complications, which may influence the choice of treatment available to her. It is therefore important to bear this in mind when recommending
treatment options. In the first instance, urinary tract infections (UTIs) have to be excluded by

a midstream specimen of urine (MSU) if this investigation has not already been done. The presence of a UTI will be associated with symptoms of urgency and urgency incontinence, and these are more common in cases associated with genital prolapse. Treating associated infections may lead to an improvement in the symptoms. The presence of genital tact prolapse will alter the treatment that the patient may have. This can be excluded by asking for symptoms of prolapse, such as the feeling of a lump or a dragging sensation in the vagina. This will need to be confirmed by a vaginal examination which, in addition to assessing the presence and severity of the prolapse, will evaluate the mobility around the urethra – an important factor, especially if surgery is to be considered.

Following this examination, the patient's general health needs to be assessed to determine how suitable she will be for any surgical treatment. This assessment must involve a physician and an anaesthetist. The physician will assess her asthma and hypertension. If the patient is not suitable for surgery, conservative management must be the first option while her medical problems are being addressed. This will be in the form of pelvic floor exercises. Pelvic floor exercises are not very effective in the treatment of urodynamic (genuine) stress incontinence, but they may improve the severity of the condition. The success rate of pelvic floor exercises will depend on the patient's motivation. In addition, if the patient is postmenopausal, oestrogen may be offered, locally or systemically. In this hypertensive patient, oestrogens may increase the risk of endometrial carcinoma unless she has had a hysterectomy.

The next treatment option will be surgery. This could take the form of a Burch colposuspension, Stamey operation or tension free vaginal tapes (TVT). The choice will be influenced by the patient's suitability for surgery and the expertise available. The most effective surgical procedure for urodynamic (genuine) stress incontinence is either colposuspension or TVT. Colposuspension is associated with increased morbidity and, for a patient with two medical complications, morbidity may be more severe. In this situation, this will not be the treatment of choice. If the patient's medical conditions are well-controlled, this will be the surgical treatment of choice as it has the best five-year survival rate of approximately 80 per cent. Morbidity following an open colposuspension may be reduced by laparoscopic colposuspension but the success rate of this procedure is not as high as that following the open procedure. The advent of TVT, with a success rate similar to that of colposuspension and a lower morbidity, makes it a better option for this patient.

Another surgical option would be a Stamey operation. This will reduce hospital stay and, therefore, morbidity. Postoperative recovery is quicker, but the success rate is less than that of a colposuspension.

In the presence of genital prolapse, an anterior repair will be the treatment of choice if the prolapse is severe. This procedure is associated with a 60 per cent five-year cure rate for urodynamic (genuine) stress incontinence. The morbidity following an anterior repair is, however, less severe compared to that following a colposuspension. In the presence of a mild to moderate prolapse, unless the patient's medical conditions are severe, the treatment of choice will still be a colposuspension. However, where the prolapse is severe and the patient is unsuitable for surgery, a pessary may be inserted to correct the prolapse and hopefully improve the symptoms of urodynamic (genuine) stress incontinence. The success rate for this conservative approach to treatment is low, however.

2. A 65-year-old woman has returned to the urogynaecology clinic with recurrent urinary incontinence four years after as successful colposuspension. Justify your subsequent management.

Common mistakes

- Listing all the causes of urinary incontinence and detailing their treatment
- Assuming that she has recurrent urodynamic (genuine) stress incontinence
- Offering surgery for prolapse without confirming its presence
- Assuming she has already had a hysterectomy
- Failure to justify (that is, giving reasons for any step taken in her management)

A good answer will include all or some of these points

- This patient has recurrent incontinence, therefore failure of previous treatment must be recognized in her management
- There is need to obtain more information to help characterize the type of incontinence
- A physical examination is necessary: to exclude prolapse; to assess mobility around the urethra as she may require surgery
- Investigations: midstream specimen of urine (MSU); blood-glucose; frequency and volume chart; urodynamics
- Treatment – depends on the cause of the incontinence: conservative – pelvic floor exercises or physiotherapy; drugs for detrusor instability – tolterodine/detrusitol, oxybutynin; surgery – repeat colposuspension – need to be referred to urogynaecologist; TVT; collagen implants

Sample answer

This patient has recurrent urinary incontinence and her management must start with obtaining more information to help identify the type of incontinence. Following the history, an appropriate physical examination and relevant investigations must be performed. Important questions to ask include associated symptoms, such as nocturia, urgency and urge incontinence. The presence of these symptoms will suggest either an associated detrusor instability or genital prolapse. If the patient has genital prolapse, she will in addition present with symptoms such as the feeling of a lump or a dragging sensation in the vagina. The type of incontinence is also important. If it is often precipitated by conditions that raise the intra-abdominal pressure, such as coughing, sneezing, etc., it is more likely to be genuine stress incontinence. This will even be more so if there is no associated increased frequency of micturition and nocturia. The presence of dysuria will suggest an associated urinary tract infection (UTI). Other symptoms, which may not directly influence the diagnosis but may affect the results of treatment, include coughing and constipation. In the presence of these symptoms, the urinary symptoms may become worse and response to surgical treatment may not be as successful.

Following the history, a general and pelvic examination must be undertaken. This is aimed to, first, ensure that the patient is fit for any surgical therapy if that is the correct option, and second, to rule out genital prolapse. The examination therefore must exclude chest signs and abdominal masses. A pelvic examination will exclude atrophy of the genital tract, associated urethrocele, cystocele, uterine prolapse if the patient has not had a hysterectomy, and an enterocele and a rectocele. Although only a cystocele may explain her symptoms, the presence of other types of genital prolapse may alter her treatment or may require additional procedures during surgery for the incontinence. A bimanual pelvic examination will identify any pelvic masses that could not be identified on abdominal examination. It will also enable the paraurethra vagina to be assessed for mobility, a factor that is extremely important if further surgery is necessary.

Relevant investigations to be performed include a midstream specimen of urine (MSU) to exclude UTIs. This is common in women with prolapse and may make the symptoms of urinary incontinence worse. A random blood-glucose will exclude diabetes mellitus, which is not uncommon in this age group and may present with symptoms mimicking urinary incontinence.

Urodynamic investigations will confirm the type of incontinence. Before this, however, a frequency and volume chart will provide additional information on the possible causes of the patient's incontinence. It may, for example, suspect detrusor instability, a recurrent genuine stress incontinence or a combination. Rarely, the patient may have a low compliance bladder. The treatment will depend on the findings on physical examination and the results of the urodynamic investigations. In the first instance, if the investigations only demonstrate a UTI and minimal prolapse, the patient could be offered physiotherapy and a local oestrogen cream to apply sparingly. For more severe forms of incontinence (genuine/urodynamic), repeat surgery will be advisable. This must be performed by a urogynaecologist if possible. Alternatively, a sling operation may be performed. The complications should be discussed before surgery, with emphasis on the poorer success rate compared to that after a primary procedure. Surgical options include a repeat colposuspension or a tension free vaginal tape (TVT). Whatever the treatment, the patient needs to be followed up for at least five years as the recurrence rate of incontinence following repeat surgery is of the order of 60 per cent after five years.

Where the cause of the incontinence is detrusor instability, the treatment of choice consists of anticholinergic drugs, e.g. tolterodine (detrusitol or oxybutynin), or calcium channel blockers. If the idiopathic detrusor overactivity (detrusor instability) co-exists with genuine stress incontinence, surgery and medical treatment have to be offered. It may be advisable to initiate treatment for idiopathic detrusor overactivity (detrusor instability) prior to surgery, although surgery for urodynamic (genuine) stress incontinence may actually make idiopathic detrusor overactivity (detrusor instability) worse. If the diagnosis is a low compliance bladder, treatment will consist of collagen implants, bladder distension and clamp cystoplasty. The success rate of these procedures in the treatment of this type of incontinence is not good.

3. A 26-year-old woman with one child presents with genital prolapse. Critically appraise your management of this patient.

Common mistakes

- Take a history and perform a physical examination – this is too vague. You need to be more specific
- Offer vaginal hysterectomy and pelvic floor repair
- Insert a pessary to treat her prolapse
- Offer investigations by electromyography
- Colposuspension and hysterectomy

A good answer will include some or all of these points

- This is an unusual presentation in a young woman
- More information is required about associated features of the prolapse, such as urinary symptoms
- Physical examination to determine the degree of prolapse
- Ascertain the patient's wishes for future pregnancies
- Further investigations of urinary symptoms, for example midstream specimen of urine (MSU)
- Conservative management until family is complete
- Surgical management – options depend on the type of prolapse: Manchester repair; hysterectomy and repair; repair only
- Counselling about the future

Sample answer

In this young patient the difficulties arise if she has not completed her family. The fact that she has developed genital prolapse at such a young age indicates that the support of her pelvic organs is weak. However, trauma from childbirth must not be discounted. The first important step is therefore to obtain an adequate history about the onset of the prolapse and the precipitating factors. A recent traumatic delivery will be suggestive of a possible cause. It is unlikely to be the main reason for the prolapse. In addition, further questioning may reveal a history of prolapse in other members of the family. This will suggest a familial tendency. However, the absence of any precipitating factor or an affected family member does not exclude congenital weakness of the pelvic muscles. Other aggravating symptoms, such chronic cough, constipation, abdominal swelling and an at-risk occupation, must be excluded.

A thorough general examination will exclude a chest infections, hypertension and abdominal masses or ascites. During a pelvic examination, the perineum and its tone will be assessed as well as the type of prolapse (cystocele and rectocele or enterocele). These will determine to a large extent the management the patient will be offered. It is very likely that in this young woman the perineum will be demonstrated to be deficient.

Definitive management will depend on the examination findings. Management will be tailored to the patient's needs. Where her family is incomplete, surgery may have to be deferred until she has completed it. In that case, a pessary may be inserted after the pelvic examination as an interim measure. Retention of pessaries depends on a relatively intact perineum and pelvic muscle tone. If she has a defective perineum but the pelvic muscles are of a relatively good tone, a ring pessary may retained. Once the patient has completed her family, definitive corrective surgery should be offered. In some cases, she may have to complete her family early to enable corrective surgery to be offered and in the long term this may result in regret if she later felt than her family was incomplete.

Another option is to offer the patient corrective surgery in the form of a Manchester operation. The operation consists of amputation of the cervix, shortening of the transverse cervical (Mackenrodt) ligament, anterior colporrhaphy and a colpo-perineorrhaphy. Which of these components will be offered will depend on the type of prolapse. This procedure must only be undertaken after adequate counselling as its complications, such as cervical stenosis, infertility and cervical weakness (incompetence), may affect the patient's ability to have children.

The long term management of this young woman is extremely important. It is most likely that she will become symptomatic in her later years even if corrective surgery is offered now or at a later date. An important part of her management should therefore include counselling about the prognosis and chances of success after corrective surgery and physiotherapy.

4. Evaluate your management options of a 67-year-old woman with vault prolapse.

Common mistakes

- Take a history and do a physical examination – this is too vague. You need to be more precise and relate this to the patient
- Offer a vaginal hysterectomy and pelvic floor repair!!
- Offer a repair for enterocele
- Anterior and posterior repair
- Conservative surgery for urinary incontinence – you are making an assumption without explaining why

A good answer will include some or all of these points

- Exclude other associated symptoms
- Examine to rule out anterior and posterior wall prolapse
- Treatment – mainly surgical: vaginal; abdominal
- Complications of both procedure
- Success rate of both procedures
- If surgically unfit and not sexually active, colpocleisis (obliteration of the vagina)
- Treatment of addition symptoms, for example detrusor instability

Sample answer

Vault prolapse is a complication that commonly occurs after a hysterectomy. The treatment will depend on the severity of the prolapse and associated symptoms. These have to be excluded from a history and the severity of the prolapse assessed by a vaginal examination.

Obtaining a history from this patient is one of the most important steps in her management. It is essential to establish the type of hysterectomy she had and whether it was associated with any repair procedures. If this information cannot be obtained from the patient, then her previous surgical notes must be reviewed, and if these are not available, contacts have to be made with the unit where her hysterectomy was performed for this additional information.

Associated factors of the vault prolapse should be determined. These include constipation and symptoms of a cystocele, such as frequency, nocturia and urinary incontinence. Urinary incontinence, for example, must be investigated before surgery. The history should exclude symptoms of cardiorespiratory and gastro-intestinal disorders that may aggravate the prolapse. Following the history, a physical examination will be performed to define the degree of prolapse and the presence of an associated cystocele or rectocele. Mobility of the para-urethral vagina must also be assessed if the patient is to have any incontinence surgery as part of her treatment.

The investigations that will be performed will depend on the associated symptoms. In the presence of urinary symptoms, a midstream specimen of urine (MSU) must be sent for microscopy, culture and sensitivity. This test should be performed even if there are no urinary symptoms but the patient has a cystocele. It is extremely valuable as treatment of any urinary tract infections (UTIs) will not only improve the symptoms of frequency, nocturia and urgency but will reduce operative and postoperative morbidity. The treatment of UTIs with antibiotics to which the responsible organism is sensitive is inexpensive and does not require hospitalization. In the presence of urinary incontinence, the most important investigation that will be performed on the patient will be a urodynamic assessment. This test is precise and available in most units. Uroflometry will identify the type of incontinence to which subsequent management will be tailored.

Once a complete assessment has been made, the patient will fall into one of several categories: no associated prolapse; associated with no urinary incontinence; associated prolapse with urinary symptoms with or without a prolapse of the walls of the vagina. Where there is no associated prolapse or symptoms of incontinence, treatment is either vaginal or abdominal. The vaginal treatment of choice is a simple repair or a sacrospinous fixation. The latter is not easy to perform. It may be associated with deviations of the vagina, haemorrhage from pudendal artery injury, pudendal nerve injury, stress incontinence and an enterocele. In experienced hands the success rate is good and, unlike the repair, it does not compromise the size of the vagina. A simple repair procedure involves isolation, excision and closure of the hernia sac at the vault and then closure of the vagina after excising the redundant part. Any associated cystocele and or rectocele may then be corrected by either an anterior and or posterior repair, respectively. The procedure has poor success rate and, additionally, may result in a considerable shortening of the vagina.

The next operation of choice is a sacrocolpopexy. This is an abdominal operation in which the vault of the vagina is anchored to the anterior longitudinal ligament of the first sacral vertebra with a non-absorbable mesh. This has the advantage of correcting a cystocele, a rectocele and the vault prolapse. It is, however, associated with a high incidence of urodynamic (genuine) stress incontinence and backache. The incidence of urinary incontinence following this procedure is approximately 10–30 per cent. Appropriate counselling must therefore be offered before surgery.

In the presence of idiopathic detrusor overactivity (detrusor instability), treatment will include anticholinergic drugs, but this must be offered as additional treatment as the patient's main symptom is prolapse. If she is surgically unfit, a pessary may be inserted, but the success of this conservative approach is poor. When intercourse is not intended the vagina can be obliterated (colpocleisis) by purse-string sutures. Unfortunately, this procedure is also associated with a recurrence.

5. Mrs AB had a colposuspension operation 12 months ago. She comes to see you again complaining of stress urinary incontinence, urgency and urge urinary incontinence. Justify the steps you will take in her management.

Common mistakes

- Candidates must resist discussing the following: why did the operation fail? She had an incorrect operation or it was poorly performed; no need to describe the operation of colposuspension; do not treat patient based on investigations performed 12 months ago; do not state that if only detrusor instability, should not have had surgery

A good answer will include some or all of these points

- Review notes, surgery and symptoms (history): are her symptoms new? any associated prolapse?
- Physical examination: mobility of the paraurethra vagina; prolapse?
- Investigations: midstream specimen of urine (MSU); frequency and volume chart; urodynamics; blood sugar
- Treatment: urinary tract infections (UTIs); idiopathic detrusor overactivity (detrusor instability) – anticholinergic agents, oestrogens, other; urodynamic (genuine) stress incontinence – pelvic floor repair, transvaginal tension free tape (TVT), colposuspension
- If both conditions, treat accordingly

Sample answer

The initial management of this patient will involve enquiring after additional relevant information. It is important to determine whether these are new symptoms or persistence of the symptoms she had before surgery. If the former is the case, surgery may have been ineffective in the first instance. If they are new symptoms, she may have developed another type of urinary incontinence or the problems may have re-occurred in a different way, for example a mixed type of incontinence. It is also possible for the patient to have been cured of stress urinary incontinence only to progressively develop symptoms of idiopathic detrusor overactivity (detrusor instability). The timing of the symptoms in relation to the previous surgery will suggest the relationship between surgery and her new symptoms. The symptoms need to be characterized. For example, associated frequency, nocturia, urgency and urge urinary incontinence will be suggestive of idiopathic detrusor overactivity (detrusor instability). However, the type of urinary incontinence can only be diagnosed with certainty from uroflometry. It is also important to exclude symptoms of genital tract prolapse, such as a feeling of a lump in the vagina and or a dragging sensation in the lower abdomen.

A physical examination would identify any signs of obstructive airway disease and masses in the abdomen, both of which may contribute to genital prolapse. During a pelvic examination, genital prolapse has to be excluded. Bimanual palpation for masses and ascertaining of the mobility of the tissues around the urethra is essential. The latter may influence the type of surgical treatment the patient may be offered.

Investigations include a midstream specimen of urine (MSU) to exclude urinary tract infections (UTIs), a frequency and volume chart which she could keep for about three to four days before attending for urodynamic investigations. This will provide additional information about how much fluid the patient is taking, but more importantly, how severe her symptoms are. The most vital investigation is uroflometry. This will not only diagnose the type of urinary incontinence but will provide some information about the likelihood of success if surgery is the treatment of choice. In some cases a random blood-glucose should be performed. This may identify patients with diabetes mellitus.

Treatment will depend on the type of incontinence and other associated factors. If the patient has urodynamic (genuine) stress incontinence, she will be referred to a urogynaecologist. In the absence of this, a repeat colposuspension will be offered provided the paraurethral vagina is relatively mobile The complications of this repeat operation must be explained to the patient. In addition, the lower success rate compared to that following primary surgery must be discussed. If the urinary incontinence is attributable to genital prolapse, this will be dealt with accordingly. Surgery for genital prolapse is often difficult if a colposuspension has been performed previously. Again, great care must be taken during surgery as it may be associated with severe complications. For a mixture of urodynamic (genuine) stress incontinence and idiopathic detrusor activity (detrusor instability), anticholinergic agents such as oxybutynin should be initiated first and surgery performed later. Where there is a large cystocele, it may be possible to perform an anterior repair alone, however, the success rate of this operation in correcting urodynamic (genuine) stress incontinence is not as high as that following colposuspension and tension free vaginal tapes (TVT). TVT is likely to be the best option for this patient if she has recurrent urodynamic (genuine) stress incontinence. It is associated with a lower morbidity and a high success rate.

6. Critically appraise your management of a 57-year-old fit patient with a low compliance bladder.

Common mistakes

- Assume that she has urodynamic (genuine) stress incontinence or idiopathic detrusor activity (detrusor instability)
- Perform a urodynamic investigation to confirm the diagnosis
- Keep a frequency and volume chart
- Examine to exclude genital prolapse
- Suggest cause for this complication

A good answer will include some or all of these points

- Recognize that this is a clinically difficult condition to treat
- The diagnosis has already been made
- Treatment options: physiotherapy – bladder distension – incontinence pads and counselling by an incontinence advisor/nurse; collagen implants; artificial sphincter; clamp procedure (vesico-caecoplasty); urinary diversion

Sample answer

The diagnosis of a low compliance bladder can only be made after urodynamic investigations. It will, therefore, be assumed in this case that the patient has already had them. A low compliance bladder is one of the most difficult urogynaecological problems to treat. This patient is likely to have presented with symptoms of urinary incontinence, frequency and nocturia. In this condition, the bladder capacity is reduced and during filling the intravesical pressure rises steadily. Following the diagnosis, neurological causes must be excluded. In addition, the patient must be screened for diabetes mellitus. Some patients with a degenerative motor disease may present for the first time with this condition. It is therefore advisable to screen the patient for this.

Treatment has to aim to increase the uteri-vesical junction pressure in order to overcome the intravesical pressure. Therapeutic options for this patient will start with physiotherapy. Unfortunately, this is not often successful and it may only be temporary whilst definitive surgery is arranged. Before surgery, she needs to have a cystoscopy to exclude interstitial cystitis. At the same procedure, a bladder distension should be performed. This procedure has a poor success rate, but some patients find it beneficial. Since she is fit, it should not be the treatment of choice. It may be part of a temporary treatment, which may also include incontinence pads and counselling from an incontinence nurse advisor.

The definitive treatment is surgery. Different surgical procedures have been suggested for this condition. The first and easiest to perform is insertion of collagen implant at the urethra-vesical junction. This will cause fibrosis and therefore improve the urethra-vesical junction resistance against a rise in intravesical pressure. The implants are available in mainly urogynaecological units. Indeed, this patient is best managed in such a unit. The advantages of this include ease with which implants are inserted, fewer complications and the option of offering further surgery if necessary.

For a more effective treatment, an artificial sphincter will be surgically created around the urethro-vesical junction. Such a device may have the controls inserted under the patient's abdomen in a position where she can control them whenever she feels like voiding. This artificial mechanism is effective if tolerated by the patient. However, there is the risk of infection or the device malfunctioning. If this happens with a full bladder, it may become exceptionally uncomfortable to the patient. The other disadvantage is that these devices are not readily available. They have to be inserted by very skilled individuals and the day-to-day management of complications within the patient's environment may be difficult if these experts are unavailable.

The third surgical option is a clamp operation. In this type of surgery, an artificial bladder is created with a portion of the patient's bowel. This is a very specialised surgical procedure, which also has severe complications. It is offered mainly by urologists and therefore the patient will have to be referred to one. The last resort will be diversion of urine. Again, this is a urological procedure in which the ureter or urethra is diverted into the colon. This can either be achieved through an ileal conduit or the ureters could be brought out through the abdomen and into an ileostomy. Whatever the case, this type of treatment is less likely to be acceptable to the patient.

13

Cervical malignancy

1. The introduction of universal screening for cervical cancer has failed to drastically reduce the incidence of cervical cancer. Justify this statement.

2. All women with abnormal cervical smears should be referred for colposcopy. Debate this statement.

3. A 25-year-old nulliparous woman has been referred for colposcopy on account of a severe dyskaryotic smear. Evaluate your management options.

4. Justify your management of a 25-year-old woman with invasive carcinoma of the cervix.

5. What steps will you take to minimize the side-effects of radiotherapy in a 26-year-old woman with carcinoma of the cervix?

1. The introduction of universal screening for cervical cancer has failed to drastically reduce the incidence of cervical cancer. Justify this statement.

Common mistakes

- Discussing the aetiology of cervical cancer
- Detailing the screening programme and how to take a cervical smear
- Emphasizing the success of the screening programme in the reduction of mortality from cervical cancer

A good answer will include some or all of these points

- The objective of screening – to reduce incidence and mortality from disease
- Brief introduction of the ideal criteria (WHO, 1968) for a screening programme
- Vital elements of a successful programme: wide coverage of population at risk
- Effective action when cytological abnormality is discovered
- Objective can only be achieved therefore by identifying premalignant conditions and treating them (studies indicate progression to cervical cancer despite treatment of CIN III – McIndoe *et al.* (1984) – 36 per cent after 20 years' follow-up. Campion *et al.* (1986) – 26 per cent of CIN I progress to CIN II within two years)
- False negative rates vary from 2.4 per cent to 26 per cent
- Sensitivity – 0.52 and specificity 0.94 (Kesic *et al.*, 1993) – low sensitivity and high specificity
- Imprecision of cervical cytological – 50 per cent of women with CIN II–III or invasive disease on cytology only have mild dyskaryosis (Flannelly *et al.*, 1994)
- Mild dyskaryotic smears – annual incidence of cervical cancer 208 per 100,000 compared to nine per 100,000 in UK women of similar age (Soutter and Fletcher, 1994)
- At-risk population aged 25–35 years – highest risk group for abnormal smears (CIN II–III)
- Cytological screening has no effect on the incidence of adenocarcinoma of the cervix (Nieminen *et al.*, 1995)
- Satisfactory sampling must include the squamocolumnar junction, cytologist must scan slides carefully to identify one of a small number of abnormal cells. Process is laborious and tiring with considerable scope for operator error
- Need to educate population being screened of the benefits of the programme

Sample answer

Cancer of the cervix is the second most common gynaecological cancer in the UK. Despite the introduction of screening, the incidence has not fallen drastically, although mortality from the disease has been falling. Several factors are responsible for this disparate position.

An ideal screening programme for any condition is applicable if the condition is sufficiently common in the target population for the number of cases identified and treated as a result of the screening to be significant, the condition has a well-defined latent period, a relatively slow progression from onset and a well-understood natural history; there is a suitable test available for the condition, the screening test is reliable, sensitive and specific; there is a effective treatment for the condition and the detection of the condition substantially improves the prognosis. In addition, the screening test itself should not be harmful and the cost must be justified (Wilson and Jungner, 1968; Davis *et al.*, 2001).

Within the context of the screening programme for cervical cancer certain important issues arise, which may account for the failure of the programme to drastically reduce the incidence of the condition. The first issue is availability of screening to the population at-risk. Although there are incentives for general practitioners (GPs) to screen all at-risk age groups (20–65 years), call/recall tends to concentrate on those willing to be screened. Failure to screen the entire population at risk, especially the highest age group (25–35-year-olds) is certainly one reason for the failure of the programme.

Although a premalignant state of carcinoma of the cervix is well-recognized, the treatment of this does not completely prevent the subsequent development of carcinoma. For example, McIndoe *et al.* (1984), in a 20-year follow-up of women treated for CIN-III, reported that 36 per cent developed cervical cancer. Screening for, and treating, the premalignant condition does not therefore entirely prevent the subsequent development of the disease. In addition, progression of CIN I to CIN III within two years has been reported in up to 26 per cent of cases (Campion *et al.*, 1986), yet the interval of screening recommended by the programme is three to five years. Additionally, screening has been shown to have no effect on the incidence of adenocarcinoma of the cervix (Niemeinen *et al.*, 1995).

Where screening is undertaken, many potential problems remain. Cervical cytology, for example, is recognized to be imprecise. It has been shown that as many as 50 per cent of woman reported as having CIN II–III or invasive disease have mild dyskaryosis (Flamelly, 1994). Even when an abnormality has been identified, there is no agreed protocol for treatment. For example, whereas mild dyskaryosis may be observed and a follow-up smear repeated in some centres, others will refer the woman for colposcopy. Unless there is an agreed protocol for managing these premalignant conditions, the success of the screening programme will vary from region to region. Screening may therefore do more harm than good in some women as it may frighten some of them away from the programme.

The collection of the sample for cytology is imprecise in some cases. A good smear must contain cells from the squamocolumnar junction. Often, this is not the case. In addition, reading the smear is laborious and time-consuming. The combined effect is a false negative rate between 2.5 per cent and 26 per cent. Sensitivity and specificity of the programme are 0.52 and 0.94, respectively (Kesic *et al.*, 1993).

As far as the natural course of the disease is concerned, whilst it may take years for cancer to develop, the incidence of cervical cancer in women with mild dyskaryosis is approximately 200 per 100,000 per annum compared to 10 per 100,000 in women of similar age (Soutter and Fletcher, 1994). Failure to understand the natural course of this disease has therefore been a limiting factor for the efficacy of this screening programme.

Failure of the programme to reduce the incidence of cancer of the cervix is therefore multi-factorial. It has certainly reduced mortality from the condition. Until the entire at-risk population at risk is screened, the sensitivity of the test is improved, the time course of the disease is well mapped out, screening the premalignant forms of adenocarcinoma is possible, uniform treatment protocols of the premalignant forms are agreed upon and implemented, the incidence will remain high. Education of the at-risk population is important and efforts should be doubled to increase the uptake of the screening programme.

References

Campion MJ, McCance DJ, Cuzick J, Singer A. The progressive potential of mild cervical atypia: a prospective cytological colposcopic and virological study. *Lancet* 1986; ii: 237–240.

Davis JPL, Crombie IK, Davis HTO. Understanding screening: requirements for a successful programme. *Hospital Medicine* 2001; 62: 104–107.

Flannelly G, Anderson D, Kitchener HC et al. Management of women with mild and moderate cervical dyskaryosis. *British Medical Journal* 1994; 308: 1399–1403.

Kesic VI, Soutter WP, Sulovic V, Juznic N, Aleksic K, Ljubic A. A comparison of cytology and cervico-graphy in cervical screening. *International Journal of Gynaecological Oncology* 1993; 3: 395–398.

McIndoe WA, McLean NM Jones RW, Muflins PR. The invasive potential of carcinoma *in situ* of the cervix. *Obstetrics & Gynecology* 1984; 64: 451–458.

Nieminen P, Kallio K, Hakama M. The effect of mass screening on incidence and mortality of squamous and adenocarcinoma of cervix uteri. *Obstetrics & Gynecology* 1995; 85: 1017–1021.

Soutter P. Premalignant diseases of the lower genital tract. In: Shaw RW, Soutter PW, Stanton SL (eds). *Gynaecology* (2nd edition). London: Churchill Livingstone, 1997; 523–524.

Wilson J, Jungner F. Public Health Papers No 34: Principles and Practice of Screening for Diseases. Geneva: World Health Organization, 1968.

2. All women with abnormal cervical smears should be referred for colposcopy. Debate this statement.

Common mistakes

- Only extorting the virtues of cervical screening
- Discussing the cervical screening programme
- Details of colposcopy
- Discussing the local treatment of abnormal cervical smears

A good answer should include some or all of these points

- Cervical screening programme aimed at reducing the incidence of carcinoma of the cervix
- Screening itself does not identify cancer, but a precancerous state
- Cytology is different from histological diagnosis
- Need for further assessment of the women with abnormal smears
- Current thinking – opinion divided: colposcopy recommended mainly to women with repeated mild dyskaryosis and moderate to severe dyskaryosis; based on the premise that progression to carcinoma from mild dyskaryosis takes a long time; most mild smears will revert to normal on observation only; the burden on resources if all had colposcopy
- Progression of CIN I to CIN III within two years in up to 26 per cent of cases. Some may have been within six months
- Cervical cytology an imprecise science – 50 per cent of women with CIN II–III have mild dyskaryosis on cytology
- Conclusion – ideal for every woman with an abnormal smear to be offered colposcopy. This may frighten women with mild abnormality and put enormous strain on manpower and other resources. Ultimately, will significantly reduce the progression of mild dyskaryosis to CIN II and CIN III

Sample answer

The cervical screening programme introduced into the UK in the 1980s, aimed at reducing the incidence and mortality from cervical cancer. For this programme to be successful it must exist alongside a colposcopy service. This is primarily because although cytology may identify abnormality, it does not define the histological grade of the abnormality, the extent of the lesion and the need for further treatment. In fact, there is evidence to suggest that cervical cytology could be unreliable in up to approximately 50 per cent of cases. In one study, it was shown that approximately 50 per cent of patients with CIN II or CIN III had mild dyskaryosis on cervical cytology. The logical argument, therefore, is that all women with abnormal cervical smears should be offered colposcopy and directed biopsies to ensure that all those with inaccurate reports are identified and treated.

How realistic is this approach? Opinion is divided among the experts. Currently, the most common approach is for those with moderate to severe dyskaryosis to be offered colposcopy, directed biopsy and treatment, whereas those with mild dyskaryosis have a repeat smear six months later and only after a repeat abnormal smear are they referred for colposcopy. Such an approach has been questioned, especially in view of the imprecise nature of the cytological reports. Counter-arguments put forward are that only 26 per cent of women with CIN III progress to cancer after 20 years' follow-up. The precancerous stage of the disease is therefore very prolonged. This may not necessarily be the case as there are patients who develop cancer soon after normal smears. In such cases, either the cytology is unreliable or the disease manifests an unusually quick progression through to cancer from a precancerous state. Those who advocate colposcopy for all women with abnormal smears argue that since cytological examination of smears are not very precise the best results can only be achieved if all women with abnormal smears are further screened by colposcopy. Such an approach would place a significant burden on already stretched resources and manpower.

Another argument for not offering colposcopy to all women with abnormal smears has been that a large proportion of women with abnormal smears undergoing colposcopy do not have any significant pathology that warrants treatment. Such an approach may therefore frighten the women and could become counterproductive, a point, which the authors of an ideal screening programme ought to have considered before it was set up. It could be counter-argued that if the screening were only to be for the abnormal cases, it would no longer be a screening programme, but a selective investigation. Currently, there are some data to support colposcopy for every woman with an abnormal cervical smear. There are also data to support limiting colposcopy to those with moderate to severe dyskaryosis. In an ideal world, all these women ought to have colposcopy to reassure them and to also provide an opportunity to identify those cases where cytology is incorrect and offer more specific treatment. Although such an approach may reduce the incidence of progression to cancer, it is impracticable as rationing which governs contemporary practice is an integral part of the National Health Service.

3. A 25-year-old nulliparous girl has been referred for colposcopy on account of a severe dyskaryotic smear. Evaluate your management options.

Common mistakes

- Details of colposcopy
- Complications of colposcopy
- Relating management to pregnancy and desire for more babies
- Cone biopsy and laser as outpatient procedures

A good answer will include some or all of these points

- Reassure patient that she does not have cancer
- Explain the procedure to her – in layman's language to calm her
- Performing the colposcopy – no need for details. Use of acetic acid
- Degree of abnormality defined and treatment offered: if satisfied, colposcopy – large loop excision of the transformation zone (LLETZ); inconclusive or other features – cone biopsy under general anaesthesia (GA)
- Malignancy found – treat accordingly
- Need for follow-up after management of abnormal cervical smears

Sample answer

This young woman will no doubt be exceptionally anxious and worried about cancer when confronted with an abnormal smear. In the first instance, therefore, an explanation of the findings must be given to her. She must be reassured that cancer has not been diagnosed and that the findings suggest the need for further investigation to be able to define the abnormality accurately and offer adequate treatment. She needs to be told that abnormal smears are common and their presence is the *raison d'être* for the cervical cytology programme.

The patient must next be referred for colposcopy. This should be performed at the next available time. The importance of minimizing delay is purely on the basis of the psychological consequences of a long delay on the patient. At colposcopy, five per cent acetic acid will be applied to the cervix to identify the abnormal cells. In addition, the vascular pattern of the cervix will be studied as well as other tell-tale features of severe abnormality or frank malignancy.

At the colposcopic examination, a biopsy would be performed. For most patients, this can be performed under paracervical block by use of a local anaesthetic. Where the colposcopy is complete, that is, the colposcopist is satisfied, treatment may be offered in the form of a large loop excision of the transformation zone (LLETZ). This will usually be sufficient for the treatment of the abnormal areas on the cervix. Complications of this procedure include haemorrhage and infections. The advantages of this inexpensive procedure are that it is performed on an outpatient basis, and that there is material for histology. The histology will also determine whether the margins of the excision were well clear of the abnormal areas on the cervix. If any of the following are present, LLETZ may not be the most appropriate method of treatment: suspicion of invasion, which can usually be obvious from the vascular pattern before the application of acetic acid; any suspicion of glandular abnormality; failure to visualize the squamocolumnar junction and, in some cases, a history of previous cervical surgery or adenocarcinoma *in situ*. For any of these, the treatment of choice will be cold knife cone biopsy, which is preferably performed under general anaesthesia (GA) and on an inpatient basis because of the complications of intraoperative and postoperative haemorrhage.

Lastly, it must not be forgotten that, in some cases, colposcopy may identify frank malignancy, which needs to be confirmed on histology. In this case, the treatment of choice will be a Wertheim hysterectomy followed by adjuvant radiotherapy if indicated, although there is now evidence to suggest that radical tachelectomy and node dissection may be able to preserve her fertility.

4. Justify your management of a 25-year-old woman with invasive carcinoma of the cervix.

Common mistakes

- Assuming that the patient has a defined stage of disease, for example stage I, and discussing only the management of this stage
- Failure to discuss treatment according to stage of disease
- Other treatment options, for example cisplatin. Chemoreduction is the treatment of choice now
- Advocating colposcopy – no place once carcinoma has been diagnosed
- Considering fertility as a factor in determining treatment of choice – this is at a very early stage and should be mentioned only for early stage disease
- Listing cone biopsy as treatment determined by complete or incomplete family
- Radical surgery – what does it stand for?

A good answer will include some or all of these points

- Staging to an extent determines management
- Radiological investigations to exclude distant metastases – chest X-ray (CXR), magnetic resonance imaging (MRI), ultrasound scans of the abdomen and urinary tract Examination under anaesthesia (EUA) (parametrial, vaginal and rectal), cystoscopy
- Only 25 years old – therefore surgery is preferred if possible. Preserves ovaries and avoids acquired gynaetresia
- For stage I and IIa – offer Wertheim hysterectomy and adjuvant therapy for positive nodes
- For advanced disease (stages IIb–IIIa), radiotherapy – external and intracavitary. Node involvement, complete excision of tumour possible?
- More advanced disease – palliative care, for example exenteration
- Multidisciplinary approach – gynaecological oncologist, radiotherapist, oncologist
- Possible role of chemotherapy
- A good candidate should mention tachelorrhaphy, laparoscopic surgery and node dissection and recognize the limitations of these new techniques

Sample answer

The management of any gynaecological cancer, especially that of the cervix, is best undertaken by a gynaecological oncologist. This is to ensure that the patient is offered the best chances of survival after five years. Therefore, if this patient were diagnosed in a unit without a gynaecological oncologist, it would be ideal to refer her to a large unit where there is one. Often, the gynaecological oncologist will be working in a team consisting of an oncologist, radiotherapist and gynaecologist. This is because adjuvant therapy or primary therapy may be radiotherapy, which will be offered by the oncologist rather than the gynaecologist.

Investigations to be performed before the initiation of treatment include a full blood count (FBC) and a renal function test. These will determine the patient's haemoglobin, as she could be anaemic if the presenting symptom is bleeding. In the presence of anaemia surgery will be more risky and, if radiotherapy is the primary therapy, response to radiation will be poor. In addition, blood must be grouped and save as the patient may require blood transfusion either to correct anaemia or following haemorrhage, which is a very common complication of surgery in such patients. An abnormal renal function test may indicate more advanced disease. An ultrasound scan or magnetic resonance imaging (MRI) of the renal tract can confirm this.

In the management of this patient, an important step is to stage the cancer as this will determine the type of primary treatment to be offered. In addition, it will facilitate counselling the patient about the five-year survival rate. The staging process will include a radiological examination of the chest and the liver for secondaries and the urinary tract for obstruction to the ureters. If there are secondaries in the chest or the liver, or the ureters are obstructed, the disease is advanced and surgery will not be the best option. If these have been excluded, clinical staging must be performed. Ideally, this should be by means of an examination under anaesthesia (EUA), cystoscopy and rectal examination. During this procedure, the parametrium must be assessed to exclude involvement.

Treatment will depend on the stage of the disease. For stages I to IIa, the treatment of choice in this young woman will be a Wertheim hysterectomy. This involves an abdominal hysterectomy, removal of the parametrium and pelvic nodes and also a cuff of the vagina (usually the upper third of the vagina). Subsequent management will depend on the presence of positive nodes. If the nodes are negative, there is no need for adjuvant therapy but if they are involved, radiotherapy, usually in the form of external beam radiation is the preferred adjunctive treatment. The advantage of surgery in this woman is that is allows the ovaries to be preserved and therefore avoids the complications of premature menopause. In addition the complication of radiation gynaetresia are absent.

For advanced stage disease (stages II to stage III) the treatment is radiotherapy. This is usually a combination of external and intracavitary radiotherapy. The most commonly used source of radiotherapy is Caesium 137. This is the chosen method because complete excision of the disease is impossible. In the more advanced disease, curative treatment is not an option. The therapy in this case is palliative. This may consist of anterior exenteration, posterior exenteration or complete exenteration. This therapy is often accompanied by supportive and psychological terminal care, which may best be offered in a hospice. The complications of radiotherapy and surgery must always be borne in mind when discussing these treatment options.

Recent developments in the treatment of carcinoma of the cervix are worth considering especially in this nulliparous young woman. If she has early stage disease and wishes to have children, radical trachelorrhaphy and dissection of pelvic lymph nodes may be an acceptable treatment option. It is important to stress that although preliminary results in some centres are encouraging, long-term follow-up in a large series is not yet available. Before considering this option, therefore, the patient must be properly counselled. The place of chemotherapy as adjuvant treatment for carcinoma of the cervix is increasingly being recognized and this may be the adjuvant treatment of choice in this young woman if she has positive nodes. The advantage of this is that it bypasses the complications of radiotherapy.

Whichever option is offered, it must be remembered that the treatment of carcinoma of the cervix is multidisciplinary and adequate follow-up must be offered to the patient for about five years before she may be considered cured.

5. What steps will you take to minimize the side effects of radiotherapy in a 26-year-old woman with carcinoma of the cervix?

Common mistakes

- Not asked about the success of radiotherapy
- What are the reproductive ambitions of the patient – stating that these will influence therapy
- Discussing the indications for radiotherapy
- Detailing how radiotherapy is administered
- Not asked for the various methods of treating carcinoma of the cervix

A good answer should include some or all of these points

- What are the side-effects of radiotherapy
- Systemic and psychological – rectal, bladder, bowel, skin and vaginal
- Treating systemic side-effects: analgesics; antidiarrhoeal agents; evacuate bowel before radiotherapy; full blood count (FBC) – correct anaemia before radiotherapy – improves responsiveness to radiotherapy and general well-being of the patient
- How can they be minimized: systemic – antiemetic agents; rectal and bladder – packing/ shielding these from applicators – ovoid in the vaginal fornices; bowel – adequate dose/shielding; perineal skin – shielding; vaginal – stenosis – dilators and regular inter-course when feasible; psychological – support and education

Sample answer

Radiotherapy is a treatment option for carcinoma of the cervix, either as a primary procedure or as an adjuvant therapy. As a primary therapy, it is commonly administered as intracavitary and external radiation, whereas as adjuvant therapy it is administered as external radiation. The complications of radiotherapy are systemic, local and psychological. Before and during therapy, therefore, all attempts must be made to minimize these side-effects to alleviate the pain and distress that such therapy may cause.

In the first instance, therefore, these side-effects must be recognized in order to minimize them. Systemic side-effects include radiation cystitis and colitis, skin radiation, nausea and vomiting. Often, radiation to the bowels will result in diarrhoea, whereas that to the bladder will result in frequency and dysuria. The psychological effects of radiotherapy are difficult to specify, but most patient will be anxious, irritable, have sleepless nights and palpitations.

The first step to minimize these effects is to ensure that the patient is not anaemic before radiotherapy. This will ensure a general improvement in her health and a feeling of well-being will lead to a better psychological tolerance of radiotherapy. Urinary tract infections (UTIs) should be treated to minimize the risk of cystitis. A midstream specimen of urine (MSU) should be performed and appropriate antibiotics given before radiotherapy. Since diarrhoea is a recognized effect of radiotherapy, it is often advisable to evacuate the bowels before the treatment. In addition, nausea may be minimized by the administration of antiemetic agents – usually systemically.

During the radiotherapy itself, side-effects may be minimized by ensuring that exposure of the bladder and bowels to radiation is kept to minimum. To achieve this, the bladder and bowel are packed away from the radiation source. The ovoids, which support the applicator for the Caesium are kept well away from the bladder by gauze packs. Shielding the perineum from the radiation will also reduce the complication of radiation burns to the skin. The bladder should be catheterized during radiation to ensure that it is constantly empty.

Psychologically, the patient needs to be supported and before therapy she should be seen by a nurse oncologist who will educate her on the entire process and the possible complications. Adequate preparation will minimize the psychological complications. After radiotherapy there is an increased risk of vaginal stenosis. To minimize this, the vagina may be dilated or, once it is possible, regular sexual intercourse is resumed. It must be remembered that once a patient is diagnosed as having cancer, psychotherapy becomes an important therapeutic modality. This is even more important in one receiving radiotherapy, especially because the cancer is advanced.

14

Uterine malignancy

1. What factors affect the prognosis of endometrial carcinoma in a 45-year-old woman and how may her survival be improved?

2. Evaluate the options for the treatment of a woman with atypical endometrial hyperplasia presenting with abnormal uterine bleeding at 56 years of age.

3. Critically appraise your management of a 65-year-old woman with a diagnosis of endometrial carcinoma.

4. During surgery for endometrial carcinoma, you discover that the tumour has extended to the cervix. Justify your subsequent management of the patient.

1. What factors affect the prognosis of endometrial carcinoma in a 45-year-old woman and how may her survival be improved?

Common mistakes

- Take a history and do a physical examination of the patient
- Discussing the management of endometrial cancer
- Listing the risk factors for endometrial cancer
- Diagnosis of endometrial cancer – this will not improve survival
- There are two arms to the question so answer both – do not ignore the other

A good answer will include some or all of these points

- Common presentation – early stage
- Prognostic factors
  - Stage of the disease – myometrial invasion? Cervical extension?
  - Grade of disease – well or poorly differentiated
  - Histological type – adenocarcinoma, adenoacanthoma, adenosquamous? – serous, clear (papillary – poor prognosis)
  - Ploidy state
  - Type of surgery: total abdominal hysterectomy + bilateral salpingoophorectomy + ? Nodes (ASTEC)
  - Surgeon (oncologist)?
  - Radiotherapy – preoperatively or postoperatively
  - Chemotherapy – progestogens
- Follow-up to detect early recurrences and persistence of disease
- Endometrial cancer prognostic index. For stage I – depth of invasion, DNA ploidy and morphometric parameters, such as mean short axis

Sample answer

Carcinoma of the endometrium commonly presents early. It has the best five-year survival of all gynaecological malignancies. Despite this early presentation, however, there are many factors that may affect prognosis. These vary from the clinical stage of the disease to histological types and distant metastases. In the management of a patient with carcinoma of the endometrium these factors must be considered in assessing prognosis and also when planning management.

Early stage disease is associated with a better prognosis. This is one of the most important prognostic factors in this patient. If the carcinoma has invaded less than 50 per cent of the myometrium then it is early stage and the prognosis is considered to be good. Extension to the cervix, invasion of blood vessels and spread to other pelvic structures, the liver or chest are poor prognostic factors. Stage I disease has the best prognosis, whereas stage IV disease has the worse The five-year survival for stage I disease is 86 per cent and this falls to 16 per cent for stage IV.

Another important prognostic factor is the grade of the disease. Well-differentiated carcinomas tend to have a better prognosis than poorly differentiated ones. Histological type is also significant. Adenocarcinomas have the best prognosis followed by adenoacanthoma, whereas adenosquamous carcinomas have the worse prognosis. Other prognostic factors include the age of the patient, the ploidy and the endometrial prognostic score. The older patient has a poorer prognosis. In this case her age may, therefore, be a good prognostic factor. The ploidy status of the cancer can only be determined cytogenetically. It is also important to determine whether the patient's carcinoma is serous, clear or papillary. The last variety has the worse prognosis compared to the serous type, which has the best prognosis. For stage I disease, the endometrial prognostic index can be used to gauge prognosis. This index includes the depth of myometrial invasion, DNA ploidy and morphometric parameters, such as mean short axis.

The prognosis of the carcinoma may be improved in a variety of ways ranging from the most appropriate treatment to adjuvant therapy. The best prognosis is obtained if the patient's surgery is performed by a gynaecological oncologist. The surgery of choice is a hysterectomy and bilateral salpingoophorectomy. The role of adenectomy in the surgery for carcinoma of the endometrium is yet to be substantiated. This is currently being assessed by the ASTEC trial, the results of which are eagerly awaited.

For early stage diseases, surgery is enough for a good outcome. However, for advanced disease, adjuvant radiotherapy improves the prognosis. What is uncertain is whether pre-operative or postoperative radiotherapy has a better effect on the prognosis. For most people, postoperative radiotherapy seems to be the best option as it is only offered to those in whom histology reveals significant myometrial invasion and or invasion of blood vessels. Chemotherapy with progestogens has been used in adjuvant therapy, although their value in improving prognosis is uncertain. They are certainly of value in recurrent disease. In this patient, though, radiotherapy will be the first option if adjuvant therapy is required.

After surgery, follow-up must be meticulous to identify early recurrences and institute therapy. This will be in the form of regular clinical examinations and identification of signs of secondaries or metastasis.

2. Evaluate the options for the treatment of a woman with atypical endometrial hyperplasia presenting with abnormal uterine bleeding at 56 years of age.

Common mistakes

- Discussing the aetiological factors of endometrial carcinoma
- Discussing the management of endometrial carcinoma
- Treating endometrial hyperplasia rather than atypical hyperplasia
- Offer hysteroscopy and ultrasound to make a diagnosis
- Treatment depends on the age of the patient and her desire for more children
- Chemotherapy is the treatment of choice

A good answer will include some or all of these points

- Endometrial atypical hyperplasia is a premalignant condition – risk of progression to malignancy up to 22–88 per cent in some cases
- Co-existent carcinoma in 25–50 per cent of cases
- Expectant management, therefore, is not an option
- History to exclude exogenous oestrogens, tamoxifen and physical examination to exclude ovarian masses. Investigations to exclude possible causes of the hyperplasia
- Treatment options need to be discussed and depend on the general health of the patient, that is, how fit she is for surgery
  - Total abdominal hysterectomy + bilateral salpingoophorectomy
  - Progestogens – high doses (duration of treatment not uniformly agreed)
  - Intrauterine contraceptive device (IUCD) (progestogens only)
  - Long-term follow-up after treatment
  - Radiotherapy – disadvantage
- If not treated by surgery, need for close follow-up

Sample answer

Atypical hyperplasia of the endometrium is a premalignant condition with the risk of progression to frank malignancy reported to vary from 22 to 88 per cent (Soutter, 1998). In the management of this patient it is essential to exclude a co-existent carcinoma of the endometrium, which may be present in between 25 and 50 per cent of patients with atypical hyperplasia of the endometrium. Important causes of this diagnosis may be excluded from a history. These include unopposed exogenous oestrogen therapy as hormone replacement therapy (HRT) or tamoxifen for breast cancer. Following this, a hysteroscopy and a thorough pelvic examination should be performed. This is only necessary if the patient has not already had such investigations. An ultrasound scan will identify an ovarian tumour, which may be the source of oestrogens responsible for the atypical hyperplasia. A CA125 will be performed if there is a suspected ovarian tumour or this has been confirmed on ultrasound scan. An abnormally high CA125 will raise suspicion of ovarian malignancy.

In view of the increased risk of progression to malignancy or the high co-existence risk of carcinoma, there is no place for expectant management of this patient. The options available to this 56-year-old woman are surgery, systemic progestogens or locally administered progestogens. The best option will be a hysterectomy and bilateral salpingoophorectomy. This ensures that the endometrial pathology is removed as well as a possible source of oestrogens (the ovaries). This option provides cure and removes any occult carcinoma, which may not have been identified from an endometrial biopsy. After surgery, there will be no need to follow up the patient, and even if she had a malignancy, (which does not usually involve more than a superficial invasion of the myometrium) this treatment will be effective.

The second option is treatment with progestogens. These can be administered systemically or locally. Systemic progestogens should be given in high doses and for about three to six months. There is no generally agreed duration of therapy with systemic steroids. However, after the treatment, the patient needs to be followed up for a long time as the recurrence of atypical hyperplasia and malignancy has been reported after a long interval following such therapy. This is not the preferred option unless the patient is unsuitable for surgery or she does not wish to have surgery. If she does not wish to have systemic steroids, the levonorgestrel intrauterine contraceptive device (IUCD) may also be used. This delivers progestogens locally and avoids some of the systemic effects of progestogens. Since progestogen therapy (systemic and local) may be associated with irregular vaginal bleeding, the occurrence of this complication may be confused with persistence/recurrence of the atypical hyperplasia.

Two other options worth considering if none of the above are applicable include danazol and intrauterine radiotherapy. Danazol is an anti-oestrogen and will therefore counteract the effects of oestrogen on the endometrium. It is, however, associated with severe side-effects, which may affect compliance. Radiotherapy will induce endometrial atrophy and will be effective, but it is associated with radiation complications and may induce vaginal stenosis. The recurrence of the disease may therefore not be easily recognized. This option will be offered if the patient is surgically unfit and cannot tolerate progestogens and danazol.

Reference

Soutter WP. Premalignant disease of the lower genital tract. In Shaw RW, Soutter WP and Stanton SL (eds) *Gynaecology* (2nd edition). London: Churchill Livingstone, 1997; 521–40.

3. Critically appraise your management of a 65-year-old woman with a diagnosis of endometrial carcinoma.

Common mistakes

- Take a history and perform a physical examination
- Hysteroscopy/ultrasound to make diagnosis
- Listing the treatment options for endometrial carcinoma
- Wertheim hysterectomy
- Vaginal hysterectomy and pelvic floor repair
- Chemotherapy/radiotherapy
- Progestogens only

A good answer will include some or all of these points

- Diagnosis already made but investigations need to be performed to define extent of disease
- Clinical assessment to determine whether she is suitable for surgery
- Planned surgery with oncologist or involve gynaecological oncologist
- Total abdominal hysterectomy + bilateral salpingoophorectomy with or without lymphadenectomy
- Postoperative radiotherapy
- Preoperative radiotherapy
- Chemotherapy with progestogens
- Follow-up clinically with general practitioner (GP) or hospital?
- Conclusion

Sample answer

Endometrial carcinoma is the second most common gynaecological cancer but has the best prognosis of all genital tract malignancies. The main stay of treatment is surgery and this is more so with early stage disease. In late stage disease, surgery has to be supported by adjuvant chemotherapy or radiotherapy. The first step in the management of this 65-year-old woman, therefore, is to try to define the extent of the disease.

A clinical assessment is paramount to determine the extent of the disease but also to exclude systemic diseases (for example, chest infections) which may affect her fitness for surgery. An abdominal and pelvic examination may demonstrate masses arising from the pelvis (uterine or ovarian) and ascites, which may indicate the presence of peritoneal secondaries. Although examining the abdomen is important, it is often negative and, indeed, does not define the true extent of the disease. This is better done at surgery and, most importantly, will have to be confirmed following histological examination. Clinical examination is also unlikely to identify metastases to nodes, the liver and other distant sites unless they are symptomatic.

Ancillary investigations such as a chest X-ray (CXR) and an ultrasound scan will be more useful in identifying secondaries in the liver and the chest. These may not, however, identify lymph node secondaries but magnetic resonance imaging (MRI) may. Urea and electrolytes (U&Es) and serum creatinine are essential to assess renal function. Since endometrial carcinoma is more common in women with diabetes mellitus, urinalysis for glucose is important. A full blood count (FBC) and group and save serum will establish the patient's haemoglobin level and will also ensure that if she requires transfusion during surgery or due to anaemia caused by vaginal bleeding (a possible primary symptom of the patient), blood is easily cross-matched.

The treatment of choice is a total hysterectomy and bilateral salpingoophorectomy. Although the hysterectomy is commonly performed abdominally, there is no evidence to suggest that mortality and morbidity are greater after a vagina hysterectomy. An abdominal approach is, however, preferred if lyphadenectomy is to be performed. If her disease is considered to be early stage, a laparaoscopically assisted vaginal hysterectomy and bilateral salpingoophorectomy will be effective treatment; offering benefits of reduced morbidity, shorter hospital stay and recovery. However, if there is any suspicion of extension beyond the uterus, this approach will be unsuitable. At surgery, peritoneal washings have to be performed and lymph nodes either removed or biopsied. Management after surgery will depend on the histological diagnosis, myometrial invasion and the presence of positive nodes. Positive nodes or myometrial invasion of more than 50 per cent, or a poorly differentiated tumour, will be an indication for radiotherapy. This is preferred to preoperative radiotherapy as it is restricted to women with nodes and other poor prognostic factors. About five per cent develop complications of radiotherapy and restricting postoperative radiotherapy therefore limits the number of women exposed to these complications.

Apart from radiotherapy, chemotherapy with progestogens may be considered for advanced disease. This is often given for recurrent cases. There are no randomized controlled trials to evaluate the efficacy of progestogens in the adjuvant therapy of endometrial carcinoma, but it is the treatment of choice for recurrent disease since over 80 per cent of progestogen receptor-positive and 70 per cent of oestrogen receptor-positive tumours respond to progestogen therapy. After surgery, this patient will need to be followed up for a least five years. During this time any recurrence will be treated with progestogens or radiotherapy for vault disease. Her follow-up would be provided by her general practitioner (GP) and the gynaecologist.

4. During surgery for endometrial carcinoma, you discover that the tumour has extended to the cervix. Justify your subsequent management of the patient.

Common mistakes

- Counsel the patient and obtain consent about more extensive surgery
- Total abdominal hysterectomy and bilateral salpingoophorectomy and offer radiotherapy
- Abandon surgery and treat with radiotherapy
- Take a history and perform an examination
- Review the notes and the results of all the investigations

A good answer will include some or all of these points

- This is an unexpected finding – ought not to have been if a thorough examination had been performed before surgery
- Once carcinoma has extended to the cervix, it must be treated as cancer of the cervix
- Involve gynaecological oncologist – Wertheim hysterectomy
- Postoperative radiotherapy after counselling
- Follow-up
- Combination of radiotherapy and chemotherapy with progestogens?
- Conclusion

Sample answer

Treatment of choice for endometrial carcinoma is hysterectomy and bilateral salpingo-oophorectomy. This is usually with the assumption that the disease has not spread to the cervix or other abdominal viscera. The current recommendation is that only ovarian and cervical cancers should be treated by gynaecological oncologists. This patient may therefore be having surgery performed by a general gynaecologist. Once the disease has spread to the cervix the treatment must then become that for carcinoma of the cervix. This is because involvement of the cervix would imply possible spread to the parametrial tissues and vessels, which may have implications for the prognosis of the disease. The finding of cervical involvement suggests an inadequate assessment before surgery.

Once an extension has been identified, the gynaecological oncologist must be involved if there is one available. The subsequent management will consist of a Wertheim hysterectomy and bilateral salpingoophorectomy. The removal of the parametrium, dissection of the lypmh nodes and removal of the upper cuff of the vagina will be the minimum. This will be on the assumption that the cancer of the cervix is restricted to stages I and IIa. If it is more advanced, the surgery will be inadequate. After surgery, subsequent management will be tailored according to the histological extent of the disease (that is, positive nodes).

337

If the pelvic nodes are involved, radiotherapy in the form of external beam will be the adjuvant treatment of choice. This must be offered by a team consisting of a clinical oncologist and a gynaecological oncologist. Endometrial cancer is not as sensitive to radiotherapy as squamous carcinoma of the cervix. The prognosis for this patient after adjuvant radiotherapy will therefore not be as good as that following squamous carcinoma of the cervix. If distant metastases are suspected, chemotherapy with progestogens should be administered. This will be effective in 80 per cent of progestogen receptor-positive and 70 per cent of oestrogen receptor-positive tumours. The duration of chemotherapy is uncertain but careful follow-up is necessary to identify recurrent disease. Any recurrence in the vagina should be treated by radiotherapy.

15

Ovarian malignancy

1. What factors govern the prognosis of ovarian cancer?

2. Screening for ovarian cancer is not as effective as that for cervical cancer. Justify this statement.

3. How will you determine whether an ovarian mass in a 56-year-old woman is benign or malignant?

4. An 18-year-old girl presented with intermittent right-sided abdominal pain and a mass of rapid onset. Ultrasound scan demonstrated a unilocular large ovarian cyst measuring $10 \times 12 \times 14$ cm with no associated ascites. The serum alpha feto-protein (AFP) was described as raised. Justify your management of the patient.

1. What factors govern the prognosis of ovarian cancer?

Common mistakes

- Monitoring serum markers for ovarian cancer
- Diagnosis of ovarian cancer
- History and physical examination
- Discussing the management of ovarian cancer
- Listing the risk factors for ovarian cancer

A good answer will include some or all of these points

- Ovarian cancer – the most common cause of mortality from gynaecological cancer
- Presentation often in stage III
- Prognostic factors
- Histological type
- Treatment
- Adjuvant therapy
- General state of health of the patient
- Follow-up and institution of necessary therapy when there is recurrence

Sample answer

Ovarian cancer is the most common cause of mortality from gynaecological cancer in the UK. The overall five-year survival rate is approximately 23 per cent. This is because most present late usually in stage III. The prognosis of ovarian cancer is guided by several factors. These vary from the histological type to the treatment that the patient is offered.

The five-year survival for ovarian cancer varies with the stage of the disease. For stage I disease, the five-year survival is 60–70 per cent, whereas for stages III–IV it is 10 per cent. The fact that the overall five-year survival is only between 15 and 23 per cent suggest that most patients present with advanced disease.

The histological type and grade of the disease influence prognosis significantly. For example, in stage I disease, five-year survival in those with grades I or II disease is 90 per cent compared with lower rates for poorly differentiated diseases. This is an important factor in early stage disease. For more advanced tumours, stage is a more important prognostic factor than grade, even for well-differentiated tumours. In addition to the histological type, ploidy is an important prognostic factor. This is an important prognostic factor in early and advanced stage disease. Diploid tumours tend to have a better prognosis than aneuploid tumours in both early and advanced stage disease.

The younger patient has a better prognosis that the older woman. However, age tends to be associated with other factors. In addition, another important prognostic factor is the surgeon.

It is now well-recognized that the prognosis is better if surgery is performed by a gynaeco-logical oncologist. More important is the size of residual disease following surgery. Where residual disease is minimal, medium-term survival tends to be longer. Adjuvant therapy is a prognostic factor for ovarian cancer. If it is offered by a team consisting of a clinical oncolo-gist, a gynaecological oncologist and an oncology nurse, the prognosis tends to be better. In addition, a combination including cisplatinum has a better prognosis than one without. Very recently, the value of oncogenes in the prognosis of ovarian cancer has been assessed. Oncogenes that have been studied include epidermal growth factor receptor, insulin-like growth factor-1 receptor, *cerb-2*, *c-ras* and *c-myc*. Overexpression of one of these oncogenes, especially epidermal growth factor receptor, was considered a poor prognostic factor. In patients with borderline tumours, the most important prognostic factor is tumour ploidy.

The prognosis of ovarian cancer is affected by the various factors. Counselling and manage-ment of women with ovarian cancer must be guided by these factors.

2. Screening for ovarian cancer is not as effective as that for cervical cancer. Justify this statement.

Common mistakes

- Not asked to describe the diagnosis of ovarian cancer or cervical cancer screening
- Not asked to discuss the risk factors for the two cancers
- Avoid treating the two screening programmes in isolation
- Focusing mainly on why cancer of the ovary cannot be screened and why cancer of the cervix has been successfully screened
- Describing the treatment of ovarian cancer and carcinoma of the cervix
- Failing to justify (that is, give reasons for what you do)

A good answer will include some or all of these points

- Ovarian cancer – most common gynaecological killer
- Screening for cancer of the cervix – has reduced mortality from it. Failure to improve five-year survival for ovarian cancer is secondary to inadequate screening
- Ideal screening – sensitive, predictive of condition, inexpensive and cost-effective, applicable to the general population
- Cervix accessible, premalignant stage defined, natural history of premalignant stage
- Ovary – inaccessible, natural history (premalignant stage poorly defined)
- Screening methods – targeted – inapplicable to the general population: pelvic examination
- Ultrasound examination – cysts? What are the characteristics?
- CA25 and other tumour markers, for example melanocyte stimulating factor (MSF), ovarian cancer antigen (OCA), alpha feto-protein (AFP), beta-human chorionic gonadotrophin (βhCG) – not specific
- Doppler ultrasound – how useful?
- BRCA1 and BRCA2
- Conclusion

Sample answer

Ovarian cancer is the most common cause of mortality from gynaecological malignancy. There are about 5800–6000 new cases every year in the UK. Although carcinoma of the cervix used to be the most common gynaecological malignancy, the introduction of the cervical screening programme has significantly reduced mortality from cervical cancer, although the overall incidence of cancer of the cervix has not decreased significantly. If mortality from cervical cancer has fallen significantly due to screening, then screening from ovarian cancer should aim to reduce mortality from this dreadful disease. Unfortunately, screening for ovarian cancer has not been as successful as cervical cancer screening. Several factors are

343

responsible for this big difference. They vary from the screening methods and accessibility of the ovaries to early diagnosis and treatment of cancer.

The ovaries, by virtue of their location, are inaccessible to early diagnosis of pathology. In addition, there is no well-recognized premalignant stage of ovarian cancer. Even where a premalignant stage is known, as in borderline disease, the natural progression of this to malignancy is unknown. This is in contrast to the cervix, which is accessible to inspection and therefore screening, has a well-defined premalignant state and a well-understood natural progression from the premalignant state to frank cancer. This difference has been responsible for the development of a screening test and programme for carcinoma of the cervix. Failure to develop a screening programme and test for carcinoma of the ovary, therefore, has been a major contributor to the failure of any screening methods at reducing the mortality from this condition.

The screening methods for ovarian cancer themselves are insensitive, poorly predictive and, in most cases, inapplicable to the general population. In addition, they are not cost-effective and most are not cheap. These screening methods primarily fail to meet the World Health Organization (WHO) criteria for a screening test. Pelvic examination, for example, in post-menopausal women is inexpensive, but is very non-specific and depends on the clinician's ability to identify an adnexal mass. Even if the ovary is palpable in a postmenopausal woman, it will not suggest the presence of a premalignant state of ovarian cancer. Another important factor is how frequently this examination has to be undertaken. This difficulty is common to all screening tests for ovarian cancer.

Radiological screening has been advocated and is being offered to some women. Ultrasound of the ovaries and or Doppler scanning of the ovarian vessels have been shown to be of poor sensitivity and unpredictable, even in the high-risk population. Again, for these to be effective various characteristics of abnormality have to be defined and be universally acceptable. Unfortunately, there are difficulties defining these criteria. In a high-risk population, however, this may be useful as it will identify increased vascularity of ovaries and cysts. The use of biochemical screening has been tried and is still being offered to women at risk of ovarian cancer. The problem with this test is that most are non-specific and cannot be offered to the whole population. For example, CA125 is raised in all epithelial tumours, infections and endometriosis. However, other markers may be more specific but these (for example beta-human chorionic gonadotrophin (βHCG) and alpha feto-protein (AFP)) cannot be used as screening tools for ovarian cancer. Recently, genetic markers have been used to identify those at risk of ovarian cancer and subsequently to screen them. The most specific markers are the breast cancer antigens BRCA1 and BRCA2. To use these, however, two relatives must be known to have died of ovarian cancer or the patient must have one dead relative and one alive with ovarian cancer. Again these are non-specific in the general population. In affected families, the presence of these genes will indicate a high risk and may therefore increase the chances of identifying early cancer.

Although there is no acceptable screening test for ovarian cancer, the history of ovarian cancer provides a reliable means of identifying the at-risk population. The lifetime risk of ovarian cancer is 1.4 per cent in the UK. If one close family relative has ovarian cancer, this risk is increased to 2.5 per cent and for two close family relatives, it rises to 30–40 per cent. This is, therefore, probably the most useful method of identifying the at-risk group. However, it does not allow the diagnosis of the premalignant stage of the disease and only prophylactic oophorectomy offered to these high-risk women may reduce the incidence of ovarian cancer.

3. How will you determine whether an ovarian mass in a 56-year-old woman is benign or malignant?

Common mistakes

- Not asked about how to manage ovarian cancer
- No need to discuss frozen sections
- The role of CA125 is limited and so, too, is the role of Doppler ultrasound

A good answer will include some or all of these points

- Different methods of differentiating – presentation, physical examination and investigations and findings at surgery and histology
- Suspicion based on history and physical examination but definitive distinction made by histology
- Clinical
  - Rapid onset
  - Associated feature of malignancy – weight loss, anorexia
  - Examination – fixed, bilateral, irregular masses, ascites
- Radiology – magnetic resonance imaging (MRI), computerized tomography (CT) – nodes and nature of masses
- Doppler increased vascularity
- Surgery
  - Fixed, ruptured capsule, bilateral
  - Secondaries on the liver, omentum and para-aortic nodes
- Cytology
- Histology: haematoxylin and eosin stains of sections

Sample answer

Ovarian tumours, by virtue of their location, are not only difficult to diagnose but it may also be extremely difficult to ascertain whether they are benign or malignant. There are, however, some features which may increase the index of suspicion of malignancy. The most definitive means of distinguishing a benign from a malignant ovarian tumour is histology. This is, however, usually available in most cases only after surgery. There are some clinical features that may be useful in making this distinction. These include symptoms, signs and results of various ancillary investigations.

A malignant ovarian tumour is most likely to be rapidly growing and associated with features of malignancy, such as anorexia, dyspepsia and weight loss. If there is a longstanding history of a swelling in the abdomen and there are no tell-tale features of malignancy, this is unlikely to be malignant. Clinical features suspicious of malignancy include weight loss, secondaries in the chest, ascites, bilaterality of the tumour and fixity in the pelvis. Radiologically, there may be features of malignancy, such as secondaries in the chest and liver on X-ray or ultrasound scan, and adenopathy on magnetic resonance imaging (MRI) of the abdomen. Irregularly enlarged ovarian masses with mixed echogenicity demonstrating in-growths on the wall of the tumours on ultrasound scan and associated ascites will be suggestive of malignancy. A Doppler examination of the ovarian pedicle and ovary showing increased vascularity is suggestive of malignancy.

At the time of surgery, specific features, which may suggest malignancy include blood-stained ascites, ruptured capsule, secondaries on the liver surface and bowel; bilateral tumours which are partly solid and partly cystic and irregular in nature and fixed to the pelvis. Malignant cells in ascitic fluid sent for cytology will be suggestive of malignancy. The ultimate distinction between a benign and a malignant ovarian tumour will be from a histological examination. Such examinations are performed on haematoxylin and eosin stains. Since histological examinations are only of specific sections prepared for the examination, there is the possibility (though slim) that early disease may be missed. This distinction, therefore, does not completely guarantee the accuracy of diagnosis.

4. An 18-year-old girl presented with intermittent right-sided abdominal pain and a mass of rapid onset. Ultrasound scan demonstrated a unilocular large ovarian cyst measuring $10 \times 12 \times 14$ cm with no associated ascites. The serum alpha feto-protein (AFP) was described as raised. Justify your management of the patient.

Common mistakes

- History and physical examination
- Screen for ovarian cancer
- Measure various markers for malignancy
- Treatment will depend on age and desire for more children
- Diagnostic laparoscopy to determine extent of disease
- Obtain consent for ophorectomy and, if necessary, speak to parents at laparotomy on type of surgery

A good answer will include some or all of these points

- The most likely diagnosis is a germ cell tumour
- Management must take her age into consideration
- Adequate counselling is an important initial step
- A laparotomy is the treatment of choice
- Define the extent of the lesion
- Surgical removal of the ovarian tumour and consider the other side – frozen section?
- Follow-up – chemotherapy, subsequent management
- Conclusion

Sample answer

The most likely diagnosis in this young girl is a germ cell tumour. In view of the rapidly developing nature of her symptoms and the raised alpha feta-protein (AFP) levels, the most likely type of germ cell tumour she may have is an endodermal sinus tumour. This is the second most common germ cell tumour. The presence of pain suggests a complication, such as haemorrhage into the cyst or necrosis within the cyst. If she has not already had a chest X-ray (CXR) and computerized tomography (CT) scan of the abdomen, this must be performed. These are necessary to determine any spread to the chest, liver and para-aortic lymph nodes.

Once this is suspected, the definitive management is a laparotomy. In this young girl, appropriate counselling before surgery is extremely important. The counselling must include the diagnosis and the implications. An endodermal sinus tumour is typically unilateral, well-encapsulated and solid. However, in some cases, there may be spread to the contrateral ovary or other sites. In view of her age, it is essential to aim to preserve the other ovary and her uterus unless the disease is outside the affected ovary. She must be counselled about the possible surgical options and the possibility of adjuvant chemotherapy. This is preferred to radiotherapy as is does not affect future fertility. In this patient a vertical abdominal incision would be preferred as it offers better exposure and allows a more thorough exploration of the abdomen and also the possibility of extension if required.

If the tumour is confined to one ovary and the capsule is intact, an oophorectomy and biopsy of the omentum and para-aortic nodes, and the contralateral ovary should be performed. If the disease has extended to the contralateral ovary, a bilateral oophorectomy, omementectomy and lymphadenectomy will be the treatment of choice. In some cases, although the disease may be confined to one ovary, the capsule may appear breached by the tumour or there may be ascites. In such cases, a frozen section of the contralateral ovary must be performed and the ascitic fluid sent for urgent histology and cytology, respectively.

Subsequent management of the patient will depend on the presence of malignant cells on the contralateral ovary or the ascitic fluid. In most cases, the logistics of a frozen section are difficult. However, subsequent management needs to be influenced by the histological findings. Although in the past, patients with these tumours were treated by hysterectomy and bilateral salpingoophorectomy if the tumour involved both ovaries or the patient did not want to have children, there is now a place to consider bilateral salpingoophorectomy and preserving the uterus. This allows the patient an opportunity to have children at a later date by use of donated ova. It is important to discuss all these options before surgery. If the patient is certain about not wanting a family, a total abdominal hysterectomy and bilateral salpingoophorectomy may be the treatment of choice. However, at the age of 18, this may be a difficult decision to make and therefore consideration ought to be given to future regrets.

Follow-up management by an oncology team would depend on the histology of the biopsy from the contralateral ovary and the para-aortic nodes. Whatever the histology of the samples obtained at surgery, the patient would benefit from postoperative chemotherapy. In the past this consisted of vincristine, actinomycin D and cyclosphophamide. More contemporaneous treatment consists of cisplatin compounds given in combination with bleomycin and etoposide. In some case, radiotherapy may be offered but this tumour is not very radiosensitive. The disadvantage of radiotherapy is its effect on the remaining ovary and therefore the patient's future fertility. It was suggested in the past that once the patient had completed her family, she should subsequently be offered a hysterectomy and removal of the other ovary. However, this approach is being questioned by some oncologist who feel that adequate follow up with serial AFP and clinical symptoms is all that is required.

16

Gestational trophoblastic disease

1. Comment on the prognostic factors in a 27-year-old patient who has been diagnosed as having choriocarcinoma.

2. When will you initiate chemotherapy in a 27-year-old woman who is being followed up after a miscarriage of a complete hydatidiform mole?

3. A 28-year-old woman presented with an incomplete miscarriage, for which an evacuation was performed. Histology of the products of conception concluded that she had a hydatidiform mole. Justify your subsequent management of this patient.

1. Comment on the prognostic factors in a 27-year-old patient who has been diagnosed as having choriocarcinoma.

Common mistakes

- Discussing the genetics of molar pregnancy
- Discussing chemotherapy
- Increased risk of prophylactic chemotherapy
- Details of chemotherapy

A good answer will include some or all of these points

- Prognostic factors are important in categorizing patients into low-, medium- or high-risk groups for the purpose of chemotherapy
- The various risk factors include: age; antecedent pregnancy; interval between antecedent pregnancy and start of chemotherapy; beta-human chorionic gonadotrophin (βHCG) level at the time of initiation of chemotherapy; blood group; largest tumour; uterine tumour; site of metastases; number of metastases identified; prior chemotherapy

Sample answer

Choriocarcinoma follows a hydatidiform mole in about 50 per cent of cases. The remaining 50 per cent may follow a normal pregnancy (live or stillbirth), a miscarriage or an ectopic pregnancy. The prognosis depends on various factors. Bagshawe et al. (1976) devised a classification system based on various risk factors. This system, which categorizes patients into low-, medium- and high-risk groups, has now been adopted by the World Health Organization (WHO) to assess the stage of disease and, therefore, the type of chemotherapy appropriate for the patient.

The patient's age is an important prognostic factor. Women over the age of 39 are of a higher risk than those who are younger. The antecedent pregnancy is one of the most important prognostic risk factors. The prognosis of choriocarcinoma after a normal pregnancy is worse than that following a miscarriage and this, in turn, is worse than that after a hydatidiform mole. Since intensive monitoring is often initiated only after a molar pregnancy, progression to choriocarcinoma is most likely to be identified early. However, after a normal delivery, there is usually no follow-up and the diagnosis of choriocarcinoma is therefore unlikely to be made until after a prolonged interval when secondaries might have developed.

It follows that the shorter the interval between the antecedent pregnancy and the initiation of chemotherapy, the better the prognosis. The longer the interval, the more likely it is that secondaries will have developed, especially in the chest, brain and the liver. Traditionally, this interval has been classified as: less than four months carrying the best prognosis; four to 12

351

months an intermediate prognosis and more than 12 months the worst prognosis. The patient's blood group, as well as that of the father of the antecedent pregnancy, are also considered important prognostic factors. The exact reasons for this are uncertain. Patients with blood group B (female) and AB (male) have the worst prognosis, whereas those with blood group O (female) and O (male) have a better prognosis.

Closely related to this interval are the beta-human chorionic gonadotrophin (βHCG) levels prior to the commencement of chemotherapy. The higher the levels, the poorer the prognosis. Levels below 1000 IU/l are associated with the best prognosis and those above 100,000 IU/l with the worse prognosis. The largest tumour, including the uterine tumour, the number and sites of metastases are prognostic factors. These are invariably linked to the βHCG levels prior to the initiation of chemotherapy. Tumours measuring between three and five centimetres have the best prognosis, whereas those greater than five centimetres have a poor prognosis. Secondaries in the brain have the worst prognosis, whereas those in the gastro-intestinal tract and liver have a moderate effect on prognosis. Where the number of metastases is fewer than four, a prognostic score of one out of four is awarded to the patient; if the numbers of secondaries are between four and eight, the score is two and for more than eight secondaries, the score is four. Prior chemotherapy is an important prognostic risk factor, with single-agent chemotherapy having a better prognostic influence than two or more chemotherapeutic agents.

Each prognostic factor in the WHO scoring system is assigned a score of 0, 1, 2 or 4 and where the total score is less than four, the patient is at low risk, scores between five and seven place the patient at medium risk and those scoring more than seven in the high-risk group. This categorization allows for easy determination of the type of chemotherapy needed and for comparison of the response to therapy between various centres. For those in the low-risk category, chemotherapy is usually with a single agent at the outset. As the prognostic score increases, the chemotherapy is modified.

Reference

Bagshawe KD. Risk and prognostic factors in trophoblastic neoplasia. *Cancer*, 1963; 38: 1373–85.

2. When will you initiate chemotherapy in a 27-year-old woman who is being followed up after a miscarriage of a complete hydatidiform mole?

Common mistakes

- Discussing chemotherapy in patients with choriocarcinoma
- Details of the different types of hydatidiform mole
- Monitoring procedure – referral to tertiary centres and routine ultrasound scan of the ovaries as follow-up
- Details of the World Health Organization (WHO) categorization of patients requiring chemotherapy into various risk groups and details of the different chemotherapeutic combinations to use
- Monitoring of various therapeutic protocols

A good answer will include some or all of these points

- High level of beta-human chorionic gonadotrophin (βHCG) four weeks after evacuation of mole (serum βHCG >20,000 IU/l; urine levels >30,000 IU/l)
- Progressively increasing βHCG values at any time after evacuation
- Histological identification of choriocarcinoma at any site, or evidence of central nervous system (CNS), renal, hepatic, gastro-intestinal metastases or pulmonary metastases >2 cm in diameter or more than three in number
- Persistent uterine haemorrhage with an elevated βHCG levels stationary for two, three or more conservative weeks? Others levels elevated after eight to 10 weeks?

Sample answer

Hydatidiform moles occur in about 1.54 per 1000 pregnancies in the UK. Once diagnosed, the patient must be followed up, as the risk of progression to choriocarcinoma or invasive mole (which will require chemotherapy) is significantly greater than after a normal pregnancy or a miscarriage. During follow-up, various factors determine when to commence chemotherapy. In most cases, this is initiated before the development of choriocarcinoma. It is often very difficult, if not impossible, to differentiate between choriocarcinoma and an invasive mole as both present with persistently high beta-human chorionic gonadotrophin (βHCG) levels and symptoms of metastases. The only means of differentiating is by histology, which is often not available.

The follow-up of this patient will consist of a combination of βHCG measurements in her urine and her general clinical condition (which may be indicated by persistent disease or the development of invasive disease). During follow-up, chemotherapy will be indicated if serum βHCG levels are more than 20,000 IU/l or urine levels are more than 30,000 IU/l four weeks after the evacuation. Occasionally, the levels may not be this high but may continue to rise after the evacuation, even though the uterus is empty. This indicates persistent trophoblastic disease and is therefore an indication for chemotherapy.

If there is histological evidence of choriocarcinoma from the tissue obtained from an evacuation (a primary evacuation or a repeat evacuation), chemotherapy will be initiated irrespective of the βHCG levels. The histological distinction is made from the absence of chorionic villi in choriocarcinoma.

Although these biochemical and radiological factors are the common indications for the initiation of chemotherapy, clinical evidence of secondaries in the central nervous system (CNS), the liver, kidneys or the presence of more than three secondaries in the lungs measuring more than 2 cm are also considered an indication for chemotherapy. Other indications for chemotherapy include persistent uterine bleeding with elevated βHCG or stationary βHCG levels on at least two occasions. Just when to commence chemotherapy in such patients with persistently high or static βHCG levels remains controversial. Some units, for example, recommend chemotherapy when the levels are elevated eight to 10 weeks after evacuation, whereas others initiate chemotherapy when levels are static for two, three or more consecutive weeks after evacuation.

Irrespective of the indications for chemotherapy, this must not be treated in isolation. It is important that, for this patient, the whole clinical picture is kept in perspective. A combination of factors will certainly affect the indication for chemotherapy more than each of them singly.

3. A 28-year-old woman presented with an incomplete miscarriage, for which an evacuation was performed. Histology of the products of conception concluded that she had a hydatidiform mole. Justify your subsequent management of this patient.

Common mistakes

- The chromosomes of the parents must be determined
- Management should be by the local oncology centre
- Follow-up must be for a defined period of two years
- Offer evacuation as hydatiform moles always need evacuation!
- Bleeding may require surgery
- Quoting incorrect incidences, for example recurrence risk, and risk of progression to cancer if untreated
- Cross-match blood

A good answer will include some or all of these points

- Review the report for the type of mole – prognosis and length of follow-up will be determined by this –complete or partial mole?
- Explain the diagnosis to the patient and her partner
- Discuss need for follow-up – persistent disease, invasive disease, choriocarcinoma – all treatable
- If untreated, risk of progression to choriocarcinoma is less than 3 per cent
- Register patient with one of three centres: Sheffield, Dundee or London
- Follow-up process
- Postal samples – frequency, if uncertain please do not quote
- Need to avoid pregnancy – why?
- Complete mole – six months? Partial mole six months
- Contraception – avoid hormonal until beta-human chorionic gonadotrophin (βHCG) levels return to normal. Avoid intrauterine contraceptive device (IUCD) – risk of bleeding. Best method – barrier methods (not too reliable though). Depo-Provera – avoid – risk of irregular vaginal bleeding. May be confused with recurrence of disease
- Subsequent pregnancies: early ultrasound scan – why? – to rule out recurrence. What is the recurrence risk? postdelivery – follow-up sample. Why?

Sample answer

Hydatidiform mole has a risk of progression to choriocarcinoma in less than three per cent of cases in the absence of follow-up and chemotherapy for persistent trophoblastic disease. The risk of developing choriocarcinoma depends on the type of molar pregnancy. It is higher after a complete than a partial hydatiform mole. The first step in the management of this patient, therefore, is to determine the type of hydatidiform mole.

This diagnosis, and the need for prolonged follow-up, should be explained to the patient. This is mainly to prevent the development of chriocarcinoma by the early identification of persistent disease, which may be treated effectively with chemotherapy. Where chorio-carcinoma has developed but is identified early, chemotherapy is effective without affecting fertility. For this follow-up, the patient needs to register at one of three centres in the UK – Sheffield, Dundee or Charing Cross in London. These centres will then send sample bottles to her through the post. The frequency with which these bottles are sent for urine collection will be determined by the centre. Briefly, this is every fortnight until beta-human chorionic gonadotrophin (βHCG) levels from the samples reach the limit of detection and thereafter every month until it is back to normal, and for another three months after it has returned to normal.

The minimum follow-up period has traditionally been six months for a partial hydatiform mole and one year for a complete mole. However, since progression of a partial mole to chori-ocarcinoma is uncommon, this may no longer be the best advice. The reasons why patients are advised to avoid pregnancy during the follow-up period is to ensure that rising levels are not confused with pregnancy and therefore delay treatment. During the follow up period, a bar-rier method of contraception is offered until three months after βHCG levels have returned to normal. This is because the combined oral contraceptive pill slows the return of the βHCG levels to normal values. An intrauterine contraceptive device (IUCD) is inadvisable as it may perforate the uterus and may also cause irregular vaginal bleeding which may be confused with features of persistent disease.

Once the patient has been followed up, subsequent pregnancies must be confirmed early to exclude a recurrence of a molar pregnancy. This patient has a 20-fold increase in the risk of recurrent hydatidiform mole following one molar pregnancy. Even after the pregnancy has been completed she will need to be followed up as the risk of a placental site trophoblastic tumour is higher in this patient. Avoiding pregnancies for at least six months is the least that is required of this woman.

17

Operative gynaecology

1. Critically comment on the types of abdominal incisions that gynaecologists use.

2. A 47-year-old woman, who is protein S deficient, is scheduled for a hysterectomy and bilateral salpingoophorectomy. Justify your perioperative management.

3. During a vaginal hysterectomy and repair on a 67-year-old obese woman, you discover (after the hysterectomy) a large partly solid, partly cystic (10.0 × 8.0 cm) ovarian mass. Justify your subsequent management of the patient.

4. During an abdominal hysterectomy, you suspect that the ureter has been damaged on the right side. Outline the steps you will take in your subsequent management of the patient.

5. How might bladder injuries be prevented during gynaecological surgery?

1. Critically comment on the types of abdominal incisions that gynaecologists use.

Common mistakes

- Discussing different types of major and minor gynaecological procedures
- Details of how to make the various surgical incisions
- Complications of the incisions

A good answer will include some or all of these points

- The types of incisions
- Advantages and disadvantages of these incisions

Sample answer

Abdominal incisions for gynaecological surgery are, to a large extent, determined by the type of operation. The fundamental principles governing the type of incisions used are adequate surgical exposure and cosmetic acceptability. Whether surgery is laparoscopic or laparotomy also influences the type of abdominal incisions; therefore, they may vary from small to large.

The most common incision for major gynaecological surgery is the Pfannenstiel incision. This is a transverse incision above the pubic symphysis. Exposure of the pelvis with this incision is considered adequate for most benign gynaecological operations. There are, however, some limitations of this type of incision. It does not provide adequate exposure to large pelvic masses. In addition, it is not easily extendable and therefore when indicated to facilitate surgery, this is either not possible or the extension is inadequate. The advantage of this incision is the associated lower risk of incisional hernia. It heals properly and is more cosmetically acceptable to patients. This type of incision is considered inadequate for ovarian cancer surgery.

The vertical incision is the second most common approach for major gynaecological surgery. It offers a better exposure for the surgeon and is also easy to extend. Vertical incisions are commonly used for gynaecological cancer surgery and surgery for large pelvic masses, such as large fibroids and ovarian cysts. Where there is the risk of bladder damage during entry into the abdominal cavity (as in cases of severe adhesions), this incision allows superior entry and therefore minimizes this risk. Disadvantages include the high risk of burst abdomen, especially in obese patients in whom postoperative infections are more likely. It is also associated with an increased risk of incisional hernia.

Other incisions that may be used are those for laparoscopic surgery. These tend to be infraumbilical or oblique incisions in the iliac fossae. Occasionally, a small suprapubic incision may be employed. These incisions have the advantage of being very cosmetic. However, they are very small and are unsuitable for any other type of surgery. If not closed properly, these incisions may be complicated by Reichter's hernia.

Although these are the most common types of abdominal incisions in gynaecological surgery, occasionally, other types may be used. These include an oblique abdominal incision in the iliac fossa. This does not permit good access and also is not cosmetically acceptable to patients.

2. A 47-year-old woman, who is protein S deficient, is scheduled for a hysterectomy and bilateral salpingoophorectomy. Justify your perioperative management.

Common mistakes

- Discussing deep vein thrombosis (DVT) or pulmonary embolism (PE) – investigations, diagnosis and treatment
- Discussing alternatives to surgery in this patient
- Discussing the indications for surgery
- History and physical examination
- Past medical history of DVT and PE

A good answer will include some or all of these points

- Increased risk of DVT and PE
- Bilateral salpingoophorectomy requires hormone replacement therapy (HRT) – which is associated with an increased risk of DVT/PE
- Reduction of DVT risk: involve haematologist; assess and modify other risk factors, such as obesity, smoking, concurrent infections; prophylactic heparin/fragmin/tinzaprin pre-operatively and postoperatively; pneumatic stockings and thrombo-embolic deterrent stockings; early mobilization; good hydration at the time of surgery; prophylactic antibiotics to minimize the risk of postoperative infection
- HRT – if ovaries removed – need for HRT; benefits versus side-effects and risk of DVT; on balance will need HRT
- Need to monitor for warning signs of DVT/PE
- Preoperatively, counsel patient about these risks and educate on warning signs
- If taking warfarin, change to heparin before surgery is undertaken

Sample answer

This patient, by virtue of her thrombophilia, is at an increased risk of venous thrombo-embolism (VTE). This risk is further compounded by the need to consider hormone replace-ment therapy (HRT), by virtue of her having a bilateral salpingoophorectomy. HRT is associated with an increased risk of thrombo-embolism. In this patient, the focus on her management must be to reduce her risk of VTE perioperatively and postoperatively. In addition, adequate counselling must be offered in order to further reduce her chances of developing deep vein thrombosis (DVT) if she has HRT.

From the outset, a haematologist should be involved in her perioperative care. Although this is unlikely to significantly alter her planned surgery, advice on the most effective thrombo-prophylaxis will be provided. This will take the form of heparin or low molecular weight heparin (LMWH) before surgery. Preoperatively, risk factors for DVT need to be identified and attempts made to modify them. Such risks include obesity, smoking and concurrent infections. At the time of surgery, pneumatic stockings should be used. The duration of surgery must be kept to a minimum, whilst blood loss must be carefully controlled. Adequate hydration must also be maintained at the time of surgery and prophyhlactic antibiotics prescribed to reduce the risk of postoperative infection.

Postoperatively, adequate hydration and early mobilization are essential. The patient should have compression stockings during her time in hospital and the anticoagulants initiated perioperatively should be continued for at least five days after surgery.

An important aspect of the management of this patient will involve HRT. This will take the form of oestrogens since she will have had a hysterectomy and oophorectomy. The need for HRT, with emphasis on its risks versus its benefits, should to be discussed before initiating it. On balance, it may be more beneficial for the patient to start HRT as she is only 47 years old. The early warning signs for DVT and pulmonary embolism (PE) need to be discussed in a careful and non-frightening manner and advice given on the need to report early if they occur.

In some cases, the patient might have already been taking warfarin before surgery. If this is the case, this oral thrombo-prophylaxis should be converted to a parenteral form before surgery. This switch is preferably done a day before surgery.

3. During a vaginal hysterectomy and repair on a 67-year-old obese woman, you discover (after the hysterectomy) a large partly solid, partly cystic (10.0 × 8.0 cm) ovarian mass. Justify your subsequent management of the patient.

Common errors

- Take a history
- Investigate – BRCA1, CA125, ultrasound, etc.
- Obtain consent for more extensive history
- Perform a laparoscopy
- Wrongly managed and therefore a serious mistake
- Management will depend on her age and desire for further pregnancies
- Staging laparotomy and then planned definitive surgery
- No further action for now as patient cannot consent
- Not asked to outline management of patient with ovarian cyst
- Preoperative information given: not legal to remove ovary without patient's consent
- Heavy periods – indication for a vaginal hysterectomy and repair?

A good answer will include most or all of these points

- The operation of vaginal hysterectomy and repair is most likely for prolapse in a woman who is over the age of 50 years
- Appearances of the ovarian pathology are highly suspicions of malignancy (that is, malignancy needs to be ruled out). This can only be achieved by an adequate exploration, which cannot be offered vaginally
- Proceed to a laparotomy (and involve gynaecological oncologist if uncertain or if a malignancy is the working diagnosis): midline incision; explore and take peritoneal fluid for cytology; bilateral salpingoophorectomy and omentectomy if suspicion of malignancy; palpate para-aortic and pelvic nodes and biopsy if necessary
- Postoperatively, explain findings and procedure to patient
- Counsel appropriately and wait for histology
- Histology: benign – no need for follow-up unless for the prolapse; malignant – chemotherapy with oncologist
- Conclusion

Sample answer

This patient's surgery is most likely to be for a uterovaginal prolapse. Prior to this procedure, a pelvic examination ought to have been performed. However, in an obese patient, this examination may not be very informative. It is assumed that this examination in this patient was not informative, otherwise, this adnexal mass would have been recognized and the type of surgery reassessed. The appearances of this ovarian mass require an exclusion of a malignancy. Indeed, this tumour must be considered malignant until proved otherwise. Subsequent management must be geared towards this tentative diagnosis and must aim to provide the best results for the patient. The only way this can be achieved is by a laparatomy and subsequent surgery.

The next stage is to perform a laparotomy by use of a midline incision. This incision will allow a better assessment of the tumour, its bilaterality, associated secondaries to the liver, omentum and lymhphadenopathy. It will also allow completion of the surgical treatment for ovarian cancer. This consists of bilateral salpingoophorectomy, omentectomy, lymphadenectomy and other necessary surgery. If there are any secondaries the ultimate aim must be to ensure that the residual disease is minimal (less than 1.5 cm if possible). Peritoneal fluid and washings must be collected and send for cytology.

Postoperatively, the patient must be offered adequate counselling about the findings and the nature of the surgery she has undergone. Whatever the case, the ultimate counselling will have to await histology on the ovarian tumour and other tissues removed at surgery. Further management will depend on the type of cancer, if she does have cancer, and the need for adjuvant chemotherapy. If the histology is benign, there is no need for chemotherapy. However, if it is a malignancy then adjuvant chemotherapy should be offered by a team consisting of a gynaecological oncologist and a medical oncologist. The patient should be followed up for at least five years to identify early recurrence.

It is very likely that where the prolapse was the reason for the surgery in the first instance, the abdominal surgery would not have corrected it. In this case, it may be necessary to reassess the symptoms and plan further treatment, especially if the histology of the ovarian tumour is benign. If the ovarian tumour was an aetiological factor in the occurrence of the prolapse, removing it may be enough to alleviate the symptoms.

4. During an abdominal hysterectomy, you suspect that the ureter has been damaged on the right side. Outline the steps you will take in your subsequent management of the patient.

Common mistakes

- Bladder/kidney injury
- Postoperative suspicion of ureteric injury
- Description of the procedure of a hysterectomy
- Prevention of ureteric injury, do not discuss: preoperative intravenous urogram (IVU) or ultrasound to outline course of ureters; the value of intraoperative IVU to outline the course of the ureters; postoperative catherization of the bladder; complications of vesico-vaginal fistula; what steps will you take to minimize bowel injury during gynaecological surgery

A good answer will include some or all of these points

- Ureteric injuries are difficult to recognize, but common in difficult gynaecological cases. Index of suspicion must therefore be high
- Suspicion is during surgery – therefore: call for help – senior gynaecologist or urologist; ensure left kidney is present and left ureter is normal
- Has any injury or damage actually occurred?: trace ureter; identify site of possible injury or damage; may need the help of cystocopic retrograde catherization of the ureter – IVU may be useful – where cystoscopic retrograde catherization is not possible
- Management of injury if confirmed: end-to-end anastomosis; reimplantation; raising a Boari flap; splint with ureteric catheter
- Postoperative management: complications – urinary peritonitis?; IVU later
- Counsel patient appropriately

Sample answer

Ureteric injuries are rare and very difficult to identify, both at the time of surgery and afterwards. A high index of suspicion is therefore important in patients at risk of ureteric injury during surgery. This injury is likely to occur in patients with adhesions, large uterine fibroids and ovarian tumours, especially malignancies, and in those undergoing Wertheim hysterectomy.

Once a ureteric injury is suspected, a key step in the management of the patient is to call for help if the surgeon does not have the expertise to recognize these lesions. The contralateral ureter must be identified to ensure that this is present. Sometimes this may be absent, in which case very great care must be exercised during the repair of the damaged side.

The next stage is to confirm that an injury has indeed occurred. This can be confirmed by observing urine welling in the operative field. However, this may not be easy. Ancillary

365

measures may be taken to confirm the diagnosis. These include retrograde catherization of the ureter, retrograde cystoureteroscopy and dye injection. The advantage of a dye injection is it allows the site of the lesion to be localized. Intraoperative intravenous urography (IVU) has a role in defining the site and nature of the injury but this is time-consuming.

Once the damage has been confirmed, various procedures may be undertaken to repair the injury. These will depend on the type of injury. Immediate anastomosis will be ideal if this is possible. In addition to end-to-end anastomosis, a ureteric stent is essential to splint the site of anastomosis. In some cases, this may not be easy. Another option is to raise a Boari flap. This ensures that the ureter remains functional and reduces the chances of kidney damage. In some cases, reimplanatation of the ureter into the bladders may be the treatment of choice. In others, however, an ileal conduit may be the best approach. Most of these procedures need to be performed by a urologist. Where the injury is a crushing type or the ureter was transfixed, simply removing the stitch and stenting it may be considered adequate. However, if the crushed segment is judged to be necrotic, it has to be excised and end-to-end anastomosis undertaken as described above.

Postoperatively, the patient should be placed on antibiotics and monitored for the early warning signs of urinary peritonitis. Once the ureteric stent has been removed, it will be advisable to offer the patient an IVU to confirm the patency of the ureter and a functioning kidney.

5. How might bladder injuries be prevented during gynaecological surgery?

Common mistakes

- Describing the operative procedures in detail
- Discussing renal tract abnormalities
- Radiological investigations

A good answer will include some or all of these points

- Injuries most likely to occur at laparoscopy, laparotomy, during dissection with distorted pelvic anatomy and at the time of vaginal surgery
- Preoperative precautions – empty bladder or intraoperative needle emptying
- Identification of at-risk patients – previous difficult pelvic surgery, history of pelvic inflammatory disease, review notes for these
- Surgical technique – laparoscopy/dissection/vaginal/abdominal – meticulous approach
- Expert help if bladder adherent
- Good knowledge of anatomy
- Entry to abdomen – modify incisions depending on anticipated difficulties
- Recognition: at the time of surgery – urine welling up; suspect but uncertain – methlyene blue into the bladder; postoperatively – incontinence – haematuria

Sample answer

Bladder injuries are not uncommon during gynaecological surgery. These are most likely to occur either during introduction of the laparoscopic port or dissection of the bladder away from the uterus, from adhesions and during a colposuspension abdominally or vaginally during a hysterectomy or anterior repair. Prevention of these injuries must start with recognizing those patients who are at risk of such injuries, followed by meticulous surgery and early recognition and management when they occur.

The patients at risk of bladder injuries during gynaecological surgery include those with large abdomino-pelvic masses undergoing surgery, pelvic adhesions from infections and endometriosis or from previous pelvic surgery, such as Caesarean section. Patients undergoing laproscopic surgery and those undergoing a vaginal procedure are also at risk. In these patients, various important steps need to be taken to prevent bladder injuries. For all abdominal procedures, the most important single step to take is to empty the bladder. This must be done before laparoscopy. For other operations, this may be done once the abdomen has been opened. The only disadvantage with this approach is that if the patient's bladder is already very full, it may actually be damaged during entry into the peritoneal cavity. Those advocating this approach argue that suprapubic drainage with a needle reduces the risk of urinary tract infections (UTIs).

The surgical technique itself must be systematic and meticulous. During laparoscopy, it is important to direct the Verre needle and the trocar towards the pelvis but away from the bladder. Similarly, if adhesions are suspected, a more superior approach to entering the abdomen will bypass an adherent bladder. Blunt dissection will be safer than sharp dissection. If there is any bleeding around the bladder base, this must be clearly identified before haemostasis is secured. Blind diathermy or suturing may result in bladder injuries. The best weapon available for avoiding bladder injuries (apart from surgical skill) is in-depth knowledge of the anatomy of the pelvis. An understanding of the relationship of the bladder to the uterus and the anterior abdominal wall is essential to minimize the risk of injury. If the surgeon encounters adhesions and lacks the expertise to deal with them, prudence demands that senior help is summoned.

Prevention of injuries must not be limited to inflicting the injury itself but early recognition and correction when it occurs. Once an injury is suspected, it must be confirmed. This could be done by filling the bladder with a dye, such as methylene blue. Alternatively, the operation site welling with clear fluid must raise the suspicion of a bladder or ureteric injury. During colposuspension, filling the bladder with methylene blue before dissecting the paraurethra tissues away from the proximal urethra and neck of the bladder will allow for early identification of any injuries and repair. The closure of the peritoneum during a vaginal hysterectomy and buttressing of the bladder base must be done with extreme caution as injuries are more likely to occur at this time. Postoperatively, the injuries may be recognized from haematuria or incontinence. These must be investigated and early treatment offered to prevent further deterioration.

18

Ethics, medico-legal

1. It has been suggested that *in vitro* fertilization (IVF) may be used to provide organ or marrow donors to siblings suffering from diseases that require transplantation. Can you debate this statement?

2. What steps will you take to reduce the rising litigation in gynaecology in the UK?

3. Selective fetocide is unjustified in the twenty-first century. Debate this statement.

4. Treatment for infertility should not be offered on the National Health Service (NHS). Do you agree with this statement?

5. How will you set up a risk management team in your unit?

1. It has been suggested that *in vitro* fertilization (IVF) may be used to provide organ or marrow donors to siblings suffering from diseases that require transplantation. Can you debate this statement?

Common mistakes

- Extolling the virtues of *in vitro* fertilization (IVF) or the history of IVF or the indications for IVF
- Discussing human rights and how the fetus and newborn have rights
- Discussing killing babies so others can survive
- Cloning of humans
- Research on embryos
- Avoid being emotional and depersonalize your answer

A good answer will include some or all of these points

- This debate crosses ethical, moral, religious and legal boundaries
- Advantages: long waiting lists for donors – overcome; risk of incompatibility – reduced; family is the source of donor and therefore feels involved in the cure of patient
- Disadvantages: expensive; complications of IVF to the mother; failure of IVF and attendant disappointment; even if successful, no guarantee of compatibility; legal and other obstacles; may be abused
- Conclusion: well-defined role to avoid abuse

Sample answer

This is a problem that crosses ethical, religious, moral and legal jurisdictions. The radical developments in assisted reproductive techniques will no doubt continue to cause an increasing number of demands on the techniques. The use of *in vitro* fertilization (IVF) to produce tissues or organs for siblings must be examined from the different perspectives above.

There are consistent problems with donor organs. These include a long waiting times for suitable donors, the problem of compatibility and often the psychological feeling by the recipient that he or she has an organ of no genetic or biological relationship. The provision of organ donors from family members, even if these were from IVF programmes, would overcome some of these obstacles. For example, they would significantly reduce the problems of rejection or compatibility. In addition, the donor would be a member of the recipient's family. This latter advantage overcomes the psychological problems of recipients never knowing any details of their organ donor. The family is the source of the donation and so feels involved in the treatment that requires the donation.

There are, however, several disadvantages of such an approach. The IVF procedure is expensive and fraught with complications, especially to the mother. There is the risk of multiple pregnancy and consequently the problems of prematurity and its possible sequelae of neurodevelopmental disability. Embarking on a pregnancy mainly to provide a donor for a sibling may be perceived as morally unjustified. In addition, such actions may have significant effects on both the donor and recipient siblings.

There is no guarantee that if IVF is successful, there would be compatibility between the donor and the recipient. The family may raise their hopes just to have them dashed. Although such an approach may be extremely beneficial to some families, there is the risk of it being abused for other non-medical reasons. There are various legal, ethical and religious obstacles that must be overcomed before this technique is made available. An important aspect of this treatment is counselling. This needs to be undertaken before treatment.

Although there is a place for offering such treatment to families with no other options, it must not be seen as the primary approach to obtaining donor organs. In most cases, the procedure has to be highly regulated to ensure that it is not abused. In addition, the process of counselling must be extensive and tailored to the needs of the family before and after the donor process.

2. What steps will you take to reduce the rising litigation in gynaecology in the UK?

Common mistakes

- Discussing the legal aspects of OBGYN
- Details of audit
- Concentrating on structures to counteract litigation claims

A good answer will include some or all of these points

- Litigation costs rising. Obstetrics – 60 per cent of the total cost in the National Health Service (NHS)
- Causes of litigation
- How to minimize risks: training; audit; openness; documentation; risk management teams; incident reporting; more senior input in care of patients

Sample answer

Litigation is increasingly becoming an important problem in gynaecology. Although there is more litigation in obstetrics than gynaecology, there is no doubt the problems exist. The principles involved in reducing litigation in any discipline are essentially the same. Increasing litigation is an important drain on resources and causes untold stress to staff. Significantly, in most cases this is preventable. The process of reducing litigation must include training, adequate communication between patients and documentation. Most of these principles are well-expounded in the clinical governance document.

Adequate training is an important first step in reducing the rising incidence of litigation. Training programmes must be set up to identify the needs, or rather deficiencies, of all gynaecologists and to ensure that these deficiencies are rectified. Training must be patient-focused and should address the concerns of patient care, the aim being to improve dialogue/communication between patients, staff and between careers.

Most problems resulting in litigation are easily identified. Poor communication between patients and hospital staff is a major constituent. In this regard, adequate training sessions for junior doctors and nurses, and other members of the team, must be undertaken. Communication must be transparent and directed to the right person and at the right level. Communication between general practitioners (GPs) and hospitals should be detailed enough to ensure that GPs are able to relate to the patient information emanating from the hospital.

In parallel with communication must be appropriate documentation in patients' notes. All discussions with patients, colleagues and others involved in patient care should be well-documented. Efforts to write contemporaneous notes will eliminate the potential difficulties of recall and obvious bias in documentation.

Patients who often complain are those likely to seek legal redress. Early recognition of these patients and prompt action to minimize the consequences of any accidents or lack of communication will significantly reduce the numbers doing so. Although a few patients set out to seek monetary compensation, a large proportion want to ensure that mistakes are not repeated and that there is some one to take responsibility and apologize for errors. Transparency in dealing with at-risk patients is therefore very important. In this regard, there is a need for a risk management team, which will deal with potential complainants and offer adequate explanations and apologies when necessary. In addition, incident reporting protocols will ensure that incidents are recognized early and dealt with, in some cases pro-actively.

If the unit does not have a transparent patients' complaints procedure, this must be established. This will ensure that patients see the transparency and speed with which their complaints are dealt. It is important to make sure that these processes are not seen as witch-hunting, as this may drive a wedge between good and responsible practice, and defensive medicine.

3. Selective fetocide is unjustified in the twenty-first century. Debate this statement.

Common mistakes

- Discussing the procedure of fetocide
- Criticizing the process itself on moral or religious grounds
- Failure to debate but simply stating the indications for fetocide

A good answer will include some or all of these points

- Advantages: reduces the risk of prematurity; complications of pregnancy; beneficial when one fetus is abnormal; more acceptable to parents – financial constraints on bringing up more than one child
- Disadvantages: complications; how do you select the fetus to kill? complications of the retained intrauterine death on the surviving fetus; ethics of this; abuse – selection of ideal sex and genetic make-up?
- Conclusion: well-balanced cases, with adequate counselling may be a procedure to be offered

Sample answer

Selective fetocide has increasingly become an important procedure in obstetrics, especially in the early stages of pregnancy. This procedure involves the killing of one or more fetuses to offer a greater chance of survival to the other(s). Although the HFEA 1991 guarantees that not more than three embryos are replaced in any assisted reproduction technique to reduce the problems of multifetal gestations, these still occur. Selective reduction may also be offered in natural pregnancies or in those following ovulation induction for various reasons.

The primary indication for selective fetocide is to reduce the number of fetuses in multifetal gestations and therefore significantly reduce the incidence of prematurity and its complications. It has been shown that by reducing the number of fetuses, the pregnancy can be prolonged significantly and increase the survival of the fetus (es). Selective fetocide may be performed as early as seven to eight weeks. It is, however, advantageous to do this in the late first trimester as most of the fetuses that will not survive for other reasons would naturally have been miscarried or died *in utero*.

Another indication for fetocide is if one fetus is abnormal. However, there is increasing social demand for fetocide where the parents are unable to cope with a twin or triplet pregnancy. There have been some cases where it has been performed for sex selection. The justification of this procedure may not be morally or religiously acceptable to some patients. The introduction of this topic, therefore, must be made with extreme caution and sensitivity.

The procedure itself has several disadvantages. It results in the retention of a dead fetus during pregnancy, which may cause problems, especially of coagulopathy and neuropathy in the surviving fetus(es). During the procedure, if there is anastomosis between the fetuses, the drug administered to effect the fetocide may be transferred to the other fetus and may cause its demise as well.

An important difficulty is which fetus(es) to select in the absence of an obvious abnormality. Moralist will argue that we have no right to select one fetus on the basis of chance. This argument is buttressed by the recent cases of a wealthy family choosing fetocide of a twin pregnancy as the parents did not want two babies to cause a significant inconvenience to their lifestyle. Such an attitude may be perceived as an abuse of the system. There is, therefore, a need for tougher regulation of selective fetocide. Abuse may extent to the choice of the sex of the baby or babies not conforming to various physical characteristic desired by the parents. With the unmapping of the human gene, it is conceivable that parents may start studying the characteristics of their future offspring and use selective fetocide to chose the right babies.

On balance, therefore, selective fetocide has an important role to play in modern day obstetrics and gynaecology. However, it must be offered in a well-regulated environment where ethical, religious, moral and legal considerations are always taken into account. Without tight regulation and moderation, this may be subject to significant abuse.

4. Treatment for infertility should not be offered on the National Health Service (NHS). Do you agree with this statement?

Common mistakes

- Details of infertility treatment
- Complications of infertility treatment
- Rationale for treating infertile couples
- Centres for treatment
- The law on infertility treatment

A good answer will include some or all of these points

- Infertility is a disease
- Treatment is both necessary and important
- World Health Organization's (WHO) definition of disease (not only the absence of infirmity)
- Cost implications deter ready availability of this treatment on the National Health Service (NHS)
- Other mundane conditions being treated – stripping varicose veins, plastic surgery, sex change operations, etc.
- Rationing in other disciplines
- Problem of making it available to all on the NHS
- Abuse
- Diverting scarce resources from other important areas to infertility
- Ideal – combining funding?
- Conclusion – may be a place for investigating and treating, but not for all cases, and not every unit should offer advanced assisted reproduction techniques – to ensure compliance with the law and improved success

Sample answer

Infertility affects about 15 per cent of couples in the UK. There are many causes of this condition, most of which can be corrected at the primary and secondary levels. In some cases, however, more extensive and advanced investigations, and treatment are required. The controversy about treating couples with infertility is often focused on these advanced therapeutic modalities. Infertility is a disease and deserves to be treated like any other disease. The World Health Organization (WHO) defines a disease as not merely the absence of an infirmity but complete psychological, physical and mental well-being. Couples with infertility, although they may not have a physical disability, have a psychologically disabling condition which deserves the same treatment offered to others with depression, anxiety and physical disorders.

377

The arguments for or against treating patients with infertility concentrate on the absence of physical disability and, therefore, failure to conform with the definition of disease. More importantly, because of the rapidly advancing technology in this field, cost implications for various health authorities are quite enormous. Another point often advanced against offering treatment is the low success rates, especially that following the advanced infertility treatments. Are these really justified?

Not all cases of infertility require advanced treatment methods. For those cases where the cause can easily be identified and adequate treatment offered, the results are very good. In fact, the treatment is often considered by most as being cost-effective. However, for the advanced therapies, the success of the regimens varies, but is usually in the region of approximately 15–25 per cent 'baby take home' rate. The suggestion that all infertility treatment should not be offered on the National Health Service (NHS) is therefore not valid for the cases that can be managed at the primary and secondary levels. For the cases requiring advanced treatment, the cost argument needs to be supported.

Within the NHS, rationing is an important process and allows prioritization of treatment because of inadequate resources. However, there are many minor medical conditions which are treated despite the need for rationing. For example, treatment for mundane conditions, such as stripping varicose veins, cosmetic plastic surgery and sex change operations. It could be argued that most of these treatments are not essential and are unnecessary. However, the reasoning behind treating these conditions is the severe psychological consequences failure to treat may have on patients. Infertility is known to consume the whole life of couples, affecting their work, relationships with colleagues and families, and has been known to cause marital disharmony and psychiatric illness. Treating couples with infertility, certainly indirectly treats these associated problems.

The NHS aims to treat all, irrespective of the problem. Infertility is a disease and therefore deserves to be treated within the NHS. But is it life-threatening compared to other conditions, such as cancer and cardiac diseases? This argument is unsubstantiated as many other illnesses being treated in the NHS are not life-threatening. If the arguments against offering tertiary treatment for infertility are that limited resources for important health conditions will be diverted to the treatment of this condition, a similar argument could be advanced for the treatment of other non-debilitating conditions.

The argument about treatment, therefore, must be similar to that for other conditions. In an ideal world where resources are limitless, this would not arise. It is important to acknowledge that rationing is an integral part of the NHS and will remain so for a long time to come. Where resources are limited, then there may be a place to limit the treatment of couples with infertility to that offered at primary and secondary levels. Tertiary treatment must, however, be made available but in a few designated centres where expertise and wide experience exists in order to improve the success rates. Regulating practice is important to prevent abuse. The principles of rationing require that all cases are assessed on merit and treatment offered when it is considered to be necessary. Couples with infertility being refused treatment on the NHS are being treated unfairly and that undermines the fundamental principles of the NHS.

5. How will you set up a risk management team in your unit?

Common mistakes

- Details of what a risk management team consists of
- Role of risk management team
- Audit cycle and risk management
- The process of risk management

A good answer will include some or all of these points

- What is a risk management team?
- Who should be in the team?
- What should be the remit of the team?
- How should it work?
- Description of the role of the team?
- Effect of the team on care
- Integration with other aspects of perinatal care
- Assessment/evaluation of the effectiveness of the team

Sample answer

Risk management is increasingly being recognized as an important component of clinical governance. This is more so in the light of the rising cost of litigation in medicine. In obstetrics and gynaecology, this is even more important in view of the fact that although the discipline contributes only a small proportion of cases, its litigation bill comprises about 60 per cent of the National Health Service (NHS) litigation bill. It is, therefore, not surprising that the Clinical Negligence Scheme for Trust (CNST) requires all units to have risk management teams. Setting up these teams is imperative. How these units are set up will define their effectiveness.

In setting up a risk management team, the first consideration must be the composition of the team. Within each unit, there should be a risk manager working within the team with the remit of minimizing risk. Team membership should reflect the multidisciplinary nature of patient care within the unit. It should include a midwife/nurse, physicians (junior and senior) and an anaesthetist. This will ensure that all members of staff feel represented. The members of the team should have an interest in risk management and must be educated on the importance of risk management as a means of improving care rather than as a punitive process.

The remit of the team must be clearly defined. The team should aim to identify risk management issues within the unit, set up guidelines on how to deal with these and, importantly, how to minimize risk management issues within the unit. There may be a place for the introduction of incident reporting so that various risk management issues could be identified and a process set in place on how to deal with any deficiencies. The role of the team within the unit must be clear. In addition, there must be channels of communication between the team, members of staff and management. This communication must be two-way and efforts made to ensure that the staff in the unit do not perceive the team as a fault-finding and blame team but one whose role is constructive aiming for a risk-free service within the unit.

Once the team has been established, there has to be a mechanism by which information is disseminated to the unit. This may be through meetings and other fora where education on risk management issues are presented. The ultimate objectives of the risk management team are to ensure that complaints are dealt with quickly and early, that potential problems are identified early, dealt with and that members of staff are educated where weaknesses are identified in their practices. Members of risk management teams must be seen to work in collaboration with all aspects of the services provided within the team.

Section Four
Practice papers for revision

1

Introduction

This section of the book is aimed to help you with your preparation for the examination. It is divided into two parts:

- Ten sample short essays questions (five obstetrics and five gynaecology)
- Three hundred multiple-choice questions (MCQs)

You should use this section to help you practise for the examination. It is advisable to time yourself as if you are sitting the real examination and only afterwards should you check the answers – both to the short essays and the MCQs. The MCQs are of an equivalent standard to those in the MRCOG Part 2 examination.

To pass the examination, you will need to score 183 out of 300 marks. You should remember that there is no pass mark for the MCQ or short essay papers. It is a pass mark for the written examination. Most candidates who pass the examination score at least 100 in the short essays. However, if you only concentrate on the essays, it will be difficult to compensate for a poor performance in the MCQs. You must aim to score at least 80 in the MCQ paper. If you have any doubts about the answers, you are advised to cross-check them in your textbooks.

2

Multiple-choice questions (MCQs)

Answer true or false

Concerning autosomal recessive inheritance

1. If the carrier has an affected partner, there is a 50 per cent chance of the children being affected.
2. There is an association with consanguinity.
3. The recessive gene may be expressed in individuals heterozygous for the abnormal gene.

Concerning X-linked inheritance

4. More females than males show the recessive phenotype.
5. The disease is transmitted by a carrier female, who is usually asymptomatic.
6. A carrier mother will have a 50 per cent chance of her sons being affected and a 50 per cent chance of her daughters being carriers.
7. Affected males may have unaffected parents but will often have an affected maternal uncle.

The following disorders are correctly associated with the mode of inheritance

8. Tay–Sachs disease	Autosomal recessive.
9. Marfan syndrome	Autosomal recessive.
10. von Willebrand disease	Autosomal dominant.
11. von Recklingausen disease (neurofibromatosis)	Autosomal dominant.

Which of the following dietary supplements are associated with congenital malformations?

12. Vitamin A.
13. Liver extracts.
14. Vitamin C.

In adolescent pregnancies

15. Biological immaturity results in more Caesarean sections.
16. The incidence of sudden infant death syndrome is higher than in older women.
17. The interval between pregnancies is influenced by whether or not the first pregnancy is planned.
18. Breech presentation is more common than in older women.

Concerning pregnancies in ethnic minorities

19. Sickle cell disease only occurs in women of African origin.
20. When there is non-engagement of the head in a Black British woman at 38 weeks' gestation, cephalo-pelvic disproportion must be excluded.
21. Gluycose-6-phosphate dehydrogenase deficiency is more common in women from the Mediterranean and African region than in those from south-east Asia.

With regards to miscarriages

22. Disseminated intravascular coagulation (DIC) is not a recognized complication.
23. Gas gangrene is a complication of septic miscarriages.
24. The treatment of an incomplete miscarriage should include a broad-spectrum antibiotic.
25. *Clostridium welchii* is a recognized cause of the recurrent variety.
26. Misoprostol may be used to medically evacuate the uterus successfully in 90 per cent of cases with incomplete miscarriages.

Recognized causes of recurrent miscarriages include

27. Sheehan syndrome.
28. Exposure to video display screens.
29. Factor XI deficiency.

A 36-year-old woman was admitted at 36 weeks' gestation with vaginal bleeding and abdominal pain. An ultrasound scan performed at 20 weeks' gestation had located the placenta to be posterior and fundal.

30. The diagnosis of placental abruption is confirmed by the presence of abdominal pain.
31. An ultrasound scan is unnecessary as placenta praevia has been excluded.
32. The risk of congenital malformations in the fetus is higher than if she had not had an antepartum haemorrhage.
33. If DIC is suspected, she should be delivered by Caesarean section.
34. If she develops a bleeding diasthesis, an epidural is not contraindicated.

Concerning ultrasound in pregnancy

35. The finding of an echogenic bowel suggests a high risk of Down's syndrome.
36. The presence of two or more soft markers increases the risk of aneuploidy.
37. When undertaken at 20 weeks' gestation, more than 70 per cent of cardiac anomalies are detected.
38. When performed repeatedly, it is associated with an increased risk of intrauterine growth restriction (IUGR).

Human immunodeficiency virus (HIV) infection in pregnancy

39. The median time between exposure to the virus and the development of detectable antibody is about two months.
40. Transplacental transfer to the fetus is reduced by Caesarean section.
41. Breastfeeding is contraindicated.
42. Without treatment, in Europeans, about 20 per cent of infected children will develop the symptoms of autoimmune deficiency syndrome (AIDS) within the first year of life.

With regards to neural tube defects

43. Recurrence tends to be concordant.
44. They may be associated with Meckel–Gruber syndrome.
45. A previously affected child increases the risk of recurrence to about one to three per cent.
46. The presence of acetylcholinesterase in amniotic fluid is diagnostic of an open defect.

Which of the following may be associated with an abnormally large nuchal translucency?

47. Diaphragmatic hernia.
48. Scarococcygeal teratoma.
49. Gastroschisis.
50. Severe IUGR.
51. Cardiac abnormality.

Soft markers for chromosomal abnormalities include

52. Cerebellar hypoplasia.
53. Pyelectasis.
54. Cerebral ventriculomegaly.
55. Choroid plexus.

Complications of chorionic villus sampling (CVS) include

56. Transverse limb reduction deformities.
57. Preterm labour.
58. Placental abruption.

Amniocentesis

59. Is associated with an increased risk of orthopaedic deformities.
60. Is complicated by chorioamnionitis in five per cent of cases.
61. May result in platelet isoimmunization.

The following are true of stillbirths

62. Most occur in labour.
63. At least 50 per cent of them are preventable.
64. Poor antenatal care is a risk factor only in developing countries.

Maternal smoking in pregnancy is associated with:

65. Reduced blood flow to the fetal brain.
66. Diminished fetal breathing movements.
67. Fetal hypoglycaemia.
68. An increased incidence of amniorrhexis.

Neonatal complications of IUGR include

69. Respiratory distress syndrome (RDS).
70. Neonatal jaundice.
71. Polycythaemia.
72. Superior sagital sinus thrombosis.

With regards to polyhydramnios, which of the following are correct?

73. The cause is identifiable in more than 60 per cent of cases.
74. The diagnosis can only be made on ultrasound scan.
75. Acute cases are more likely in twin-to-twin transfusion syndrome.
76. The incidence of unexplained stillbirth is higher when the aetiology is unexplained.

Oligohydramnios:

77. Is associated with renal agenesis in most cases.
78. May be due to fetal renal failure.
79. Is associated with congenital malformations in about 15 per cent of cases.
80. When its onset is before 25 weeks' gestation, neonatal mortality is of the order of 90 per cent.

Complications in the surviving twin of a monozygotic pregnancy with one intrauterine fetal death include

81. Bilateral renal cortical necrosis.
82. Multicystic encephalomalacia.
83. Hydrocephalus.

With regards to fetal hydrops

84. The diagnosis is based on the presence of fluid within at least one fetal cavity.
85. Non-immune hydrops is five times more common than the immune type.
86. The prognosis depends on the cause and the time of diagnosis.
87. Perinatal mortality is of the order of 30 per cent.

Concerning the detection of alloimunization

88. The colloid test is able to distinguish between IgG and IgM antibodies.
89. Indirect Coombs test assesses the presence of antibodies in the serum.
90. Direct Coombs test detects the presence of antibodies on the red cells from the patient.

Maternal autoimmune thrombocytopenia

91. Complicates seven to eight per cent of all pregnancies.
92. Is associated with an increased risk of fetal thrombocytopenia if it is symptomatic.
93. Splenectomy increases the risk of neonatal thrombocytopenia to about 40 per cent.
94. Haemorrhagic complications arise if the fetal platelet count is $30 \times 10^9/l$.
95. Is a contraindication to instrumental vaginal deliveries.
96. Fetal blood sampling should be avoided.

Fetal bradycardia

97. Uncomplicated is most likely to be secondary to hypoxia.
98. May result in hydrops.
99. If unprovoked should be managed by immediate delivery.

Congenital heart diseases

100. Complicates about one per cent of all pregnancies.
101. The best time for antenatal diagnosis is at 20 weeks' gestation.
102. Most are diagnosed from the four-chamber view of the heart.

With respect to parvovirus B19 infection

103. It causes fetal hydrops.
104. Viraemia develops one week after exposure.
105. It is an RNA virus.

Congenital infection with cytomegalovirus (CMV)

106. Is associated with cerebral calcifications.
107. Is a recognized cause of microcephaly.
108. May be detected by culture of the infant's urine.
109. Is associated with polyhydramnios.
110. Is associated with IUGR.
111. Is associated with thrombocytopenia.

Concerning tuberculosis in pregnancy

112. It is a notifiable disease.
113. Breastfeeding is contraindicated.
114. Infected patients must be screened for HIV.
115. The miliary form is more common.

Malaria infection in pregnancy

116. Is most commonly due to *Plasmodium falciparum*.
117. Congenital malaria is common.
118. May present as convulsions.
119. Placental infestation occurs in as many as 40–50 per cent of cases.

Neonates of drug-addicted mothers

120. Have withdrawal symptoms classically after four to five days.
121. Should be offered methadone.
122. Breastfeeding may worsen the symptoms of withdrawal.

The following drugs are considered teratogenic

123. Lithium.
124. Amphotericin B.
125. Zidovudine.
126. Thiazide diuretics.

Use of diethystilboestrol in pregnancy is associated with the following in the offspring

127. Clear cell carcinoma of the vagina.
128. Vagina agenesis.
129. Incompetent cervix.
130. Ovarian hypoplasia.

In a woman with severe pre-eclampsia

131. Creatinine clearance is raised.
132. Fibrinogen degradation products (FDPs) are normal.
133. Calcium levels are elevated.

Recognized effects of the administration of beta-sympathomimetic drugs in the third trimester include

134. Increased maternal pulse pressure.
135. Decreased maternal blood insulin concentration.
136. Increased surfactant production.
137. Reduced urine output.

Concerning shoulder dystocia

138. It occurs more frequently in macrosomic fetuses of diabetics.
139. Erb palsy is a recognized complication.
140. Brachial plexus injury involves nerve roots 5 and 6 more frequently than 7 and 8.
141. May be avoided by a generous episiotomy.

Pregnancy exacerbates the clinical features associated with

142. Sickle cell haemoglobinopathy.
143. von Recklingausen disease.
144. Peptic ulceration.
145. Bronchial asthma.
146. Eisenmenger syndrome.

Regarding peripartum cardiomyopathy

147. The mortality rate within the first year is more than 80 per cent.
148. Cardiac transplantation is inappropriate.
149. Anticoagulation is required.
150. Prophylactic antibiotics are required.

Endometrial ablation

151. Is effective in the treatment of menorrhagia secondary to adenomyosis.
152. Has a better patient satisfaction compared to that after hysterectomy.
153. Should only be performed in women who have completed their families.

After an abdominal hysterectomy, there are difficulties in waking up the patient from general anaesthesia (GA). Which of the following may be responsible?

154. Use of hypotensive agents.
155. Pulmonary oedema.
156. Myocardial infarction.

Concerning damage to viscera during gynaecological surgery

157. A crushing damage of the urethra should be corrected by resecting the damaged portion and re-anastomosis.
158. Damage to the bladder should be repaired with a non-absorbable suture material and a catheter left *in situ* for seven to 10 days.
159. A defunctioning colostomy is required after repair of damaged small bowel.
160. Following suspected perforation of the uterus, a laparotomy must be performed.

Incisional hernias

161. Are more likely after a Pfannenstiel incision than a midline incision.
162. Most occur within one year of surgery.
163. The best treatment is achieved by repairing with non-absorbable material.

Following massive haemorrhage.

164. Hyperkalaemia may be a complication of blood transfusion.
165. Fresh frozen plasma which contains the protein constituents of plasma, including the clotting factors, should be given.
166. Oxygen delivery is only impaired if the patient's haemoglobin drops below 22 per cent.
167. Hypothermia is a recognized complication of treatment.
168. Cryoprecipitate should be given if the fibrinogen level is less than 1.0 g/dl.

Testicular regression syndrome

169. Is familiar.
170. Is associated with normal testes at birth.
171. Provides evidence that other autosomally located genes play a role in testicular development.

In a fetus with 5-α reductase deficiency

172. There is failure of conversion of testosterone to dihydrotesterone in target tissues.
173. Masculinization at puberty is secondary to high circulating levels of androgens.
174. Partial androgen insensitivity may be associated with partial masculinization and breast growth.
175. There is no need to remove the gonads.

During the menstrual cycle

176. The luteinizing hormone (LH) surge begins at the same time as the follicle-stimulating hormone (FSH) surge.
177. Oestradiol 17-β peaks during the early luteal phase.
178. The mean duration of the LH surge is 36 hours.
179. Ovulation occurs 24 hours after the LH surge.
180. Endogenous opioids play a role in the regulation of the hypothalamic pituitary axis.

The following are recognized causes of precocious puberty

181. Hypothyroidism.
182. Craniopharyngioma.
183. McCune–Albright syndrome (polyostotic fibrous dysplasia).
184. Neurofibromatosis.

A child presents with labial adhesions

185. Reassure the mother and leave the child alone.
186. Prescribe topical oestrogen preparations after separating the labia.
187. Exclude congenital malformations of the upper genital tract.

A 21-year-old presented with primary amenorrhoea. She is one of three sisters – the others attained menarche at 11 and 13 years, respectively. On examination, the secondary sexual characteristics are normal. Some investigations were undertaken and the results are as follows: FSH = 7 IU/1, LH = 5 IU/l, 17-β oestradiol = 350 pmom/l, testosterone = 0.7 nmol/l, prolactin = 350 IU/l, chromosomes = 46XX. Which of the following are correct?

188. An obstruction to the lower genital tract is a likely cause of her amenorrhoea.
189. If she suffers from clyclical pain, the diagnosis is an imperforate hymen.
190. Ultrasound scan of the pelvis is more reliable than a magnetic resonance imaging (MRI) in diagnosing the cause.
191. The progesterone challenge test is an option in the evaluation of the cause of the amenorrhoea.

Concerning precocious puberty

192. Treatment with gonadotrophin-releasing hormone (GnRH) analogues results in atrophy of the breast.
193. May be associated with short stature.
194. Cyproterone acetate is an acceptable treatment option.
195. Radiotherapy should be considered if medical treatment fails.

The following are recognized causes of galactorrhoea in a 36-year-old woman

196. Phenopthiazines.
197. Haloperidol.
198. Metoclopramide.
199. Cimetidine.

Bromocryptine treatment

200. Causes postural hypotension.
201. Improves libido.
202. Will restore fertility in all cases of hyperprolactinaemia.
203. May be combined with the combined oral contraceptive pill in some patients.

Premature ovarian failure

204. Is defined as ovarian failure before the age of 35 years.
205. Is associated with a negative progesterone challenge test.
206. Occurs in 10–15 per cent of women presenting with secondary amenorrhoea.
207. Is best treated with hormone replacement to induce ovulation.

In unexplained infertility

208. Spontaneous conception rates close to 80 per cent are achievable if the duration is less than three years.
209. Treatment with clomiphene will improve conception rates.

A 26-year-old woman undergoing super-ovulation for infertility presents with severe ovarian hyperstimulation syndrome

210. She is at an increased risk of venous thrombo-embolism (VTE).
211. Renal function is normal in most of such patients.
212. In view of the haemoconcentration, she should be given isotonic fluids, such as normal saline.
213. The presence of a pleural effusion is an indication to abandon the infertility treatment.
214. If she becomes pregnant, she should be given human chorionic gonadotrophin (HCG) to support the pregnancy.

Antisperm antibodies can be detected by

215. Mixed aggluninin reaction (MAR) test.
216. Immunobead test.
217. Postcoital test.
218. Immunoabsorbent assay of the antibodies in semen.

Which of the following statements regarding male reproduction are correct?

219. Testosterone administration improves semen quality when there is oligozoospermia.
220. *Ureaplasma urealyticum* infection does not impair fertility.
221. Chronic renal failure is associated with impaired fertility.
222. Cystic fibrosis is a recognized cause of infertility.

Recognized regimens for super-ovulation include:

223. Clomiphene citrate and human menopausal gonodotrophin (HMG) and/or pure FSH.
224. HMG and/or pure FSH.
225. Tamoxifen and pure FSH.
226. GnRH analogues and oestrogens and progestogens.
227. Bromocryptine and pure FSH.

Ovarian hypersimulation syndrome

228. The risk is related to the total number of mature and immature follicles.
229. The incidence does not correlate with conception cycles.
230. Avoidance of sexual intercourse when there is a significant risk is an acceptable advice.
231. Spontaneous resolution will occur without treatment if there is a successful pregnancy.

Features associated with a missed abortion (failed pregnancy) include

232. Breast tenderness.
233. A brown vaginal discharge.
234. An empty amniotic sac.

A four-year-old presented with a persistent vaginal discharge that causes significant vulval irritation and staining of the underwear. The following statements about her management are correct

235. Sexual abuse should be considered as a cause.
236. Most cases are characterized by recurrence until puberty.
237. A broad-spectrum antibiotic should be prescribed.
238. Examination under anaesthesia (EUA) is indicated if the discharge is bloodstained.
239. Threadworm infections are unlikely if there is no associated itching.

Patients with polycystic ovary syndrome are more likely

240. To achieve regular cycles if they significantly lose weight.
241. To have an elevated plasma oestrone concentration.
242. To have abnormal testosterone concentration.
243. To have elevated levels of dehydroepiandrosterone sulphate.
244. To be hyperinsulinaemic.

Medroxyprogesterone acetate

245. Is effective in the treatment of endometriosis.
246. Is associated with breakthrough bleeding.
247. Induces endometrial hyperplasia.
248. Induces hypertension.

A pelvic abscess is associated with

249. Diarrhoea.
250. Bacteraemia.
251. Swinging pyrexia.

Carcinoma of the cervix

252. Is characteristically preceded by human papilloma virus (HPV) infection.
253. Characteristically originates from the transformation zone.
254. Is adenocarcinoma in less than 10 per cent of cases.
255. Stage II is commonly associated with ureteric obstruction.

The diagnosis of premenstrual syndrome may be confidently made from

256. Symptom diary chart.
257. A gonadotrophin analogue therapeutic trial test.
258. General health questionnaire.
259. Blood hormone assays performed throughout the ovarian cycle.

With regard to the menopause

260. Premature menopause is defined as cessation of menstruation before the age of 40 years.
261. Hypothalamic–pituitary activity changes are not obvious until two to three years before menopause.
262. During the phase of ovarian failure, the ovarian stroma ceases production of hormones.
263. The symptoms of menopause are related to the levels of FSH and LH.

Risk factors for osteoporosis include:

264. Cortisol therapy.
265. Hypothyroidism.
266. Chronic renal failure.
267. Prolonged lactation.

Hormone replacement therapy (HRT)

268. Increases the risk of VTE by two- to four-fold.
269. The combined form should be given to women with an intact uterus.
270. Is contraindicated in patients with previous VTE.
271. Increases the relative risk of breast cancer after five years.

If a woman on the combined oral contraceptive pill experiences breakthrough bleeding

272. Reassure her if the bleeding occurs within the first six months on the pill.
273. Exclude a co-existing gynaecological disorder if it persists.
274. Change from a 50 μg containing pill to a 30 μg containing pill.
275. Stop the pill immediately and observe for persistence of the bleeding as a means of excluding a co-existing cause.
276. Change the pill to one containing a different progestogen.

Concerning female sterilization:

277. The failure rate with Fishie clips is higher than with diathermy.
278. Up to 10 per cent of women regret their decision to undergo the procedure.
279. The failure rate is three per 1000.
280. There is an increased gynaecological consultation for menstrual problems following sterilization.

There is an increased incidence of postoperative burst abdomen with

281. Steroid therapy.
282. Mass closure.
283. The use of catgut to close the sheath.
284. Smoking.
285. Non-closure of the peritoneum.

The following procedures have been shown to significantly reduce the risk of adhesion formation after myomectomy

286. Plication of the round ligament.
287. Removal of posterior fibroids through an anterior uterine wall incision.
288. Instillation of concentrated solutions of dextran after surgery.
289. Use of oxidized regenerated cellulose in the peritoneal cavity after surgery.

With regards to cervical intra-epithelial neoplasia (CIN)

290. It rarely affects the gland crypts.
291. Cellular atypia is the most important abnormality when assessing CIN.
292. The squamocolumnar epithelium must be present for an adequate diagnosis to be made.
293. The proportion of the thickness of the epithelium showing differentiation is important in assessing the degree of severity.

Which of the following provisions of the Abortion Law in the UK are correct?

294. An abortion may only be performed by a medical practitioner.
295. Termination after the gestational age of 24 weeks must be after a fetocide.
296. Two gynaecologists or obstetricians must consent for a termination after 24 weeks' gestation.
297. Selective fetocide in a woman with triplets falls outside the bounds of the Abortion Law.
298. All terminations must be registered at the Office of Population and Censuses.

Concerning surgery for urethra sphincter incompetence

299. Anterior colporrhaphy is associated with a five-year cure rate of 70 per cent.
300. Colposuspension is commonly complicated by detrusor instability.

Answers to the multiple choice questions

1. T   2. T   3. T

Automsomal recessive (AR) genes or traits are only expressed in homozygotes for the gene. Horizontal inheritance occurs and affected individuals usually have normal parents. Mating between heterozygotes will produce individuals with a 25 per cent risk of being affected. Both sexes are equally affected, although AR genes may show a sex influence, for example haemachromoatosis is autosomal recessive but has a higher incidence in males due to a lower dietary iron intake and menstruation in females. There is an association with consanguinity.

4. F   5. T   6. T   7. T

Sex-linked defects are located on either the X or Y chromosomes. Y-linked inheritance is very rare. For X-linked inheritance, more males than females show the recessive phenotype, the disease is transmitted by a carrier female, who is usually asymptomatic. Sons of a carrier mother will have a 50 per cent chance of being affected while her daughters will have a 50 per cent chance of being carriers. Affected males usually have no affected offspring but all the daughters will be carriers and, in turn, 50 per cent of their sons will be affected.

8. T   9. F   10. T   11. T

Autosomal recessive conditions include cysic fibrosis, phenylketonuria, Tay–Sachs disease, sickle cell disease, Gaucher disease, thalassaemia and congenital adrenal hyperplasia. Autosomal dominant conditions include achondroplasia, retinoblastoma, tuberous sclerosus, Marfan syndrome, von Willebrand disease and familial hypercholesterolaemia.

12. T   13. T   14. F

Vitamin A in large doses is associated with congenital malformations and fetal growth restriction. Dietary supplementation is therefore restricted to 5000 IU. Folate supplementation is associated with a reduced incidence of neural tube defects. Periconception, multivitamin supplementation is associated with a reduction in the occurrence of hypertrophic pyloric stenosis, congenital cardiac defects, renal and obstructive uropathies. Liver extracts should be avoided in pregnancy. Vitamin C supplementation is not associated with congenital malformations.

15. F   16. T   17. F   18. F

In adolescent pregnancies, the incidence of sudden infant death syndrome is higher and the Caesarean section rates are not significantly higher. Whether or not the pregnancy is planned does not influence the interval between pregnancies. Anaemia is more common. The incidence of abnormal presentations is not different from that in older women.

19. F   20. F   21. T

Sickle cell disease is more common in Blacks but may occur in other races. The fetal head commonly enters the pelvis during labour in Blacks. G-6-PD deficiency is more common in the Mediterranean and Africa than south-east Asia.

22. F   24. F   26. F   28. F
23. T   25. F   27. F   29. F

Clostridiume welchii is not a recognized cause of recurrent miscarriages. However, gas gangrene is a recognized complication of incomplete miscarriages, especially those that become septic. Other complications of septic miscarriages include disseminated intravascular coagulation (DIC) and septicaemia. Medical management of failed pregnancies is about 80–85 per cent of cases.

30. F   31. F   32. T   33. F   34. F

Placental abruption present with abdominal pain. The diagnosis cannot be excluded by ultrasound scan and it is associated with an increased risk of congenital malformations. DIC is a recognized complication and in its presence, regional anaesthesia is contraindicated.

35. F   36. T   37. F   38. F

Most babies with echogenic bowels on ultrasound scan are normal. Other associated soft markers need to be excluded. This may be associated with cystic fibrosis, bowel obstruction, cytomegalovirus (CMV) infection and aneuploidy. In isolation, it is not an indication for karyotyping. The presence of two or more soft markers is an indication for karyotyping. Routine anomaly scans are able to identify on between 40 and 60 per cent of cardiac malformations.

39. F   40. F   41. T   42. F

Transplacental transfer of the HIV virus to the fetus can be minimized by antiviral treatment. Delivery by Caesarean section and the avoidance of breastfeeding will also reduce the risk of vertical transmission.

43. T   45. T   47. T   49. F   51. T   53. T   55. F
44. T   46. T   48. F   50. F   52. F   54. T

An abnormal nuchal translucency may be associated with thoracic malformations, cardiac malformations, aneuploidy and various poorly defined syndromes. However, most fetuses with a value of more than 3 mm are normal. The recurrence of neural tube defects (one to three per cent) tends to be concordant. They may be part of the abnormalities in Meckel–Gruber syndrome. Others include a posterior fossa cyst and renal malformations. Amniocentesis is not indicated to diagnose neural tube defects, but the presence of acetylcholinesterase in amniotic fluid is diagnostic of an open neural tube defect. Soft markers of aneuploidy include pyelectasis, cerebral ventriculomegaly, choriod plexus cyst, echogenic focus in the chest, short femur and Sandal gap.

56. T	57. F	58. F	59. F	60. F	61. T

Chorionic villus sampling (CVS) may theoretically be complicated by transverse limb defects, miscarriages and Rhesus isomimmunization. Mosaicism is reported in approximately one per cent of cases. Amniocentesis is not associated with orthopaedic deformities. Chorioamnionitis is the most common cause of miscarriages, which complicate between 0.5 and one per cent of cases. Isoimmunization may complicate amniocentesis.

62. F	63. F	64. F

Most stillbirths occur antenatally and intrauterine growth restriction (IUGR) is a common association. Most are unexplained but in general poor antenatal care is a recognized associated factor.

65. F	66. T	67. F	68. F

Maternal smoking is associated with a reduction in the incidence of pre-eclampsia, which reduces fetal breathing movements but not blood flow to the brain. It is not associated with fetal hypoglycaemia or amniorrhexis. It is a risk factor for stillbirth and VTE.

69. F	70. F	71. T	72. T

Neonatal complications of IUGR include hypoglycaemia, polycythaemia, thrombosis, hypothermia and necrotizing enterocolitis (NEC).

73. F	75. T	77. F	79. F
74. F	76. T	78. T	80. T

Acute polyhydramnios is more likely in monozygotic twin pregnancies. Most cases of polyhydramnios are idiopathic, are associated with unexplained stillbirths and may be diagnosed clinically by the present of a fluid thrill and a uterine fundus larger than dates. Oligogyhdramnios, on the other hand, may be due to renal agenesis, renal failure or congenital infections. Mortality is over 90 per cent when it occurs early because of pulmonary hypoplasia.

81. T	82. T	83. T

Following the death of one twin, the surviving twin has an increased risk of renal cortical necrosis, multicystic encehalomalacia and hydrocephalus. The risk of neurodevelopmental abnormality is considerably higher.

84. F	85. F	86. T	87. F	88. F	89. T	90. T

Fetal hydrops is diagnosed when fluid is present in at least two fetal cavities. The non-immune type is more common and the prognosis depends to an extent on the timing of the diagnosis. The earlier the diagnosis, the poorer the outcome. Alloimmunization may be assessed by Coombs test.

91. T	92. T	93. T	94. T	95. F	96. F

Maternal autoimmune thrombocytopenia complicates about eight per cent of all pregnancies. It may be associated with haemorrhagic complications in the fetus. Instrumental deliveries are contraindicated if the count is less than 30,000.

97. F	98. F	99. F	100. T	101. F	102. F

Congenital cardiac disease complicates approximately one per cent of all pregnancies. The best time of diagnosis is 22–24 weeks. The five-chamber view will diagnose close to 60 per cent of all cases. Hypoxia will induce complicated bradycardia and tachycardia may cause hydrops from heart failure.

103. T	105. F	107. T	109. T	111. T
104. T	106. T	108. T	110. T	

Fetal hydrops may be caused by parvovirus B19, CMV and toxoplasmosis. CMV may also cause echogenic bowel, cerebral calcifications and IUGR. CMV may be detected in the urine of the infant. Most viral infections may cause polyhydramnios, IUGR and thrombocytopenia in the fetus.

112. T	113. F	114. F	115. F

Tuberculosis is a notifiable disease, caused by *Mycobaterium tuberuli*. Infected mothers may breastfeed. Although its presence should increase the risk of HIV infection, screening should only be offered after counselling.

116. T	117. F	118. T	119. T

Malaria is commonly due to *Plasmodium falciparum*. It may cause miscarriages, preterm labour and IUGR. Placental infection occurs in up to 40–50 per cent of cases and when there is severe pyrexia, the mother may present with febrile convulsions.

120. F	122. F	124. T	126. T
121. F	123. T	125. F	

Neonates of addicted mothers may suffer from withdrawal symptoms and, in most cases, breastfeeding reduces the severity of withdrawal symptoms. Teratogenic drugs in pregnancy include vitamin A, lithium, amphotericin B and thiazide diuretics.

127. T	128. F	129. T	130. F

Diethystilboestrol exposure *in utero* is associated with clear cell carcinoma of the vagina, vaginal agenesis and cervical incompetence. It does not affect ovarian development, although the incidence of endometriosis is higher in these patients.

131. F   132. F   133. F

Abnormal changes which may be present in women with pre-eclampsia include raised fibrinogen degradation products (FDPs), thrombocytopenia and abnormal liver function tests (LFTs). Most of these abnormalities are only present in severe disease. Urinary function is only altered in severe disease.

134. T   135. F   136. F   137. T

Beta-sympathomimetic agent administration is associated with hyperglacaemia, hypotension, tachycardia and increased maternal insulin levels. Concomitant administration of steroids may increase the risk of pulmonary oedema.

138. F   139. T   140. F   141. F

Shoulder dystocia commonly occurs in macrosomic babies, although most of these are of diabetic mothers. Complications include fracture of the long bones, Erb's palsy and fracture of the clavicle. It is one of the important causes of litigation.

142. T	144. F	146. T	148. F	150. F
143. T	145. F	147. F	149. T	

Sickle cell anaemia, von Recklingausen disease and Eisenmenger syndrome are exacerbated in pregnancy. Pregnancy in women with HbSS is less severe than in women with HbSC. Peripartum cardiomyopathy is associated with a high maternal mortality, especially in the pueperium. Prophylactic antibiotics are not required in the management of peripartum cardiomyopathy.

151. T   152. F   153. T   154. T   155. T   156. F

Endometrial ablation should be performed in women who have completed their families because of the complications of pregnancy after this procedure. Some practitioners perform sterilization at the time of ablation. Endometrial ablation is effective in treating menorrhagia but not the dysmeonorrhoea of adenomyosis.

157. F   158. F   159. F   160. F

Visceral injuries occurring at the time of gynaecological surgery should be managed depending on the viscera and the type of injury. If there is a crushing injury to the urethra, an indwelling catheter would be sufficient. All injuries to the bladder involved complete breach of the wall should be repaired with an absorbable material and the bladder rested for seven to 10 days. A defunctioning colostomy is required when there is large bowel injury but each case must be assessed on its merit.

161. F   162. F   163. T

Incisional hernias are more common after vertical than transverse incisions. Most occur within 12 months of the initial surgery. They are best repaired by non-absorbable material.

164. T   165. F   166. T   167. T   168. T

Transfusions after massive haemorrhage may be complicated by hyperkalaemia, hypothermia and thrombocytopenia.

169. T   171. T   173. T   175. F
170. F   172. T   174. T

5-alpha reductase deficiency is characterised by masculinization at puberty and failure of conversion of testosterone to dihydrotestosterone at the target tissues. Testicular regression syndrome is familiar and at birth, the testicles are abnormal.

176. F   177. F   178. F   179. F   180. T

Physiological changes during the ovarian cycle include an LH surge which occurs 24 hours before ovulation. The LH surge does not begin at the same time of the FSH surge and ovulation occurs 24–36 hours after the LH surge.

181. T   182. T   183. T   184. T

Precocious puberty is defined as the occurrence of pubertal changes culminating in menstruation before the age of eight years. Recognized causes include hypothyroidism, craniophyaryngioma, neurofibromastosis and McCune–Albright syndrome.

185. F   186. T   187. F

Labial adhesions in a child could be treated with oestradiol cream. They are not usually associated with congenital malformations of the genital tract.

188. F   189. F   190. F   191. F

In a patient presenting with primary amenorrhoea, constitutional factors must be excluded. Investigations should not only be initiated after this has been excluded.

192. T   193. T   194. T   195. F

Acceptable treatment options for precocious puberty include gonadotrophin-releasing hormone (GnRH) agonists and cyproterone acetate.

| 196. T | 198. T | 200. T | 202. F |
| 197. T | 199. F | 201. T | 203. T |

Hyperprolactinaemia may be cause by pheothiazines, rauwalfia alkaloids, steroids, cimetidine, metoclopramide, steroids and antidepressant agents. Bromocryptine is a recognized treatment but it may be associated with hypotension.

| 204. F | 205. T | 206. T | 207. F | 208. T | 209. T |

Spontaneous conception rates up to 80 per cent occur in unexplained infertility of less than three years. Treatment with clomiphene citrate will improve conception rates. Premature ovarian failure is associated with a negative progestrone challenge test, occurs in about 15 per cent of women presenting with secondary amenorrhoea and treatment is usually ineffective.

| 210. T | 211. F | 212. F | 213. F | 214. F |

Ovarian hyperstimulation syndrome is more likely in women undergoing super-ovulation induction. Women with polycystic ovary syndrome are at a greater risk and when it occurs treatment should include correction for haemoconcentration. Infertility treatment should not be abandoned because of ovarian hyperstimulation syndrome. However, when it occurs, the pregnancy should be supported with progestogens rather than HCG.

| 215. T | 217. F | 219. F | 221. T |
| 216. T | 218. F | 220. F | 222. T |

Male infertility may be associated with antisperm antibodies, which may be identified with either a MAR or an immunobead test. Infections with *Ureaplasma urealyticum* are a recognized cause. The administration of testosterone is ineffective treatment. Cystic fibrosis and bronchiectasis is a recognized cause.

| 223. T | 225. F | 227. F | 229. F | 231. F |
| 224. T | 226. F | 228. T | 230. T | |

Induction of ovulation may be with a variety of regimens, which include clomiphene and gonadotrophins, HMG and pure FSH.

| 232. F | 233. T | 234. T |

Missed abortions (failed pregnancies) are associated with a brownish vaginal discharge and disappearing pregnancy symptoms. Most women will report a reduction in breast tenderness. In most cases, an ultrasound scan will reveal an empty gestational sac with no fetal pole.

235. T   236. T   237. F   238. T   239. T

Causes of a vaginal discharge in a four-year-old child include foreign bodies, trauma, infections (especially with parasites, such as threadworms), malignancies and sexual abuse. Clinical examination should be limited to inspection and if there is a need for a more detailed examination, this is best performed with the patient under general anaesthesia (GA).

240. T   241. T   242. T   243. F   244. T

Patients with polycystic ovary syndrome have an elevated plasma oestrone concentration and may be hyperinsulinaemic. Some of them are anovulatory. The diagnosis may be made either by ultrasound scan alone or by biochemistry alone.

245. T   246. T   247. F   248. F

Medroprogesterone acetate may be used as an effective contraceptive and is also effective in the treatment of endometriosis. It is associated with breast tenderness and functional ovarian cysts in about 15 per cent of cases. It is a 17-C progestogen and is therefore not associated with hypertension.

249. T   250. F   251. T

Pelvic abscesses may present with diarrhoea, a throbbing pain in the lower back and a swinging pyrexia.

252. F   253. T   254. F   255. F

Carcinoma of the cervix is more common in women with multiple sexual partners, especially in women with human papilloma virus (HPV) infection. It characteristically starts in the squamocolumnar region and the most common histological type is of the sqamous type. Involvement of the ureters would be suggestive of at least stage IIb.

256. T   257. T   258. F   259. F

Premenstrual syndrome is characterized with various psychosomatic symptoms, which are best demonstrated with a symptom diary chart. The diagnosis can be made with a therapeutic GnRH agonist trial.

260. T   262. F   264. T   266. T   268. T   270. F
261. F   263. F   265. T   267. T   269. F   271. T

Risk factors for osteoporosis include cortisol therapy, hypothyroidism, chronic renal failure, prolonged lactation, early menopause and being underweight. Hormone replacement therapy (HRT) increases the risk of VTE two-fold. Women with an intact uterus would benefit from combined therapy but this is not suitable for every patient. The risk of breast cancer is increased after five years on HRT.

272. F   273. T   274. F   275. F   276. T

The contraceptive pill may induce breakthrough bleeding and when this occurs within six months of starting, reassuring the patient is enough. A change of the pill may correct the complication. When this persists, there may be a need to investigate with a hysteroscopy.

277. F   278. T   279. F   280. T

Female sterilization is associated with a failure rate of one per 200. This is higher with diathermy than with clips. Gynaecological consultation for menstrual problems after sterilization is increased and the risk of hysterectomy is higher in women who have been sterilized.

281. T   282. F   283. T   284. T   285. F

Burst abdomen is a complication that is more common in immunosuppressed patients, those having surgery for malignancy and patients on steroids. Chronic cough and smoking are risk factors for this complication.

286. F   287. F   288. F   289. F

Adhesion formation in gynaecological surgery may be reduced by the use of Adept and intercede. Various surgical procedures have been tried unsuccessfully to reduce adhesion formation.

290. F   291. F   292. F   293. T

Cervical intra-epithelial neoplasia may affect gland crypts. The most important abnormalities are the changes in the nucleus of the cells. Most cases can be treated with large loop excision of the transformation zones (LLETZ).

294. F   295. F   296. F   297. F   298. T

Termination of pregnancies in the UK must comply with the Abortion Act, which was passed in 1967 and amended in the Human and Embryology Fertilization Act of 1990. Two medical practitioners (who need not be gynaecologist) must sign the blue form before the termination is undertaken. Selective fetocide must comply with the Abortion Act. There is no requirement for the terminations to be performed only in hospitals. All terminations must be registered with the Office of Population and Censuses.

299. F   300. F

Urethral sphincter incompetence is a synonym for urodynamic (genuine) stress incontinence. The current treatment for this condition is either a colposuspension or transvaginal free vaginal tapes (TVT). Treatment with anerior colporrhaphy is associated with a five-year survival rate of 60 per cent.

Section Five

The structured oral examination (OSCE)

1

Introduction

The objective structured clinical examination (OSCE) has replaced the traditional clinical component of the MRCOG Part 2 examination. It ensures that candidates are exposed to the same scenarios, eliminates to some extent examiner and patient bias and allows a more comprehensive assessment of clinical competencies. Critics argue that the OSCE assesses clinical competences in an artificial environment, which bears no resemblance to reality. Candidates and examiners are often conscious of this and, although role-players have traditionally tried to simulate real clinical interactions, shortcomings remain. However, there is no doubt that it is a fairer examination and one that removes the problems of recruiting co-operative patients for extensive clinical examinations. Since its introduction, the assessment has continued to evolve and I believe that this is for the better. As we become more experienced with this type of examination, we will build on its strengths and modify its weaknesses to make it better.

The examination itself consists of a dozen, 15-minute stations. Two of these are preparatory stations. Each station assesses a different aspect of clinical practice. Once you have passed the written part of the examination, the Royal College of Obstetricians and Gynaecologists (RCOG) will send you information about this part of the examination. This package includes advice on how to prepare for the examination. Since it is a clinical examination, the best way is not to bury your head in books but to concentrate on your clinical skills. It is also advisable to be familiar with the themes that have been in the spotlight about four to six months before the examination.

Unfortunately for those coming from overseas for the examination, the standards required are those of practitioners in the UK. It may seem unfair on them, but it is important for consistency and the maintenance of standards that there is some clinical standard by which to judge candidates. Overseas candidates may be wise to spend a few weeks in the UK observing clinical practice, especially communication skills and attitudes towards patients. These are definitely some of the areas in which they may have difficulties.

This section of the book is aimed only at introducing candidates to the oral part of the examination. There is no point in mastering all the concepts in this section, or indeed the contents, when you have not passed the written examination. What I hope to achieve in this section is to broaden candidates' knowledge of the type of questions they may face in the examination. It is difficult, here, to provide in-depth materials for the oral examination, as the best 'book' is the patients and the environment in which they are seen. You may wish to consult a textbook on OSCEs written by the author for more practice questions. The details are given in the recommended reading list (Chapter 4 of this section).

2

Sample OSCE questions

Station 1

Despite the increased awareness of the possible consequences of improperly managed extrauterine pregnancy, it remains an important cause of maternal morbidity and mortality in the UK. How will you draw up a protocol for the management of ectopic pregnancies in your unit and how will you assess the success of your protocol?

Station 2

Mrs BAY is 40 years old. She has been referred for contraceptive advice. You are required to take a history from her and offer her the most appropriate contraceptive advice. You may wish to ask the examiner for additional information.

Station 3

You are about to see a 29-year-old woman who is scheduled for a laparoscopically assisted vaginal hysterectomy and bilateral salpingoophorectomy because of endometriosis. She had a pregnancy three years ago but miscarried at 10 weeks' gestation. Your task is to undertake the counselling before surgery on this patient.

Station 4

Mrs T is 67 years old and has attended the gynaecology clinic after urodynamic investigations for urinary incontinence, which revealed urodynamic (genuine) stress incontinence. You saw her four months ago and, on pelvic examination, found nothing. You will be required to explain the diagnosis and treatment of choice to Mrs T. Assume that she is fit and well and wants to have a Burch colposuspension. She is not interested in the tension free vaginal tape (TVT) procedure.

Station 5

You are the SpR in a unit and are about to see a 51-year-old lady who had a total abdominal hysterectomy and bilateral salpingoophorectomy by your team five days ago for atypical hyperplasia of the endometrium, having presented with postmenopausal vaginal bleeding. The histology report is available but she is yet to be informed of its contents. The histology report is enclosed.

> MARKS WILL BE AWARDED FOR CANDIDATES' ABILITY TO INFORM, DISCUSS THE DIAGNOSIS AND SUBSEQUENT MANAGEMENT WITH THE PATIENT

Specimen: uterus, Fallopian tubes and ovaries

Clinical history
Complex hyperplasia on biopsy of endometrium from endometrial biopsy. Total abdominal + bilateralsalpingoophorectomy done; appears to be a malignancy of endometrium with ? involvement of the cervix.

Macroscopic
Opened uterus and cervix and both tubes and ovaries 115 × 95 × 80 mm. Macroscopic tumour 100 × 40 × 35 mm, maximum depth 15 mm, involving endometrial cavity and invading into cervix. Left ovary 35 × 25 × 10 mm with cystic areas. Left Fallopian tube 55 mm. Right ovary 30 × 20 × 10 mm, with cystic areas. Right Fallopian tube 15 mm. The uterus was received opened with resulting contamination of the fixative with multiple pieces of tumour. This has led to problems with interpretation of the histology detailed below.

Microscopic
The endometrium is almost completely replaced by tightly packed abnormal endometrial glands forming a trabecular pattern with some villiform areas, set in a fibrous stroma. The epithelium is pseudostratified and consists of columnar cells with vesicular oval nuclei showing a low degree of nuclear pleomorphism. This endometrioid adenocarcinoma is intramucosal in some areas, but in others invades into the inner half of the myometrium. The serosa is not breached, although there are probable contaminant tumour deposits on the surface. In multiple endometrial blocks there is evidence of tumour invasion into small and large blood vessels. The cervix is invaded by tumour. The right and left cornua are not involved with tumour. In the left and right parametria, there are multiple areas of tumour deposits between tissue planes. This is difficult to interpret, but the appearance is suggestive of postoperative contamination rather than true spread of tumour. The left ovary contains a luteinized follicle. Peripheral contamination with tumour is noted in the left Fallopian tube. A Müllerian inclusion cyst is noted in the connective tissue between the right ovary and Fallopian tube. Again, probable contaminant tumour is noted in tissue planes in this region.

Conclusion
Well-differentiated endometrioid carcinoma of the endometrium, grade 1, invading cervix, inner half of the myometrium and blood vessels.

Station 6

Mrs Jones had *in vitro* fertilization (IVF) and had a twin pregnancy. She went into spontaneous labour at 39 weeks' gestation and is now fully dilated. The first twin is cephalic with the vertex at the introitus. How will you conduct the delivery of Mrs Jones?

> YOU WILL BE AWARDED MARKS ON THE CONDUCT OF TWIN DELIVERY

Station 7

A general practitioner (GP) has referred a patient to the gynaecology clinic with the following letter. Read the letter below and then obtain the relevant history from the patient. You are expected to discuss the management options with her. The examiner will provide you with additional information should you require it.

Holly Tree Surgery
Wooden House Lane
Thorpes Beast Village
Walthome WN2 SU7

Dear Dr —

Would you be kind enough to see this 38-year-old woman who has been suffering from very heavy periods for the past four years. When I examined her, I noted that her uterus was 24 weeks' size and an ultrasound scan confirmed the presence of uterine fibroids. Her haemoglobin was 7.5 g/dl and I therefore placed her on iron tablets. She has recently been diagnosed with HIV and is currently on triple anti-viral therapy. Her CD4 count has improved significantly since she was commenced on this therapy by the GUM physicians.

Thank you for your help.

Yours sincerely

Peter Bowels DRCOG, MRCGP, MBCHB (Leic)

> YOU WILL BE AWARDED MARKS FOR YOUR ABILITY TO TAKE A RELEVANT
> HISTORY, EXPLAIN THE INVESTIGATIONS, TREATMENT OPTIONS AND THE
> VARIOUS ISSUES RAISED BY THIS PATIENT'S PROBLEMS

Station 8

Mrs Potter, a 67-year-old retired teacher, presented to the gynaecology outpatient department with urinary incontinence. Various investigations were performed and she was offered Burch colposuspension on account of a diagnosis of urodynamic (genuine) stress incontinence diagnosed on uroflometry. She has attended for a preoperative assessment. You are the SpR in the unit and have been asked to obtain her consent for the operation.

Station 9

You are the SpR on call for gynaecology. You have been handed over the following problems at 0830 on Monday:

1. A 22-year-old with six weeks' amenorrhoea, abdominal pain and vaginal bleeding. She presented at 0630. Her haemoglobin (Hb) is 12.6 g/dl. She is suspected of having an ectopic pregnancy but is clinically stable.
2. Mrs Green presented 45 minutes ago at 10 weeks' gestation with vaginal bleeding. She was initially clinically stable but has been in very severe pains for the last 20 minutes and is now in shock. When she was examined on admission, the cervical os was closed.
3. Mrs BJY is 78 years old and had surgery for ovarian cancer yesterday. She is not yet eating and drinking. Her drip has tissued and it is time for her intravenous drugs.
4. Miss TTO is 14 weeks pregnant and presented in acute urinary retention. She is yet to be seen by a doctor.
5. Mrs Bailey has attended for surgery and is still to be consented. She is the first on the list, which starts at 0830 hours.

The staff available on the ward include the Senior House Officer (who is a GP trainee) and three nursing staff – one senior and the others junior).

> MARKS WILL BE AWARDED FOR YOUR ABILITY TO MANAGE THESE PATIENTS AND PRIORITIZE THEM

Station 10

Investigations and treatment for menorrhagia are an important and expensive part of most gynaecological units in the UK. There is increasing concern, however, about the variable standards of care women with this complication receive in various units. You have been mandated to undertake the process of ensuring that the best quality of care is provided to women attending your gynaecological unit with this problem. How will you set about achieving this process?

> MARKS WILL BE AWARDED ON HOW THE PROCESS IS UNDERTAKEN AND EVALUATED

Station 11

You are the SpR on the delivery suite and the midwife has crash-bleeped you for a shoulder dystocia. Describe how you will manage this complication.

Station 12

The patient you are about to see has been referred to your outpatient clinic by her GP. A copy of the referral letter is given below. Read the letter and obtain any relevant history from the patient. You should discuss any relevant investigations and treatment that you feel may be indicated. The examiner will provide you with the results of the pelvic examination when requested.

Blaston Surgery
Market Place
Blaston LE7 9JA

Dear Dr —

I would be grateful if you could see Mrs Daisy Plummer, aged 41. She has been having increasingly heavy periods over the last year and has failed to respond to medical treatment

Yours sincerely

Peter Crustmond MBBS, DRCOG, MRCGP

> YOU WILL BE AWARDED MARKS FOR YOUR ABILITY TO TAKE A HISTORY AND EXPLAIN ANY INVESTIGATIONS AND TREATMENT TO THE PATIENT

Station 13

Mrs B, a lawyer, and her husband, a business executive, had an unexplained stillbirth at 40 weeks' gestation. Mrs B has attended for postnatal follow-up. The results of the various investigations performed after the delivery, are as follows:

- HbAIC   5 per cent (normal 5 to 7 per cent)
- Thyroid function test   Normal
- Infection screen   Normal
- Autopsy   Normal external and internal structures
- Placenta   Fibrinoid areas scattered within the placenta with some areas of vascular occlusion
- Anticardiolipin Ab   (IgG) 16 (normal (0–14 IU/ml)
- Lupus anticoagulant   1.13 (0.1–1.09)
- Factor V Leiden   1.24 (>2.5)
- Other thrombophilias   Normal

Could you conduct her post-natal visit?

Station 14

A 29-year-old woman in her third pregnancy presents in labour at 39 weeks' gestation. A vaginal examination reveals an undiagnosed breech. She is 4 cm dilated and the membranes are intact. The two previous pregnancies were full-term normal deliveries and the babies weighed 3678 g and 3401 g, respectively.

Station 15

You arrive on the delivery suite and the board has 10 patients. The sister-in-charge quickly runs through the problems, telling you that it is busy and she is short of staff. The 10 patients are as follows:

- Room 1: a 27-year-old with a previous Caesarean section for failure to progress in the second stage, in labour for 12 hours and complaining of abdominal pain.
- Room 2: Mrs JT – a primigravida at 35 weeks' gestation with premature rupture of fetal membranes and having variable decelerations.
- Room 3: Mrs. James with uncomplicated twins in early labour at 37 weeks' gestation.
- Room 4: a primipara who has been fully dilated and pushing for two hours.
- Room 5: a 32-year-old primigravida with an undiagnosed breech in labour at 39 weeks' gestation.
- Room 6: Mrs PJ with abdominal pains at 26 weeks' gestation.
- Room 7: a 42-year-old primigravida at 38 weeks' gestation presenting with vaginal bleeding
- Room 8: a patient in normal labour.
- Room 9: another patient in normal labour.
- Room 10: a 28-year-old who delivered four hours ago and is being observed for a post-operative pyrexia of 37.6°C.

At the next station, you will meet the examiner with whom you will discuss your decisions and your reasoning.

> YOU WILL BE AWARDED MARKS FOR YOUR ABILITY TO MANAGE THE
> DELIVERY SUITE

Station 16

A primigravida attended for her anomaly scan at 18 weeks' gestation and the fetus was found to have a diaphragmatic hernia and bilateral talipes equinovarus. She has been informed of the abnormalities by the radiographer. How will you set about managing this patient?

Station 17

The induction rate of a unit is said to reflect the standard of obstetric care and supervision within it. You work in a unit where the induction rate is 30 per cent. Discuss the process of auditing the inductions in the unit and how you will close the audit loop.

Station 18

Mr B and his wife attended the gynaecology clinic with primary infertility. The couple were investigated and the following results were obtained from a semen analysis, which was repeated twice:

- Time of production   0930
- Time of examination   1015
- Volume   3 ml
- Count   500,000/ml
- Motility   50 per cent
- Morphology   50 per cent
- Cells   1–3/ml

The investigations on Mrs B revealed mild endometriosis, predominantly on the posterior peritoneum and the uterosacral ligaments. How will you counsel the couple on the cause of their infertility and what management will you recommend

3

Marking schemes

Station 1

Structured mark sheet

MedLine search/literature review

- Prevalence of ectopic pregnancies
- Causes of ectopic pregnancy

0   1

High-risk groups – defining them

- Previous *Chlamydia trachomatis* or *Neisseria gonorrhoea* infection
- Previous ectopic pregnancies
- Single and promiscuous/multiple sexual partners
- Intrauterine contraceptive device (IUCD) use
- Tubal surgery
- Infertility treatment

0   1   2   3   4   5

Proforma for identification of patient with a possible ectopic pregnancy

- History – pain, irregular vaginal bleeding, vaginal discharge
- Amenorrhoeic
- Shoulder tip pain
- Tenderness (abdomen and cervical, especially excitation tenderness)
- Adnexal mass fullness in the pouch of Douglas

0   1   2   3   4

Investigations

- βHCG – quantification – important cut-off levels for the identification of an intra-uterine gestation sac
- Serial measurements of βHCG
- Ultrasound – transvaginal/abdominal

0   1   2

Treatment

- Surgery
- Medical

0   1

Audit of outcome of protocol

- Diagnosis
- Treatment
- Missed cases
- Ruptured ectopics

0   1   2   3

Dissemination

- Audit outcome to members of the unit
- Implementing changes identified

0   1

Total mark is out of 20

Comments

It is important to remember that there are two parts to the question. Most candidates will go straight to the audit part. The protocol part actually carries more marks and failure to address this will result in failure. Although audit and drawing up of protocols have always been important aspects of good clinical practice, the advent of clinical governance has made it mandatory for any unit to demonstrate that these components are routinely undertaken. Such a demand means that all trainees must understand the concepts involved and, indeed, must have taken part in either activity. It is therefore only right that the MRCOG examination assesses candidates' ability in this aspect of clinical practice. Most revision courses will, no doubt, go through the routine of audit and how to conduct one. It is important to remember that examiners are aware of this and you should therefore not go into the exams prepared to regurgitate everything you know about audit without relating it to the context of the examination.

How to approach the question

A good starting point is to do a literature/MedLine search. You should be familiar with sources of information and their drawbacks. Sources include the Cochrane Reviews, Royal College of Obstetricians and Gynaecologists (RCOG) guidelines, randomized controlled trials, case-controlled studies, care reports, retrospective reviews, etc. Also remember that the National Institute for Clinical Excellence (NICE) produces guidelines. When undertaking this search, you need to focus on the relevant aspects for your protocol. For example, when drawing up a protocol for the identification and management of intrauterine growth restriction (IUGR), your search will focus on the known causes of IUGR and the populations at risk, the incidence, diagnosis and management (monitoring and timing of delivery). You would then like to produce a proforma on how to identify at-risk groups and how to monitor them to diagnose IUGR when it develops, how to monitor the fetuses, and when and how to deliver. Obviously, any protocol must demonstrate a benefit to the unit and this can only be done from data on outcome. This must be built into the protocol.

For any audit, the starting point is to define the standards to be used as benchmark for comparison. Identifying these standards can sometimes be difficult but you should once again consider the following sources:

- Cochrane Reviews
- Meta-analyses
- RCOG guidelines
- NICE guidelines
- Randomized controlled trials
- Other types of studies
- Other units
- Textbooks
- Opinions of respected colleagues

Candidates must be aware of the limitations of the different types of evidence.

Once the standards have been defined, a proforma should be designed to enable information to be gathered. There are two types of audit – prospective and retrospective. The advantages and disadvantages of each type should be familiar to candidates. It is often advisable to consult the audit unit to help with the design of the proforma and also to calculate the power for the audit. This ensures that the outcome measures are statistically acceptable and may therefore alter practice.

Once the information-gathering is complete, data should be analysed and presented to all the stakeholders. Recommendations should be discussed and agreed upon. Once everyone has bought into these recommendations, they should be implemented and a timeframe after which they are re-audited defined.

Candidates should be aware of the following questions:

- How will you ensure that everyone in the unit buys into the recommendations?
- What if, one of the consultants refuses to accept the recommendations?
- There is nothing in the literature to provide standards for the audit.
- How to disseminate the results of the audit to the stakeholders.
- How to implement the protocol without marginalizing colleagues (especially as there is often great anxiety about change).

Station 2

Role-player's instruction

You are a 40-year-old housewife and mother of three. Your last child was born three years ago. During the pregnancy, you developed a high blood pressure, which required hospitalization and treatment with methyldopa. You had once been on the combined oral contraceptive pill when you were 24 years and took it for six years until you were married. Your mother died from a stroke and your weight has been increasing. You are fit and well, and do not smoke, but drink alcohol socially. You consider yourself to be generally well-informed about women's issues and you have read a lot of information from the internet and in women's magazines about contraception. You believe that you are very clear in your mind as to what is the most effective contraception for you, and indeed, what you want (the combined oral contraceptive pill). In general, your periods are regular and the last menstruation was three weeks ago. In your past medical history, you had your gallbladder removed three years ago.

Structured mark sheet

History

- Menstrual history
- Obstetric history
- Previous contraception
- Past medical history
- Drug history
- Family history
- Gynaecological and sexual history
- Social history

0	1	2	3	4	5	6	7

Physical examination (the examiner will provide this information but must only do so when the candidates says he/she would like to examine the patient)

- Obese – weight   95 kg
- Blood pressure (BP)   145/85 mmHg (with a large cuff)
- Essentially normal pelvic organs
- No breast lumps

0	1	2	3

Advice on contraception

- Combined oral contraceptive pill – not suitable for her (obese, blood pressure high, mother died of stroke)

- Alternatives – intrauterine contraceptive device (IUCD), sterilization, Implanon, the mini-pill – discuss each and the complications
- Vasectomy as an option

0   1   2

Options

- Consider referral to family planning centre
- May require screening for thrombophilia

0   1   2

Communication

- Introduction and putting the patient at ease
- Communicating at an appropriate level
- Encourages questions and provides suitable answers

0   1   2

Total mark is out of 20

Station 3

Structured mark sheet

Review

- The notes patient's notes
- Enquire after her symptoms to ensure that they have not changed
- Confirm that she is having the surgery for which she is scheduled
- Does the patient understand what is going to have done?

0   1   2   3

Explain the surgery in layman's terms – some details of what is to be done

- Complications of surgery
- Haemorrhage
- Injury to viscera
- May be converted to an abdominal surgery
- Other complications and how they will be managed

0   1   2   3   4

Implications for taking the ovaries out at this young age

- Risk of CVS, osteoporosis

0   1

Alternative to surgery

- Mirena coil
- Cyclooxygenase inhibitors

0   1

Recovery

- Time in hospital
- Time off work

0   1

Total mark is out of 20

Station 4

Examiner's instructions

Use the structured mark sheet for the assessment of this station. You may ask the candidates direct questions aiming to ascertain whether they understand the surgical procedure and postoperative management.

Structured mark sheet

Explanations

- The diagnosis to the patient
- Ensuring that the symptoms have not changed

0   1

Description of the surgical procedure – in detail, but not to frighten the patient

- Abdominal incision under adequate anaesthesia (usually general anaesthesia, GA)
- Surgery in the retropubic area and around the urethra
- Indwelling catheter – suprapubic or urethral
- Drain if necessary
- Success rate of the procedure (~85 per cent five-year cure rate)

0   1   2   3   4

Postoperative management

- Management of the catheter
- Need for thrombo-prophylaxis
- Follow-up in the gynaecology clinic

0   1   2

Complications and how they will be managed

- Haemorrhage
- Damage to the bladder
- Difficulties with voiding after removal of the catheter

0   1   2

Others

- Duration of stay in the hospital
- Return to work
- Support at home

0   1   2

Communication

- Introduction
- Use of non-medical language

0   1

Total mark is out of 20

Station 5

Examiner's instructions

Use the structured mark sheet for the assessment of this station. You may ask the candidate direct questions about chemotherapy and why the need for adjuvant therapy.

Structured mark sheet

Explanation

- Of the diagnosis to the patient

0   1   2   3

Introduction

- Non-medical language

0   1   2

Implications for diagnosis

- Need for further treatment
- Need for further investigations
- Long-term follow-up
- Referral to oncologist

0   1   2   3   4

Adjuvant therapy

- Radiotherapy
- External and vault

0   1   2

Complications of radiotherapy

- Diarrhoea
- Nausea and vomiting
- Cystitis
- Skin burns

0   1   2   3   4

Communication

- Inviting questions
- Listens to patient and does not interrupt

0   1   2

Follow-up

- Radiotherapist/clinical oncologists
- Gynaecological oncologist/joint clinics

0   1   2   3

Total mark is out of 20

Station 6

Examiner's instructions

Score the candidate on the structured mark sheet. Candidates are expected to describe their conduct of delivery of the twins, including the management of any complications. You are at liberty to ask specific questions, especially about the retained second twin and the need for a breech extraction.

Structured mark sheet

Ensure

- Intravenous (i.v.) line
- Paediatrician is available
- Anaesthetist is available

0   1   2   3

Delivery

- Twin 1 as normal
- Abdominal examination – lie and presentation of Twin 2
- Exterior cephalic version (ECV) if necessary
- Ensure contractions; may require syntocinon
- Descent of presenting part
- Artificial/spontaneous rupture of membranes?
- Conduct of delivery

0   1   2   3   4   5   6   7   8

If fetal distress?

- Breech extraction
- Caesarean section
- Internal podalic version and breech extraction
- Ventouse/forceps delivery

0   1   2   3   4   5   6

Third stage

- Watch out for postpartum haemorrhage
- Prevention against postpartum haemorrhage

0   1   2   3

Total mark is out of 20

Station 7

Role-player's instruction

You are a 38-year-old happily married woman with very heavy periods of four years' duration. Your periods are regular, occurring every 28–30 days and lasting for six to eight days. Four years ago they were only lasting for three to four days. You have to change your heavy-duty pads every two hours on days one to five of your periods. You pass clots, and commonly bleed through the pads. At the end of each period, you feel very weak and listless. You are currently on iron tablets as your iron level was low. The bleeding is very embarrassing and you have to stay home during the heavy periods. Your GP has offered you various drugs, including ponstan, norethisterone and cyclokapron to no avail. You have no children and have been trying for a family for the past three years. You would very much like to have a child. Your last menstrual period was three weeks ago and you started menstruating at the age of 12 years.

Past medical history

- Had been an i.v. drug user (sharing needles) for six years but stopped last year
- Recently diagnosed as human immunodeficiency virus (HIV) positive and receiving three different drugs from the genito-urinary medicine (GUM) clinic
- Had appendix removed at the age of 17

Social history

- Drinks alcohol occasionally but smoke 20 cigarettes per day

Instructions to the examiner

At this station, candidates will have 15 minutes to obtain a history relevant to the patient's complaint. Candidates should then ask you for the examination findings before proceeding to discuss the investigations and treatment options they feel are necessary for the patient.

Examination findings

- General examination – pale but not jaundiced
- Looks generally healthy
- Abdominal examination – uniformly distended, obvious mass arising from the pelvis to the size of a 26-week gestation. Irregular and firm in consistency. No ascites Pelvic examination – no lower genital tract abnormality. Abdominal mass appears to be uterine in origin
- Investigations: full blood count (FBC)/iron stores; thyroid function test; ultrasound scan; semen analysis; 21-day progesterone
- Management options

Medical treatment

- Danazole – temporary but will reduce periods and maybe size of fibroids (will affect fertility and not advisable if pregnancy is planned – risk of virilizing female fetus)
- Gonadotrophin-releasing hormone (GnRH) agonists – effective in controlling periods and fibroid size but not permament (will be associated with anovulation and therefore pregnancy not possible during treatment)
- Advantage of medical treatment – will allow time for haemoglobin (Hb) to improve and HIV control to be maximized before embarking on further surgery or pregnancy

Surgical

- Myomectomy – risk of progression to hysterectomy, risk of needle injury to surgeon
- Hysterectomy – option most unlikely to be acceptable

Interventional radiological

- Uterine artery embolization

Other issues

- HIV – fertility (need counselling on HIV and fertility treatment)
- Counselling about chances of success

Structured mark sheet

Introduction

- Putting patient at ease
- Non-medical language
- Eye contact
- Listens to patient/does not interrupt
- Invites questions

0   1   2   3   4

History

- Symptoms
- Duration
- Menstrual history
- Period before onset of menorrhagia
- Infertility/obstetric history
- Past medical history – HIV and treatment
- Social history – previous drug abuser and smoking

0   1   2   3   4   5   6

Investigations

- Hb/iron stores
- Ultrasound scan
- Thyroid function test
- 21-day progesterone
- Semen analysis
- Explanation of tests

0   1   2   3   4   5

Treatment

- Medical: GnRH anallogues; danazole
- Surgery: myomectomy; hysterectomy; uterine artery embolization
- Explanation of the treatment options

0   1   2   3   4   5

Total mark is out of 20

Station 8

Examiner's instructions

Use the structured mark sheet for the assessment of this station. You may ask the candidates direct questions aiming to ascertain whether they understand the surgical procedure and post-operative management.

Structured mark sheet

Explanation

- Of the diagnosis to the patient
- Ensuring that the symptoms have not changed

0   1   2

Communication

- Introduction
- Use of non-medical language

0   1   2

Description

- Of the surgical procedure – in detail, but not to frighten the patient
- Abdominal incision under adequate anaesthesia (usually GA)
- Surgery in the retropubic area and around the urethra
- Indwelling catheter – suprapubic or urethral
- Drain if necessary
- Success rate of the procedure (-85 per cent five-year cure rate)

0   1   2   3   4   5   6

Postoperative management

- Management of the catheter
- Need for thrombo-prophylaxis
- Follow-up in the gynaecology clinic

0   1   2   3

Complications and how they will be managed

- Haemorrhage
- Damage to the bladder
- Difficulties with voiding after removal of the catheter

0   1   2   3

Others

- Duration of stay in the hospital
- Return to work
- Support at home

0   1   2   3   4

Total mark is out of 20

Station 9

Examiner's instructions

Candidates have 15 minutes to explain to you the following: the tasks that need doing on the gynaecology ward; and the order in which they would do them and which staff they would allocate to each task.

Structured mark sheet

Tasks

- Patient 1: ensure FBC, group and save, arrange ultrasound scan and book theatre for diagnostic laparoscopy ? proceed
- Patient 2: ensure i.v. line, blood grouped and saved/cross-matched. Vaginal examination, resuscitate, inform theatre and anaesthetist, arrange evacuation
- Patient 3: resite i.v. line and administer drug
- Patient 4: pass catheter and arrange ultrasound scan
- Patient 5: obtain consent and notify theatre of possible delay

0	1	2	3	4	5	6	7	8	9	10

Prioritization/delegation

- Priority is Patient 2. SHO to site venflon, whilst SpR performs a speculum/vaginal examination; remove products of conception from cervix. Nurse to phone theatre to delay list. Anaesthetist to be summoned if necessary
- Delegate nurse to catheterize Patient 4
- SHO to site venflon in Patient 4 after doing same for Patient 2
- Nurse to contact ultrasound department to arrange scan for Patient 1
- SHO to obtain blood from Patient 1 for group and save, HCG
- SpR to consent Patient 5

0	1	2	3	4	5	6	7	8	9	10

Total mark is out of 20

Station 10

Examiner's instructions

At this station, the candidates' task is to design an audit of investigations and treatment of menorrhagia within their hospital. They must demonstrate their understanding of the audit cycle and how to close the loop. You may ask specific questions to enable you assess these aspects properly.

Structured mark sheet

Standards

- Definining national/international standards
- Aware of the courses of these standards: Royal College of Obstetricians and Gynaecologists (RCOG) guidelines; journals; NICE; Cochrane Reviews
- Types of evidence: randomized controlled trials, etc.

| 0 | 1 | 2 | 3 | 4 | 5 | 6 | 7 |

Communication

- Agreeing within the unit on the need for the audit
- Deciding on an acceptable protocol for the audit

| 0 | 1 | 2 | 3 |

Definitions

- Defining the period of audit
- Type of audit (prospective/retrospective) – advantages and disadvantages

| 0 | 1 | 2 | 3 | 4 | 5 |

Presentation

- Of results
- Actions/recommendations
- Implementation
- Re-audit

| 0 | 1 | 2 | 3 | 4 | 5 |

Total mark is out of 20

Station 11

Examiner's instructions

At this station, candidates have 15 minutes to describe how they will deal with this obstetric emergency. You will score candidates based on their competence at the various techniques and their attention to detail. You may ask questions for clarification.

Structured mark sheet

Actions

- Call for the anaesthetist and paediatrician
- Inform a senior obstetrician on duty
- Ensure the fetus is alive (CTG)

0   1   2   3   4

Interventions

- Draw patient's buttocks to the edge of the bed.
- Give or extend the episiotomy
- McRobert technique (hyperflex knees and abduct at hip)
- Suprapubic pressure and moderate traction then deliver posterior arm and shoulder

0   1   2   3   4   5   6

Other manoeuvres

- Wood screw manoeuvre
- Patient to go on all fours
- Zavenelli manouevre
- Symphysiotomy
- Destructive operations

0   1   2   3   4   5   6

Complications

- Fetal
- Maternal

0   1   2   3   4   5   6

Total mark is out of 20

Station 12

Role-player's instructions

You are 41 year old and have two children, both born by Caesarean section because of fetal distress. Your periods have been getting heavier over the past year, since you were sterilized. You are happily married and work as a care assistant. Your periods are regular, coming every 30 days but lasting up to eight days, with clots and occasional soiling of the your clothes. Staining of bed linen is more frequent. For sanitary protection you need to wear maxipads most of the time. Pain during periods is mild and occurs during the period itself. You find that your social activities are restricted and you regularly take one or two days off work at the time of your period. You developed a deep vein thrombosis (DVT) whilst on the pill 18 months ago. You were subsequently sterilized and had a normal cervical smear one year ago.

Past medical history

- DVT

Previous treatment

- Progestogens
- Mefenamic acid
- Cyclokapron

Family history

- Nil relevant

Social history

- Smokes 29 cigarettes a day
- Drinks 10 units of alcohol per week

Patient's attitude

Fed up with having heavy periods and will not consider further medical treatment. Has recently read that gynaecologists are taking out the wombs of women unnecessarily and therefore is reluctant to have a hysterectomy. Has heard that there is a new operation that can cure her problem without having a hysterectomy.

Examiner's instructions

At the station candidatesl have 15 minutes to obtain a history relevant to the patient's complaint. They should also discuss with the patient any investigations and treatment they feel will be necessary. When candidates feel they has completed the history, they may ask for details of a physical examination. You should give these to them, as outlined.

Examination findings

- General examination – no abnormalities
- Pelvic examination – no abnormalities

Score candidates' performance on the structured mark sheet.

Structured mark sheet

Introduction

- Non-medical language
- Eye contact
- Listens to patient/does not interrupt
- Invites questions

0   1   2   3   4   5

History

- Symptoms
- Duration
- Menstrual history: oral contraceptive pill/DVT; sterilization
- Obstetric history
- Social history

0   1   2   3   4   5   6

Investigations

- Hb/Iron studies
- Hysteroscopy/biopsy/ultrasound scan
- Thyroid function
- Explanation of tests

0   1   2   3   4   5

Treatment

- Ablation/resection
- Local destructive procedures, for example microwave, etc.
- Levonorgestrel IUCD
- Explanation of treatment
- Advantages/disadvantages

0   1   2   3   4

Total mark is out of 20

Station 13

Examiner's instructions

Candidates have 15 minutes to conduct the postnatal visit of this patient. Award marks for thoughtfulness in approach, clarity of explanation and ability to gain the patient's confidence. You may ask the patient what she thinks of the candidate. Use the structured mark sheet to score the candidate. You may ask candidates questions as if you are either the patient or her husband.

Structured mark sheet

Introduction

- Non-medical language
- Eye contact
- Sympathy/empathy

0   1   2   3   4

Explanation of the results

- Need to repeat some of the investigations
- Relevance of explanation
- Appropriate interpretation in relation to loss

0   1   2   3   4   5

Plan for subsequent pregnancy

- Monitoring
- Combined care with haematologist/refer to centre with expertise
- Treatment if required
- Duration of treatment

0   1   2   3   ·   4   5   6   7

Counselling

- Support groups
- Menstrual cycle
- Other problems

0   1   2   3   4

Total mark is out of 20

Station 14

Examiner's instructions

Candidates should discuss the management of this undiagnosed breech presentation in labour.

Structured mark sheet

Introduction

- Explanation of the diagnosis in layman's language
- Explaining the risks of a breech vaginal delivery

0   1   2   3   4   5

Options

- Offer a Caesarean section – RCOG recommendation based on term breech trial
- Option of a vaginal breech delivery if pelvis is judged to be adequate

0   1   2   3   4   5

Interventions

- How will you conduct a breech delivery – details of the various techniques for delivering the arms and after-coming head
- Describe in detail the delivery of after-coming head

0   1   2   3   4   5

Other

- Other options for delivery of the after-coming head – forceps and being able to demonstrate how to apply them

0   1   2   3   4   5

Total mark is out of 20

Station 15

Examiner's instructions

Candidates have 15 minutes to explain to you the following: the tasks that need doing on the delivery suite; and the order in which they would do them and which staff they would allocate to each task.

Tasks

- Room 1: any vaginal bleeding? Assess maternal vital signs, reasons for failure to progress (for example, adequacy of contractions or disproportion) and fetal well-being – CTG
- Room 2: need to exclude cord prolapse or compression
- Room 3: ensure venflon is sited, blood for group and save serum, notify anaesthetist, assess fetal health
- Room 4: need to assess reasons for failure to deliver and fetal health (CTG)
- Room 5: need to discuss options of delivery and assess suitability for a vaginal delivery. Inform anaesthetist
- Room 6: assess CTG, more information about pain and associated bleeding
- Room 7: assessment of the bleeding, state of the fetus and additional information, for example contracting?
- Room 8: normal labouring patient – no action – to be managed by midwife
- Room 9: normal labouring patient – no action – to be managed by midwife
- Room 10: assess, after history and examination, consider antibiotics

| 0 | 1 | 2 | 3 | 4 | 5 | 6 | 7 | 8 | 9 | 10 |

Priority of tasks and staff allocation

- Urgent review of patients in rooms 3, 1 and 8
- A quick vaginal examination of patient in Room 2 will exclude cord prolapse. Turn patient to side to see effect. If CTG normal consider as cord compression. Will need delivering
- Patient in Room 1 requires an urgent assessment to rule out imminent rupture. Urgently assess the state of fetus and vital signs of mother. Quick abdominal and vaginal examination for signs of rupture and evidence of disproportion
- Patient in Room 8 requires urgent exclusion of abruption. Quick vaginal examination to assess state of the cervix
- SHO to see patient in Room 7 and exclude abruption and ensure fetal health is satisfactory
- Midwife to continue monitoring patient with twins in Room 3 until assessed
- Semi-urgent review of patient in Room 5 by Registrar. Needs a vaginal examination to determine why not delivered. If good contractions and head low enough, expedite delivery with forceps or ventouse. If vaginal delivery not possible, for Caesarean section. May require syntocinon if head is high and contractions are poor
- Semi-review of patient in Room 6 by Registrar
- SHO to review patient in Room 10 and start on antibiotics

| 0 | 1 | 2 | 3 | 4 | 5 | 6 | 7 | 8 | 9 | 10 |

Total mark is out of 20

Station 16

Examiner's instructions

Use the structured mark sheet to assess candidates. Marks should be awarded for candidates' ability to communicate in a language that a lay person will understand. In addition, an ability to emphathize should be awarded with extra marks.

Structured mark sheet

Introduction

- Communication with the patient
- Explanation of the diagnosis to the patient
- Putting patient at ease and empathizing
- Implications of abnormalities
- Need to exclude other associated and chromosomal abnormalities

0   1   2   3   4

Investigations

- Although other structural and chromosomal abnormalities may be excluded, baby may still be syndromic
- Further scanning at tertiary level – fetomaternal medicine unit

0   1   2   3   4

Prenatal karyotyping

- Amniocentesis + FISH – advantages/disadvantages (only for specific probes, therefore other uncommon karyotypic abnormalities not excluded) – early result – 48–72 hours. Standard amniocentesis – two to three weeks for results
- Chorionic villus sampling (CVS) (placental biopsy) – direct preparation – results within 48–72 hours. Culture – 10 days. Risk of mosaicism
- Miscarriage risk with both tests – 0.5 to one per cent with amniocentesis; one per cent with CVS

0   1   2   3   4

Options

- Karyotypy abnormal – termination of pregnancy/continue
- If termination, gestational age more than 22 weeks, consider fetocide with KCL, etc.
- If before 22 weeks, protaglandins and mifepristone (RU486)
- Other abnormalities severe enough to affect outcome – termination option

0   1   2   3   4

Others

- No karyotypic abnormality or decision to continue with pregnancy
- Counselling by geneticists
- Plastic surgeon to discuss management after of the cleft and talipes (photographs may be helpful)
- Neontalogist involvement – feeding difficulties, vocalization and complications of aspiration pneumonia
- Serial follow-up ultrasound scans for growth and complications, such as poly-hydramnios

0   1   2   3   4

Total mark is out of 20

Station 17

Structured mark sheet

Defining standards

- MedLine search/literature review
- Sources of defined standards: Cochrane Reviews; systematic reviews; RCOG standards; NICE or regional/national standards

0   1   2   3   4

Definitions

- Defining the required population sample required for a proper audit
- Audit unit/statistician to calculate requisite number from standards and previous audits

0   1   2   3   4

Proforma

- For data collection
- Indications for induction of labour: postdates; complications of pregnancy, for example breech presentation, pre-eclampsia, etc.; previous Caesarean section; others, for example social
- Decision for Caesarean section – made by whom?
- Methods of induction
- Outcome/complications

0   1   2   3   4   5

Collection of data

- Prospective
- Retrospective

0   1   2

Analysis and presentations

- Input date onto a spreadsheet or database
- Analyse – indication, staff making decision, outcome and complications

0   1   2   3   4

Recommendations, implementation and re-audit

- Discussed within unit and changes made
- Timeframe defined for implementation

- Support of all stakeholders
- Re-audit to complete cycle

0   1   2   3

Total mark is out of 20

Station 18

Structured mark sheet

Introduction

- Communication in an appropriate language
- Encouraging questions

0   1   2   3

Explanation of the results

- Semen analysis
- Diagnostic laparoscopy
- Implications of laparoscopic findings – minimal disease may not be the cause of the infertility
- Male factors needs to be rechecked – oligozoospermia needs to be confirmed
- Any need for medical or surgical treatment of endometriosis? – evidence conflicting so far –
- Endoscan trial Canada, study from Italy

0   1   2   3   4   5   6   7

Options

- Assisted reproduction techniques – AID, AIH, GIFT, IVF with husband or donor spermatozoa

0   1   2   3   4   5   6

Others

- Adoption

0   1   2

Global score

0   1   2

Total mark is out of 20

Global score =

4

Recommended reading

Dewhurst's Textbook of Obstetrics & Gynaecology for Postgraduates (6th edition). Oxford: Blackwell Scientific, 1998.

James DK, Steer PJ, Weiner CP, Gonik B. *High Risk Obstetrics – Management Options* (2nd edition). London: Harcourt Brace, 1998.

Konje JC, Taylor DJ. *Objective Structured Clinical Examination in Obstetrics & Gynaecology*. Oxford: Blackwell Science, 1996.

Monaghan JM. *Bonney's Gynaecological Surgery*. London: Baillière Tindal, 1988.

Shaw RW, Soutter WP, Stanton SL. *Gynaecology* (2nd edition). London: Churchill Livingstone, 1997 (or a newer edition).

Studd J. (ed.) *Progress in Obstetrics and Gynaecology* – all volumes. London: Churchill Livingstone.

Vignettes for the MRCOG – all volumes. Salisbury: Quay Books.

Index

abdomen, postoperative burst 397, 406
abdominal examinations 134, 335
abdominal incisions 141, 359–60, 365
abdominal masses 243–4, 296, 309–10, 335, 367
abdominal X-rays 186
ablation, endometrial 194, 196, 391, 402, 439
abnormal presentation 78, 89–94, 386, 398
    see also breech delivery
Abortion Act (UK) 397, 406
abortion, missed (failed pregnancy) 395, 404
    see also miscarriage
abscess
    Bartholin's 249, 250
    pelvic 164, 395, 405
    tubo-ovarian 283–4
acetic acid 321, 322
acetylcholinesterase 387, 399
acid-fast bacilli testing 44, 164
actinomycin D 348
acyclovir 60
Add-Back therapy 194, 202, 230, 232, 234, 236
adenectomy 332
adenoacanthoma, endometrial 332
adenocarcinoma
    cervical 316, 317
    endometrial 332
adenomyosis
    combined oral contraceptive pill for 273
    and cyclical secondary dysmenorrhoea 197,
        198
    and menorrhagia 195, 196
adhesiolysis 234
adhesions 224, 227, 234, 284
    in Asherman syndrome 200
    combined oral contraceptive pill for 274
    formation following myomectomy 397, 406
    labial 393, 403
    and surgical bladder injury 367, 368
adnexal pathologies 298, 344, 363–4
adolescent gynaecology 179–90, 386, 398
adolescent pregnancy 19–20, 188, 189, 386, 398

adoption
    and at birth diagnosis of Down's syndrome 184
    and autosomal recessive disorders 120
    for infertile couples 258, 268, 447
after-coming head, manoeuvres for 137–8, 441
age
    and endometrial carcinoma 332, 335–6
    and ovarian malignancy 341
agenesis
    of the Müllerian system 212, 251–2
    renal 80
airway management 31
alanine transaminases 30, 36
albumin 265
Alcoholics Anonymous 84
alcoholism, in pregnancy 83–4
alkaline phosphatases 30, 36
allergies 186
alloimmunization 389, 400
alpha feto-protein (AFP) 344, 347, 348
amenorrhoea 414, 435
    combined oral contraceptive pill for 274
    norethisterone for 276
    primary 211–12, 251–2, 393, 403
    secondary 199–200, 209–10
amniocentesis 388, 400, 443
    for autosomal recessive conditions 120
    and chorionic villus sampling 23–24
    complications of 24
    and diaphragmatic hernia 26
    disadvantages of 24
    for Down's syndrome 22, 184
    for exomphalus 18
    and intrauterine/intrapartum stillbirth 118
    and maternal HIV infection 62
    in response to maternal Rhesus (D) antibodies 68
amnioinfusion 80, 102
amnioreduction 100
amniotic fluid
    see also anhydramnios; liquor;
        oligohydramnios; polyhydramnios

acetylcholinesterase in 387, 399
amniotic fluid index (AFI) 75
anaemia 324
see also sickle cell anaemia
in adolescent pregnancy 386, 398
associated with fibroids 229, 230, 232, 413, 430–32
anaesthesia
see also general anaesthesia
epidural 36, 38, 111–12, 133–4
examination under 186, 253, 324
local 109, 110, 321
anaesthetic disorders, in pregnancy 105–12
anaesthetist 31, 302
and grade III cardiac disease 49, 50
and intellectually subnormal mothers 139, 140
and postpartum haemorrhage 161
and risk management teams 379
and shoulder dystocia 127, 437
and twin delivery 429
and uterine rupture 141
analgesia
epidural 109–10, 111–12
local 293
anastomosis 366
androgenicity 275–6
androgens 236
aneuploidy 399
anhydramnios 79–80
antacids 107–8
anti-D prophylaxis 65–6
administration guidelines 71–2
failure 71–2
human-derived 66, 72
monoclonal 66, 72
anti-depressants 202
anti-emetics 108
anti-hypertensive agents 30, 32, 33–4, 36, 38
anti-oestrogens
for menorrhagia 194
for ovulation induction 261–2, 264
antibiotic therapy 366
for Bartholin's abscess 250
broad-spectrum 217, 282, 283–4
for *Chlamydia trachomatis* 222, 283–4, 288
for chorioamnionitis 134
for pelvic inflammatory disease 282
to prevent preterm labour 100, 102
for septic incomplete miscarriage 217
antibodies
antisperm 394, 404
to chickenpox 59–60
chlamydial 283
Rhesus (D) 67–9

anticholinergic drugs 304, 308, 310
anticoagulants 100, 361, 362
antifibrinolytic agents 193
antisperm antibodies 394, 404
antiviral therapy 61, 62, 413
apareunia 251
apnoea 110
artificial insemination by donor (AID) 69, 120, 268
artificial insemination with the husband's semen (AIH) 258, 268
ascites 348
Asherman syndrome 199–200, 218, 274
asphyxia, fetal 143, 144
aspiration, vomiting under general anaesthesia 107–8, 111, 112
aspiration pneumonia 107–8, 112
aspirators, pipelle/vibra 293–4, 296
aspirin 34, 100
assisted reproductive techniques 447
see also specific techniques
for oligozoospermia 268
and selective fetocide 375
for unexplained infertility 258
ASTEC trial 332
asthma 302
at-risk registers 88
atrophic vaginitis 296
audits
of ectopic pregnancy management 420, 421
of labour induction 418, 445–6
of menorrhagia treatment 436
prospective 421
retrospective 421
autoimmune thrombocytopenia, maternal 389, 401
autopsy, fetal 80, 115–16, 117–18
autosomal dominant conditions 385, 398
autosomal recessive conditions 119–20, 385, 398
azithromycin 286
AZT 61–62

babies
see also neonates; newborns
and HIV 61
and hypothermia 171–2
of intellectually subnormal mothers 140
backache 110
bacterial infection 163
see also specific infections
bacterial vaginosis 98, 100, 286
bacteruria, asymptomatic 98, 100
balloon ablation 194, 196
barrier methods of contraception 215–16, 287, 356

barrier nursing 44
Bartholin's abscess 249, 250
BCG, INH-resistant 44
bed rest 98
beta human chorionic gonadotrophins (ßHCG)
    and hydatiform mole 353–4, 356
    and ovarian cancer 344
    and ovarian hyperstimulation syndrome 264,
        265
    and trophoblastic disease 224, 352, 353–4,
        356
beta-sympathomimetic drugs 390, 402
betadine douches 286
bilirubin 68, 173–4
biochemical screening
    first trimester 15–16
    for maternal hypertension 29–30, 35, 36, 38
    for ovarian malignancy 344
    for preterm labour 98, 100
    for trisomy 21 21–2
biophysical profilometry 75, 76
biopsy
    see also chorionic villus sampling
    cervical 319, 320, 321, 322
    cold knife cone 322
    endometrial 200, 208, 293–4, 295, 296, 297–8
    liver 174
    omental 244, 348
    ovarian 348
    para-aortic node 348
bladder
    distension 304, 311
    injury during gynaecological surgery 367–8
    low compliance 304, 311–12
    pre-surgical emptying 367–8
bleomycin 348
blood clots, uterine 163
blood groups 324, 336, 352
blood patches 103, 110
blood pressure 34, 36, 76
    see also hypertension; hypotension
blood transfusion
    for cervical malignancy 324
    for endometrial carcinoma 336
    fetal 68
    following massive haemorrhage 392, 403
    for septic incomplete miscarriage 217
    for uterine rupture 141
blood viscosity 170
blood-glucose monitoring 46, 47–8
blood-glucose test 46
BM stix 48
Boari flap 366
body mass index (BMI) 46

body weight
    see also obesity; weight loss
    maternal 46
bone marrow donors 371–2
bowel, echogenic 387, 399
Brace suture 160, 162
bradycardia, fetal 110, 130, 141, 150, 389, 401
BRCA1/BRCA2 344
breast cancer 276
breast examinations 164
breastfeeding 163–4
    and HIV transmission 61, 62
    and psychiatric medication 166
    and tuberculosis transmission 44
breech delivery 78
    and Caesarean section 137, 138, 152, 441
    and cord prolapse 144
    external cephalic version for 91
    incidence 91, 137
    manoeuvres for the after-coming head 137–8,
        441
    spontaneous correction 91
    undiagnosed 416, 417, 441, 442
    vaginal 137–8, 441
bromocriptine 210, 393, 404
brown fat 169, 171
buccal smears 182
Burch colposuspension 302, 411, 414, 425–6, 433
Burns–Marshall technique 137–8
buserelin 264–265

C-reactive protein 102
CA125 (carcinoma antigen) estimation 242, 244,
        333–4, 344
Caesarean section 134
    in adolescent pregnancy 386, 398
    advantages 123
    and breech delivery 137, 138, 152, 441
    classical 76, 78, 94, 130, 150, 155–6
    complications of 152
    and cord prolapse 144
    disadvantages of 123
    elective 121–2, 152, 153–4
    emergency 78
    and external cephalic version 91
    fasting for 107
    for the fitting mother 32
    for the hypertensive mother 30, 32, 36, 38
    and induction of labour 126
    for infants with diaphragmatic hernia 26
    and intrauterine growth restriction 76, 78
    inverted-T 150
    lower-segment 76, 78, 94, 149, 155, 156
    and maternal herpes simplex infection 58

and maternal HIV infection 62
and maternal Rhesus (D) antibodies 68
and Mendelson's syndrome 107, 108
modified lower-segment 78
following myomectomy 230
pain relief for 109
and postoperative infections 150
and postpartum haemorrhage 159–60
and preterm rupture of fetal membranes 103
previous
    complicated 130
    and uterine rupture 129–30, 149, 155–6
    and vaginal delivery 149–50, 155–6
sterilization during 153–4
UK rates 151–2
and unstable lie at term 94
and uterine rupture 129–30, 141, 142, 149, 155–6
Caesium 137, 324, 328
calcium channel blockers 304
Calman timescale 152
Canadian Randomized Trial 137
Candida albicans 286
carbegoline 210
carboxyhaemoglobin 85
cardiac disease
    grade III maternal 49–50
    ischaemic 207–8
cardiac failure 50
cardiac malformations *see* congenital cardiac
    abnormalities
cardiac scans 19, 20, 42
cardiologist 19, 20
cardiomyopathy, peripartum 391, 402
cardiotocography (CTG) 76, 103, 140
cardiovascular disorders 207–8
care in the community 140
catheters
    Foley's 132
    intrauterine pressure tip 130
    urinary 32, 110, 366, 433
cephalosporins 217, 284, 286
cerebrospinal fluid (CSF) 110
cervical cerclage 97, 98
cervical cytology
    imprecision 316, 319–20
    sensitivity 316, 317
cervical dilation, retrograde 98
cervical erosion (ectropion) 286
cervical incompetence/weakness 97–8
cervical intra-epithelial neoplasia (CIN) 397, 406
    CIN-I 316
    CIN-II 316, 319
    CIN-III 316, 319, 320
cervical length assessment 98, 100

cervical malignancy 313–28, 395, 405
    see also cervical intra-epithelial neoplasia
    adenocarcinoma 316, 317
    at-risk groups 316–17
    cold knife cone biopsy 322
    colposcopy 316, 319–20, 321–2
    directed biopsy 319, 320, 321
    failure to reduce the incidence of 315–17
    frank 322
    histology 322
    incidence 315, 316–17, 319–20
    invasive carcinoma 323–25
    mild dyskaryosis 316, 319
    mortality rates 315, 316, 319, 343
    natural course of 316, 320
    palliative care 324
    premalignant stage 316, 317, 320, 344
    radiotherapy 322, 324, 327–8
    screening 315–17, 319–20, 343–4
    secondaries 324
    staging 324
    survival rate 324
    Wertheim hysterectomy for 322, 324
cervical smear tests 315–17, 319–20, 343–4
cervical stenosis 197, 198
cervicitis 296
cervix
    amputation 306
    and endometrial biopsy 294, 296, 297
    endometrial carcinoma of 337–8, 412
    massaging 132
    ripe 132
    trauma 162, 219
chemotherapy 242, 243–4, 296
    for cervical malignancy 324–5
    for choriocarcinoma 351–2, 354
    for endometrial carcinoma 332, 336, 338
    for hydatiform mole 353–4, 355, 356
    for ovarian malignancy 348, 364
chest X-rays (CXRs) 43, 164, 253, 336, 346, 347
chickenpox 59–60
children
    and the combined oral contraceptive pill 273
    and domestic violence 87–8
    labial adhesions in 393, 403
    precocious menstruation in 187–8
    vaginal bleeding in 189–90
    vaginal discharge in 185–6, 395, 405
Chlamydia trachomatis 221–2
    at-risk groups 287–8
    as cause of chronic pelvic pain 282
    as cause of chronic vaginal discharge 286
    prevention measures for 287–8
    and tubo-ovarian abscess 283, 284

cholesterol 207–8
chorioamnionitis 80, 101, 102, 133–4, 400
choriocarcinoma 353, 355–6
    prognostic factors 351–2
    secondaries 352, 354
chorionic villus sampling (CVS) (placental biopsy)
        80, 443
    advantages of 23
    and amniocentesis 23–4
    and anhydramnios 80
    for autosomal recessive conditions diagnosis
        120
    complications of 23, 387, 400
    and diaphragmatic hernia 26
    for Down's syndrome 22, 184
    for exomphalus 18
    and intrauterine/intrapartum stillbirth 118
    and maternal HIV infection 62
chromosomal abnormalities 443
    and the accuracy of amniocentesis 24
    associated with anhydramnios 80
    associated with cardiac abnormalities 19–20
    associated with diaphragmatic hernias 26
    associated with exomphalus 17, 18
    identification in the first trimester 15–16
    and intrauterine/intrapartum stillbirth 118
    and primary amenorrhoea 212
    soft markers of 387, 399
    trisomy 21 21–2, 183–4
    ultrasound scanning for 22
chromosome 22, deletion of the short arm 19
cisplatin compounds 348
cisplatinum 342
clamp operations 304, 312
Clinical Negligence Scheme for Trust (CNST) 379
clinician 47
clomifene citrate 261–2, 264
clomipramine 202
Clostridiume welchii 399
Cochrane Reviews 420, 421, 436, 445
coining 98
collagen implants 304, 311–12
colpo-perineorrhaphy 306
colpocleisis 308
colporrhaphy, anterior 306
colposcopy 253, 316, 319–20, 321–2
colposuspension 304, 310
    and bladder injury 367, 368
    Burch 302, 411, 414, 425–6, 433
communication skills 373, 423, 426, 428, 431,
        433, 436, 439, 440, 443
complaints procedures 373–4
compliance 194, 206, 215, 228
compression stockings 362

computerized tomography (CT) scans 210, 242,
        347
conception rate, cumulative 261
congenital adrenal hyperplasia 181, 182
congenital cardiac abnormalities 19–20, 389, 401
    associated with diaphragmatic hernia 24
    identification in the first trimester 15–16
    major 19–20
    minor 19
    ultrasound scanning for 399
congenital malformations 13–26
    see also chromosomal abnormalities;
        structural abnormalities
    associated with Down's syndrome 183–4
    cardiac 15–16, 19–20, 24, 389, 399, 401
    and dietary supplements 385, 398
    and intrauterine/intrapartum stillbirth 117–18
    and maternal chickenpox infection 59, 60
    and maternal diabetes mellitus 46, 48
    neural tube defects 41, 42, 387, 398, 399
    and selective fetocide 375
consent 139
contact-tracing 222, 284, 288
contraception 154, 206
    see also sterilization
    in a 40 year old woman 411, 422–3
    barrier methods 215–16, 287, 356
    and hormone replacement therapy 292
    following hydatiform mole 356
    for intellectually subnormal women 140
    in the perimenopause 277–8
    following termination of pregnancy 215–16
contractions, monitoring 130, 134
contrast medium 260
Coomb's test 174
cord prolapse 93, 94, 143–4
corkscrew manoeuvre 128
corticosteroids 265
counselling
    for alcoholic mothers 83–4
    regarding amenorrhoea 200
    regarding autosomal recessive conditions
        119–20
    regarding cervical malignancy 324
    regarding chromosomal abnormalities 18
    regarding chronic vaginal discharge 286
    regarding ectopic pregnancy 223
    regarding endodermal sinus tumours 347–8
    regarding endometriosis 237, 282, 411, 424
    regarding epilepsy 42
    regarding fibroids 228
    regarding genital prolapse 306, 308
    regarding HIV screening 53–4
    regarding home births 145

regarding hormone replacement therapy 291, 292
regarding hysterectomy 160, 411, 424
regarding *in vitro* fertilization-produced organ/bone marrow donors 372
regarding infertility 257–8, 418, 447
regarding intrauterine growth restriction 76, 78
regarding maternal chickenpox infection 60
regarding maternal hypertension 30
regarding Müllerian agenesis 251
regarding neonatal death 119–20, 122
regarding ovarian malignancy 342, 347–8, 364
regarding perimenopausal contraception 278
regarding precocious puberty 188
regarding primary amenorrhoea 212
regarding maternal Rhesus (D) antibody status 68
regarding septic incomplete miscarriage 218
regarding sexually transmitted diseases 55, 56, 222
for smoking mothers 85–6
regarding sterilization 153–4
regarding sterilization reversal 272
regarding stillbirth 115, 116, 117–18, 440
regarding structural abnormalities 17, 19–20
regarding termination of pregnancy 219
regarding tubo-ovarian abscess 284
regarding unexpected diagnosis at birth 184
regarding urinary incontinence 311
following uterine rupture 142
regarding vaginal delivery following previous Caesarean section 150, 156
craniotomy 138
cranium
fractured 138
X-rays 210
creatinine 30, 32, 36, 38, 336
Creutzfeldt–Jakob disease (CJD) 66, 72
cricoid pressure 108
cryocautery 286
curettage, overzealous 218
cyclical secondary dysmenorrhoea 197–8
cyclofenil 262
cyclophosphamide 348
cyproterone acetate 188, 206, 274
cyst, ovarian 241–2, 243–4, 245–6, 347–8
cystectomy 242, 246
cystitis, interstitial 311
cystocele 304, 305, 307, 308, 310
cystoscopy 253, 304, 311, 324
cystoureteroscopy, retrograde 366
cytomegalovirus (CMV), congenital infection 389, 401

danazol
for cyclical secondary dysmenorrhoea 198
for endometrial hyperplasia 334
for endometriosis 236, 282
for fibroid treatment 228, 230, 232, 431, 432
for menorrhagia 194
for precocious puberty 188
for premenstrual syndrome 202
dating pregnancy 21–2
deep vein thrombosis (DVT) 134, 164, 361–2, 438
see also venous thrombo-embolism
degenerative motor disease 311
dehydration 133–4, 176
delegation 414, 417, 435, 442
delivery
see also breech delivery; Caesarean section; forceps delivery; labour; preterm delivery
choriocarcinoma following 351
for cord prolapse 144
for diabetic mothers 48
for the epileptic mother 42
of exomphalus infants 18
for the fitting mother 32
following previous Caesarean section 149–50, 155–6
and genital prolapse 305
and grade III maternal cardiac disease 49–50
for the hepatitis B infected mother 56
for the herpes simplex infected mother 57–8
at home 145–6
for the hypertensive mother 30, 32, 34, 35, 36, 37, 38
of infants with cardiac abnormalities 20
of infants with diaphragmatic hernia 26
and intrauterine growth restriction 75, 76, 77–8
Mendelson's syndrome in 107–8
following neonatal death 122
postpartum haemorrhage following 161–2
and preterm rupture of fetal membranes 103
in response to maternal Rhesus (D) antibodies 68
and shoulder dystocia 127, 415, 437
for tuberculosis-infected mothers 44
twin 144, 413, 429
ventouse 144
delivery suite, management 417, 442
Depo-Provera 154, 216, 277
detrusor instability 304, 308, 309, 310
dexamethasone 36, 48, 76, 98, 102
diabetes mellitus
and endometrial carcinoma 336

diabetes mellitus – *contd*
  maternal
    complications of 48
    high-risk groups 45–6
    improving pregnancy outcome 47–8
    and the neonate 169–70, 171, 175–6
    and preterm delivery 100
    screening for in pregnancy 45–6
  and ovulation induction 262
  risk factors for 45–6
  urinary symptoms 304, 310, 311
Dianette 206, 274
diaphragmatic hernia, fetal 25–6, 417
diastolic flow, absent/reverse end- 76
diathermy 286, 368
  drilling of the ovaries 262, 264
  for endometriosis 236
  sterilization by 271
diazepam 32
dietary supplements 385, 398
diethystilboestrol 390, 401
dihydrogesterone 276
dip-stick tests 30, 36
disseminated intravascular coagulation (DIC) 386, 399
documentation 373
domestic violence 87–8
dopamine agonists 210
Doppler scanning
  middle cerebral artery 30, 36, 38, 68, 75, 76
  for ovarian malignancy 344, 346
  renal artery 80
  umbilical artery 30, 36, 38, 75, 76, 102
  uterine artery 34, 100
douches 286
Down's syndrome
  see also trisomy 21
  recurrence risk 184
  unexpected diagnosis at birth 183–4
Down's syndrome Association 184
drainage 284
drug abuse, in pregnancy 81–8, 390, 401
Dublin randomized trial 194
dural tap/puncture 110, 112
dye injection 366
dysuria 303

echocardiography 19, 25, 48
echogenic bowel 387, 399
eclampsia 30, 32, 38
  see also pre-eclampsia
ectopic pregnancy 216, 223–4, 414, 435
  at-risk groups 419
  identification 419

management 411, 419–21
  recurrence risk 224
Eisenmenger syndrome 391, 402
electrolysis 206
embolism
  see also venous thrombo-embolism
  pulmonary 164, 362
embryo transfer (IVF-ET) 258
endocrinology in gynaecology 203–12
endodermal sinus tumour 347–8
endometrial ablation 194, 196, 391, 402, 439
endometrial biopsy 200, 208, 293–4, 295, 296
  and hysteroscopy 293, 294, 296, 297–8
  and ultrasound scanning 293, 294, 297, 298
endometrial carcinoma 331–2, 333
  adenoacanthoma 332
  adenocarcinoma 332
  adenosquamous 332
  age factors 332, 335–6
  at-risk groups 295
  cervical invasion of 337–8, 412
  grading 332
  histology 332, 412
  management 412, 427–8
  norethisterone for 276
  ploidy status 332
  due to polycystic ovary disease 208
  and postmenopausal bleeding 293, 295–6
  prognosis 331, 335
  radiotherapy for 332, 336, 427
  recurrence rates 332
  secondaries 276, 335, 336, 338
  serous/clear/papillary 332
  staging 331–2
  survival rates 331, 332
endometrial hyperplasia 276, 333–4, 412
endometrial prognostic index 332
endometrial resection 194, 196, 439
endometriosis
  as cause of chronic pelvic pain 282
  and cyclical secondary dysmenorrhoea 197, 198
  and infertility 418, 447
  management 273, 411, 424
  and menorrhagia 195, 196, 233–7
  and painful menstruation 233–7
  recurrent 233–4
  symptoms 233
endometritis 134, 163
endotracheal tubes, cuffed 108
enterocele 305, 308
eosin stains 346
epidermal growth factor receptor 342
epidural anaesthesia
  advantages/disadvantages 111–12

as cause of fever in labour 133–4
in hypertensive mothers 36, 38
epidural analgesia
  advantages/disadvantages 111–12
  complications 109–10
  unblocked segments 109
epilepsy, maternal 41–2
epiphyses, premature closure 188
episiotomy 127, 437
ergometrine 159
erythromycin 102
erythropoiesis 68
ethics, medico-legal 16, 76, 369–80
ethnic minorities 46, 386
etoposide 348
European Union (EU) 152
evening primrose oil 202
examination under anaesthesia (EUA) 186, 253,
    324
examinations
  failing 9
  multiple choice questions 3, 5, 383, 385–406
  oral 3, 5, 407–49
  short essay questions 5–7, 9, 11–380, 383
exenteration 254, 324
exomphalus 17–18
external cephalic version (ECV) 62, 94, 137
  timing of 91–2

Fallopian tube
  see also salpingoophorectomy
  assessment in infertile women 259–60
  and ectopic pregnancy 224
  following sterilization reversal 272
  and tubal ligation 142
  and tubo-ovarian abscess 283–4
falloposcopy 260
family planning 269–78
feeds, neonatal refusal of 175–6
fertility
  see also infertility
  and amenorrhoea 200, 212
  and cervical malignancy treatment 322, 324
  and chemotherapy for hydatiform moles 356
  and endometriosis 236–7
  and fibroids 227–8, 230, 232, 430, 431
  and genital prolapse 305, 306
  and menorrhagia 195
  and Müllerian agenesis 251, 252
  and ovarian malignancy 347–8
  and postpartum haemorrhage management
      162
  and sterilization reversal 271–2
  and tubo-ovarian abscess 284

fetal autopsy 80, 115–16, 117–18
fetal blood group 68–9
fetal blood sampling 22, 68
fetal bradycardia 110, 130, 141, 150, 389, 401
fetal cells/DNA in the maternal circulation 16
fetal death
  and induction of post-term pregnancy 125–6
  and intrauterine growth restriction 76, 78
  due to preterm labour 99–100
  twin 388, 400
fetal diaphragmatic hernia 25–6, 417
fetal echocardiography 19, 25
fetal fibronectin (FFN) 98, 100
fetal growth, abnormal 73–80
  see also intrauterine growth restriction
fetal haemoglobin (Hb) 68
fetal haemolysis 68–9
fetal hydrops 389, 400, 401
fetal hypoxia 32, 34, 36, 38, 110
fetal lie 93–4, 155–6
fetal lung development 102
fetal macrosomia 45, 46, 48, 169
fetal monitoring
  for diabetic mothers 48
  for epileptic mothers 42
  for the hepatitis B-infected mother 56
  and home births 145–6
  and intrauterine growth restriction 75–6
  for labour in intellectually subnormal mothers
      139–40
  and maternal hypertension 36, 38
  for post-term pregnancies 126
  and preterm rupture of fetal membranes 103
feto-maternal haemorrhage 66
fetocide, selective 100, 375–6
fetus
  5-α reductase deficiency 392, 403
  abnormal presentation 78, 89–94, 386, 398
  after-coming head manoeuvres for 137–8
  bilateral talipes equinovarus 417
  bilirubin levels 68
  and cord prolapse 143, 144
  effects of alcoholism on 84
  effects of dexamethasone administration on
      98
  effects of smoking on 85
  and hepatitis B infection 56
  and herpes simplex type II infection 57
  and HIV infection 61–2
  and maternal diabetes 48
  and maternal Rhesus (D) antibodies 68
fibrinogen 30, 32, 36
fibrinogen degradation products (FDPs) 30, 36,
      38

fibroids
  18-week size 231–2
  26-week size 229–30
  asypmtomatic 227
  and cyclical secondary dysmenorrhoea 198
  and endometrial biopsy 294
  and human immunodeficiency virus 231–2
  management 227–8, 229–30, 413, 430–32
  and menorrhagia 195, 196
  in a primigravida 227–8
  re-growth 228
  symptoms of 229
first trimester
  anti-D prophylaxis during 72
  in hypertensive mothers 34
  prenatal screening during 15–16, 22, 42
fits, during labour 31–2, 42
flow cytometry 71
fluid input/output charts 32
fluid overload 49, 50
fluid therapy 134
fluorescent *in situ* hybridization (FISH) 18, 24, 443
fluoxetine 202
flutamide 206
folate supplementation 41, 398
Foley's catheter 132
follicle-stimulating hormone (FSH) 262
follicles 264
follicular aspiration 265
follicular tracking 264, 265
forceps delivery
  and breech presentation 137, 138, 441
  elective 44
  and grade III cardiac disease 50
  and maternal tuberculosis 43–4
foreign bodies, vaginal 186, 189, 190
fracture
  cranial 138
  mandible 138
fragmin 50
frequency and volume chart 304, 310
full blood count (FBC) 30, 32, 38, 102, 163, 230
  for cervical malignancy 324
  for endometrial carcinoma 336
  for neonatal jaundice 173
  for ovarian cyst 245
  for septic incomplete miscarriage 217

galactorrhoea 209–10, 393
gamete intra-Fallopian transfer (GIFT) 120, 258, 268
gangrene
  gas 399
  of the ovary 246

general anaesthesia (GA) 150
  advantages/disadvantages 111–12
  for cold knife cone biopsy 322
  for endometrial biopsy 293
  for hysterectomy 391
  for hysterosalpinography 260
  for laparoscopy and dye test 260
  for laparotomy for uterine rupture 141
  Mendelson's syndrome in 107–8
  repeated 272
  for termination of pregnancy 219
general practitioner (GP) 234
  and cervical malignancy 316
  and *Chlamydia trachomatis* 287
  and communication skills 373
  and diabetes mellitus 46, 47–8
  and endometrial carcinoma 336
  and the epileptic mother 42
  and gynaecological referral 413, 415
  and intrauterine/intrapartum stillbirth 116, 118
  and maternal tuberculosis 44
  and polycystic ovary disease 208
  and postpartum psychiatric disorders 165
  and unexpected diagnosis of Down's syndrome at birth 184
genetic markers, for ovarian malignancy 344
geneticist 26, 116, 118, 184, 444
genital prolapse 299–312, 363, 364
  cystocele 304, 305, 307, 308, 310
  enterocele 305, 308
  family history of 305
  management 305–6
  rectocele 305, 307, 308
  repair 302, 308, 310
  vault prolapse 307–8
genitalia, ambiguous external in newborns 181–2
genito-urinary medicine (GUM) clinic 284, 286
genito-urinary medicine (GUM) physician 55, 62
genito-urinary medicine (GUM) team 232
germ cell tumour, ovarian 347–8
gestational trophoblastic disease 349–56
  choriocarcinoma 351–2, 353, 354, 355–6
  hydatiform mole 351, 353–4, 355–6
gestrinone (Demetrios) 236
glucagon 48
glucose tolerance test, oral 46
glucose-6-phosphate deficiency (G-6-PD) 386, 399
glycosuria 46
gonadotrophin-releasing hormone (GnRH) analogues
  for body hair reduction 206
  for cyclical secondary dysmenorrhoea 198
  depot injections 194

for endometriosis 23, 236, 282
for fibroid treatment 228, 230, 232, 431, 432
for menorrhagia 194
for ovulation induction 264
for precocious puberty 188
for premenstrual syndrome 201, 202
gonadotrophins, and ovulation induction 261, 262, 264, 265
goserelin 228
Guedel's mouthpiece 31
gynaecological oncologist 244
and cervical malignancy 323–4
and endometrial carcinoma 332, 337, 338, 428
and internal iliac artery ligation 162
and ovarian malignancy 342, 364
and vaginal carcinoma 253, 254
gynaecologist
and cervical malignancy 324
and endometrial carcinoma 336, 337
and sexual abuse 186
and surgical treatment of menorrhagia 196

H_2-antagonists 107–8
haematologist 66, 141, 161, 361
haematoma, vulval 249, 250
haematoxylin 346
haemolysis 68–9, 173
haemorrhage
see also postpartum haemorrhage
fetal intracranial 138
feto-maternal 66
massive 392, 403
haemotological analysis 30, 35, 36, 38
see also blood-glucose monitoring
hair removal 205–6
hand prolapse 93
HbA1c 46, 48
headaches 37
Heaf test 200
health worker 44
hebamate 160
Hegar dilator 98
heparin 38, 50, 361
hepatitis B, in pregnancy 55–6
hepatitis B immunoglobulin (HBIG) 56
hernia 18
fetal diaphragmatic 25–6, 417
incisional 392, 403
inguino-labial 249, 250
Reichter's 359
herpes simplex type II 57–8
HFEA 1991 375
hirsutism 205–6, 274
hormone profiles 210, 211

hormone replacement therapy (HRT) 234, 236, 396, 405
contraindications 292
and endometrial carcinoma risk 295
for the menopause 291–2
for the perimenopause 277–8
in a thrombophilic patient 361, 362
hospices 324
hospital staff 231–2
hospitalization
early 156
prolonged 126
human chorionic gonadotrophins (HCG) 262, 264
see also beta human chorionic gonadotrophins
human immunodeficiency virus (HIV)
in the gynaecology ward 231–2, 413, 430–32
high risk groups 54
mother-fetal transmission 61–2
in pregnancy 53–4, 61–2, 387, 399
screening 53–4
stigma concerning 55
transmission risk to hospital staff 231–2
human menopausal gonadotrophins (HMG) 262, 264
hydatiform mole 351, 353–4, 355–6
complete 356
partial 356
hydrallazine 32, 36, 38
hydration 362
see also dehydration; fluid therapy
hygroscopic devices 132
hyperbilirubinaemia, unconjugated 173
hyperglycaemia, in utero 169
hyperosmolar solution 224
hyperprolactinaemia 209–10, 404
hypertension
due to polycystic ovary disease 207–8
in pregnancy 27–38
and anaesthesia during delivery 112
and maternal diabetes 48
risk factors for 33
severity of 33–4, 35–6, 37, 38
and urodynamic stress incontinence 302
hypocalcaemia 169
hypoglycaemia 48, 169, 175–6
hypomagnesaemia 169
hypoplasia
nasal bone 16
pulmonary 80, 101
hypotension 109, 110
hypothermia, neonatal 169, 171–2, 175, 176
hypothyroidism 187, 188
hypotonia of the uterus 162

hysterectomy
  abdominal 365–6, 391, 412
  and bladder injury 367, 368
  for cervical malignancy 322, 324
  for chronic pelvic pain 282
  for cyclical secondary dysmenorrhoea 198
  for endometrial carcinoma 296, 332, 336, 337
  for endometrial hyperplasia 334, 412
  for endometriosis 233–4, 236, 411, 424
  for fibroid treatment 227–8, 230, 232, 431,
    432
  and hormone replacement therapy 291, 292
  for menorrhagia 19, 194
  for ovarian malignancy 348
  for ovarian mucinous cystadenoma 244
  and perioperative management of a protein S
    deficient patient 361–2
  for postpartum haemorrhage 160, 162
  and septic incomplete miscarriage 218
  and uterine rupture 142, 150
  vaginal 336, 363–4, 368, 411, 424
  for vaginal carcinoma 253
  and vault prolapse 307
  Wertheim 322, 324, 337
hysterosalpingography (HSG) 98, 200, 260
hysteroscopy 200, 208, 293, 294, 296, 297–8
hysterosonography 260

idiopathic hypersecretion 210
ileal conduit 366
ileostomy 312
iliac fossa 359, 360
immunoglobulin G (IgG) 59, 283
immunoglobulin M (IgM) 60, 283
Implanon 154, 216
in vitro fertilization (IVF) 120, 237, 284, 413
  to provide bone marrow donors 371–2
  for oligozoospermia 268
  to provide organ donors 371–2
  and ovarian hyperstimulation syndrome 265
  for unexplained infertility 258
incisional hernia 392, 403
incisions
  abdominal 359–60
    infraumbilical in the iliac fossa 359
    midline 364
    midline subumbilical 141
    oblique in the iliac fossa 359, 360
    Pfannenstiel 359
    vertical 359
incubators 171–2
induction
  see also labour, induction
  of ovulation 258, 261–2, 264, 394, 404

infections
  see also specific infections
  due to cervical incompetence testing 98
  and intrauterine/intrapartum stillbirth 115–16
  and neonatal jaundice 174
  and neonatal refusal of feeds 175, 176
  pelvic 279–88
  postoperative following Caesarean section 150
  in pregnancy 43–4, 51–62, 100, 387, 390, 399,
    401
  and preterm labour 100
  and puerperial pyrexia 163
  and vaginal bleeding in children 189, 190
  wound 164
infertility 101–3, 255–68
  incidence 377
  NHS treatment of 377–8
  oligozoospermia 267–8
  in polycystic ovary syndrome 261–2
  primary 418, 447
  tubal function assessment 259–60
  unexplained 257–8, 394, 404
Ingram's bicycle seat 252
inguino-labial hernia 249, 250
inhibin 62
insulin levels 169
insulin resistance 208
insulin therapy 47–8
intellectually subnormal mothers, labour in
  139–40
internal iliac artery ligation 160, 162
intersexual disorders 212
intracranial haemorrhage, fetal 138
intracytoplasmic sperm injection (ICSI) 268
intramyometrial prostaglandins 160, 162
intrathecal injection 109, 110
intrauterine contraceptive device (IUCD)
  for Asherman syndrome 200
  complications of 216
  for cyclical secondary dysmenorrhoea 197
  and ectopic pregnancy risk 216, 224
  for endometrial hyperplasia 334
  following hydatiform mole 356
  for menorrhagia 194, 439
  as perimenopausal contraception 277, 278
  progestogen-only (levonorgestrel) (Mirena) 194,
    202, 334, 439
  following termination of pregnancy 216, 217
intrauterine growth restriction (IUGR) 421
  age-of-onset 77–8
  and dexamethasone use 102
  ethical issues regarding 76
  and hypertensive disorders 30, 34, 36, 38
  and maternal epilepsy 42

and maternal hepatitis B infection 56
neonatal complications 388, 400
and neonatal hypothermia 171, 172
recurrence 76
severe 75–6, 77–8
and stillbirth 400
intrauterine pressure tip catheter 130
intrauterine/intrapartum stillbirth 113–22, 388, 400
and congenital malformations 117–18
fetal autopsy for 115–16, 117–18
postnatal visits following 416, 440
recurrence risk 116, 118
intravenous (i.v.) feeding 176
intravenous (i.v.) line 141, 161–2
intravenous urography (IVU) 253, 366
intravesical pressure 311, 312
intubation and ventilation
and home births 146
for infants with diaphragmatic hernia 26
for pain relief in labour 108, 110, 112
ischaemic heart disease 207–8
isoimmunization 63–72, 173, 174
isoniazid 44

jaundice, neonatal 126, 170, 173–4

kangaroo approach 172
karyotyping 80, 443
see also specific methods
and at birth diagnosis of Down's syndrome 184
and congenital cardiac abnormalities 19–20
and diaphragmatic hernia 26
indications for 399
sex 182
and stillbirth 118
kernicterus 173
ketoconazole 206
kidney compromise 230
Kleihauer test 66, 71

labetalol 32, 36, 38
labial adhesions 393, 403
labium majoram, swollen 29–50
labour 123–34
see also delivery; preterm labour
in diabetic mothers 48
dysfunctional 133–4, 152
fits during 42
in grade III maternal cardiac disease 49–50
in hypertensive mothers 31–2, 36
induction
auditing 418, 445–6
in diabetic mothers 48
in a grand multipara 131–2

mechanical methods 132
in post-term pregnancies 125–6
stabilization induction 94
and uterine rupture 129–30, 141–2, 150
in intellectually subnormal mothers 139–40
intrapartum care and complications 135–46
maternal fits in 31–2, 42
Mendelson's syndrome in 107–8
monitoring 130, 134
and mother-fetal HIV transmission 61
pain relief in 36, 38, 109–10, 111–12
pyrexia in 133–4
second stage 50, 417, 442
slow progress 133–4, 417, 442
third stage 50
lamineria tents 132
laparoscopic drainage 284
laparoscopic laser/diathermy 236, 262, 264
laparoscopic uterosacral nerve division (LUNA) 282
laparoscopy
abdominal incisions 359
and bladder emptying 367–8
and bladder injury 367
complications 223
cystectomy by 242, 246
diagnostic 198, 234, 447
for chronic pelvic pain 282
and dye test 260
for ectopic pregnancy 223–4
for ovarian cyst 242, 245
myomectomy by 227, 228, 230
sterilization by 154, 271
laparotomic drainage 284
laparotomy
abdominal incisions 359
cystectomy by 242, 246
diagnostic 245
for ectopic pregnancy 223–4
for endodermal sinus tumour 347–8
myomectomy by 227, 228, 230
for ovarian malignancy 364
for postpartum haemorrhage 162
and uterine rupture 130, 141
large loop excision of the transformation zone (LLETZ) 321–2, 406
laser ablation, of the endometrium 194, 196, 391, 402, 439
laser hair removal 206
last menstrual period (LMP) 21–2, 66
lateral suprapubic pressure 128
leg, weakness 109
lesions
benign ovarian 239–46
benign uterine 225–37

leucocytosis 163
leucorrhoea 286
levonorgestrel intrauterine contraceptive device (Mirena) 194, 202, 334, 439
ligation, internal iliac artery 160, 162
Liley charts 68
lipoma, vulval 250
liquor
    see also amniotic fluid; oligohydramnios; polyhydramnios
    absence of 79–80
    optical densitometric analysis 68
    volume estimation 102
literature/MedLine searches 419, 420–21, 445
lithotomy position 128
litigation
    in gynaecology 373–4, 379
    in obstetrics 128, 379
liver biopsy 174
liver extracts 385, 398
liver function test (LFT) 32, 38, 56, 173–4, 244
Livial 236
local anaesthetic 109, 110, 321
local analgesia 293
low molecular weight heparin (LMWH) 38, 361
lung
    chronic disease in babies 122
    embolism 164, 362
    hypoplasia 80, 101
    oedema 32
luteinizing hormone (LH) 262
lymph nodes
    para-aortic 348
    pelvic 296, 322, 324, 325, 336, 337, 338
lymphadenectomy 253, 348, 364
lymphangiography 253

macroadenoma, pituitary 210
McRobert's technique 127, 437
macrosomia 45, 46, 48, 169
magnesium sulphate (MgSO$_4$) 31–2, 38
magnetic resonance imaging (MRI) 244
    abdominal 230, 242, 324, 336, 346
    cranial 210
    endometrial 336
    ovarian 242, 346
    renal 324
Magpie trial 38
malaria, in pregnancy 390, 401
male reproduction 267–8, 271–2, 394, 404, 418, 447
malignancy
    see also cervical malignancy; ovarian malignancy; uterine malignancy

and vaginal bleeding in children 189, 190
Manchester operation 306
mandible, fractured 138
Mantoux test 43–4, 164, 200
marsupialization 250
mastitis 164
maternal mortality
    and hypertension 29, 32, 35, 37
    and postpartum psychiatric disorders 165–6
    and postpartum haemorrhage 160, 161–2
maternal weight 46
Mauriceau–Smellie–Veit manoeuvre 137, 138
Meckel–Gruber syndrome 399
medical disorders in pregnancy 39–50
medroxyprogesterone acetate 188, 276, 395, 405
mefenamic acid 193–4
membrane sweeps 132
menarche 189, 211
Mendelson's syndrome 107–8, 112
menopause 289–98, 396
    see also perimenopause
    combined oral contraceptive pill for 274
    hormone replacement therapy for 291–2
menorrhagia 193–4, 195–6
    combined oral contraceptive pill for 273
    continuous 275
    associated with endometriosis 235–7
    failure to respond to medical treatment 415, 438–9
    associated with fibroids 231–2, 413, 430–32
    idiopathic 196
    norethisterone for 275
    quality of care 415, 436
menstrual cycle 392, 403
menstrual disorders 191–202
    see also amenorrhoea; menorrhagia
    cyclical secondary dysmenorrhoea 197–8
    irregular menstruation 275–6
    painful menstruation 194, 235–7, 273
    precocious puberty 187–8
    premenstrual syndrome 201–2, 273–4, 396, 405
mesh, fetoscopic insertion 103
metabolic abnormalities 80
metformin 262
methotrexate 224
methyldopa 38
methylene blue 368
metoclopramide 108
metrodin 262
metronidazole 217, 284, 286
microprolactinoma 210
microwave ablation 194, 439
midstream specimen of urine (MSU) 163, 302, 304, 307–8, 310, 327–8

midwife 31, 442
  and Caesarean section 152
  community 30
  and the epileptic mother 42
  and grade III cardiac disease 49
  and home births 145, 146
  and intrauterine/intrapartum stillbirth 118
  and labour in intellectually subnormal
    mothers 139, 140
  and maternal diabetes mellitus 47
  and maternal smoking 86
  and maternal tuberculosis 44
  and preterm rupture of fetal membranes 103
  and risk management teams 379
  and shoulder dystocia 415
  and unexpected diagnosis of Down's syndrome
    at birth 184
mifepristone 220, 443
minipill 218, 277, 278
miscarriage
  see also abortion, missed
  and amniocentesis 24, 443
  and chorionic villus sampling 23, 443
  of a hydatiform mole 353–4, 355–6
  incomplete 217–18, 355–6, 399
  and ovulation induction 262
  recurrent 386, 399
  septic 217–18, 399
  spontaneous 16, 80
misoprostol 132, 220
mobilization 362
mortality
  see also maternal mortality
  due to cervical malignancy 315, 316, 319,
    343
  fetal 76, 78, 388, 400
  due to hysterectomy 196
  neonatal 119–20, 121–2
  due to ovarian cancer 341, 343
  perinatal 99–100, 125–6
motor disease, degenerative 311
Müllerian agenesis 212, 251–2
multigravida, undiagnosed breech delivery in
  416, 441
multipara 100, 262
  see also twin pregnancy
  grande 131–2
multiple-choice question (MCQ) paper 383
  passmark 3
  practice papers 385–406
  structure 3, 5
multivitamin supplements 398
myomectomy
  adhesion formation following 397, 406

for fibroid treatment 196, 227, 228, 230, 232,
    431, 432
myometrium 159

nasal bone hypoplasia 16
National Health Service (NHS) 54, 320, 377–8, 379
National Institute for Clinical Excellence (NICE)
    420, 421, 436, 445
nausea 37
necrotizing enterocolitis (NEC) 76
Neisseria gonorrhoea 250, 286
neonatal intensive care units (NICUs) 103, 122
neonates
  see also newborns
  accidental sedation 176
  of addicted mothers 390, 401
  who have experienced anhydramnios 80
  and chickenpox infection 60
  death 119–20, 121–2
  and hepatitis B prophylaxis 56
  and herpes simplex type II infection 57–8
  and HIV infection 61
  hypothermia in 169, 171–2
  who have experienced intrauterine growth
    restriction 76
  jaundiced 126, 170, 173–4
  and maternal chorioamnionitis 134
  and maternal diabetes mellitus 169–70
  and maternal tuberculosis 44
  refusal of feeds 175–6
  and shoulder dystocia 128
  unexpected diagnosis of Down's syndrome at
    birth 183–4
neonatologist 18, 20, 134, 444
  and ambiguous external genitalia 181–2
  and anhydramnios 80
  and home births 146
  and maternal chickenpox infection 60
  and preterm rupture of fetal membranes 102
  and stillbirth 118
  and unexpected diagnosis of Down's syndrome
    at birth 184
neonatology 167–76
neovagina 251–2
neural tube defects 41, 42, 387, 398, 399
neurodevelopmental disability 102
neurofibromatosis 188
neurosurgery 188
newborns
  see also neonates
  ambiguous external genitalia in 181–2
  transient tachypnoea of 122, 156
nicotine 85
nifedipine 32, 36, 38

non-steroidal anti-inflammatory drugs (NSAIDs)
193
norethisterone 194, 275–6
normagon 262
Norplant 154, 216
nuchal translucency (NT) 15, 16, 21, 22, 61, 62,
387, 399
nulligravida 217–18
nurse 342, 414, 435

obesity 363–4
  and diabetes mellitus 46, 47–8
  and ovulation induction 262
  due to polycystic ovary disease 208
objective structured clinical examination (OSCE)
3, 5, 407–49
obstetrician 19, 31, 66
  and elective Caesarean section 152
  and the epileptic mother 42
  and grade III cardiac disease 49, 50
  and intellectually subnormal mothers 139, 140
  and internal artery ligation 160, 162
  and laparotomy for uterine rupture 141
  and maternal diabetes mellitus 47
  and maternal tuberculosis 44
  and postpartum haemorrhage 160, 161, 162
  and shoulder dystocia 437
  and unexpected diagnosis of Down's syndrome
    at birth 184
  and vaginal delivery following previous
    Caesarean section 150
oedema, pulmonary 32
17-beta-oestradiol 132
oestradiol
  implants 202
  serum levels in ovarian hyperstimulation
    syndrome 264–5
  transdermal patches 202
oestriol, salivary 98, 100
oestrogen/oestrogens
  as AddBack therapy 236
  creams 296, 304
  and cyproterone acetate (Dianette) 206
  and endometrial hyperplasia 333
  implants 292
  for osteoporosis 210
  for urinary incontinence 302, 304
oligo-amenorrhoea 274
oligohydramnios 101, 103, 388, 400
  amnioinfusion for 80
  associated with intrauterine growth restriction
    75, 76
oligozoospermia 267–8
omental biopsy 244, 348

omentectomy 244, 296, 348, 364
oncogenes 342
oncologist 242
  see also gynaecological oncologist
  and cervical malignancy 324
  and endometrial carcinoma 338, 427, 428
  and ovarian malignancy 342, 348, 364
oncology nurse 342
oophorectomy
  bilateral 202, 348
  for endometriosis 234, 236
  for ovarian cyst 242, 246
  for ovarian malignancy 344, 348
  for premenstrual syndrome 202
  prophylactic 344
operative gynaecology 358–68, 391, 402
  see also specific techniques
operative obstetrics 147–56
  see also specific techniques
optical densitometric analysis, of liquor 68
ORACLE trial 100, 102
oral contraceptive pill
  combined
    advantages of 215
    for amenorrhoea 210, 212
    and body hair reduction 206
    and breakthrough bleeding 396, 406
    contraindications of 215, 422
    for cyclical secondary dysmenorrhoea 198
    for endometriosis 236, 282
    following hydatiform mole 356
    less androgenic 274
    for menorrhagia 193, 194
    summary of non-contraceptive uses 273–4
    as perimenopausal contraception 277, 278
    for premenstrual syndrome 201–2
    use following termination of pregnancy
     215
  progesterone-only 216, 277, 278
oral examination (OSCE) 3, 5, 407–49
organ donors 371–2
osteopenia 194, 232
osteoporosis 210, 396, 405
ova retrieval and storage 236–7
ovarian cyst 241–2, 245–6
  haemorrhage into 245
  malignant 242
  management 347–8
  torted 241, 242, 245–6
ovarian endometriomata 198, 234, 242
ovarian failure, premature 393, 404
ovarian hyperstimulation syndrome 258, 261,
  262, 394, 404
  minimization of 263–5

risk factors for 264
symptoms of 263–5
ovarian lesions, benign 239–46
ovarian malignancy 339–48, 364, 414, 435
  absence of premalignant stage 344
  assessment 345–6
  at-risk groups 344
  family history of 344
  features of 345–6
  germ cell tumours 347–8
  grading 341
  histology 345, 346, 348
  incidence 343
  mortality rates 341, 343
  of ovarian cysts 242
  of ovarian mucinous cystadenomas 243–4
  ploidy status 341, 342
  prognosis 341–2
  residual disease following surgery 342
  screening for 343–4
  secondaries 346, 364
  staging 341
  survival rates 341
ovarian mucinous cystadenoma 243–4
ovarian tumours 29
  benign 345–6, 364
  and endometrial hyperplasia 333–4
  unexpected at hysterectomy 363–4
  and vaginal bleeding in children 190
ovary
  see also oophorectomy; salpingoophorectomy
  contralateral 347–8
  examination 344
  fixing 246
  gangrene 246
  laparoscopic laser/diathermy drilling 262, 264
  preservation in cervical malignancy 324
  torted 241, 242, 245–6
  wedge resection 262
ovulation
  assessment 271–2
  induction 258, 261–2, 264, 394, 404
oxybutynin 304, 310
oxytocic agents 126, 140
  bolus doses 159–60, 162
  continuous infusion 162
  contraindications for 156
  use in grade III cardiac disease 50
  to control postpartum haemorrhage 159–60, 162
  and uterine rupture 130, 141–2
oxytocin 50

packing, of the uterine cavity 162

paediatric surgeon 18, 26
paediatrician 26
  and intellectually subnormal mothers 140
  and intrauterine growth restriction 76
  and maternal diabetes 48
  and maternal tuberculosis 44
  and sexual abuse 186
  and shoulder dystocia 127, 437
  and twin delivery 429
  and unexpected diagnosis of Down's syndrome at birth 183
pain 109
  see also anaesthesia; analgesia
  abdominal
    constant lower 245–6
    cyclical 233–4
    during pregnancy 386, 417
    intermittent lower 243–4, 245–6
    intermittent right-sided 347–8
    associated with ovarian cysts 241
  pelvic 279–88
    chronic 281–2
palliative care 324
palpation 130
PAP1 62
para-aortic node biopsy 348
paracervical block 321
parametrium 324, 337
partogram 134
parvovirus B19 389, 401
pelvic abscess 164, 395, 405
pelvic examinations
  see also vaginal examinations
  bimanual 304
  in children 186, 189
  for chronic vaginal discharge 286
  for endometrial carcinoma 335
  for endometrial hyperplasia 333
  for genital prolapse 305, 310
  for obese patients 363–4
  for ovarian cyst 242
  for ovarian malignancy 344
  for postpartum haemorrhage 162
  for slow progress in labour 134
  for urinary incontinence 304
pelvic floor exercises 302
pelvic infections 279–88
pelvic inflammatory disease
  and *Chlamydia trachomatis* 221
  chronic 282
  and cyclical secondary dysmenorrhoea 197, 198
  due to intrauterine contraceptive devices 216
  and menorrhagia 196

pelvic lymph nodes 324, 325, 336, 338
    dissection 296, 322, 324, 337
pelvic masses 304, 367
pelvic pain 279–88
    chronic 281–2
pergonal 262
perimenopause 277–8
perinatal mortality
    and induction of post-term pregnancy 125–6
    due to preterm labour 99–100
perinatologist 25
perineum 305–6
peripartum cardiomyopathy 391, 402
pessaries, prolapse-correcting 302, 306, 308
Pfannenstiel incision 359
physician 42, 47, 302, 379
physiotherapy 306, 311
phyto-oestrogens 292
pipelle aspirators 293–4, 296
pituitary macroadenoma 210
pituitary prolactinoma 210
placebos 201
placenta
    and intrauterine growth restriction 76
    and postpartum haemorrhage 162
placenta acreta 159
placenta increta 159
placenta praevia 159–60
placental abruption 88, 386, 399
placental bed 159
placental biopsy 80
    see also chorionic villus sampling
placental mosaicism 23, 24, 80, 400, 443
plastic surgeon 444
platelet levels 30
pneumonia
    aspiration 107–8, 112
    in pregnancy 60
police 186
polycystic ovary syndrome 207–8, 395, 405
    and amenorrhoea 199, 200
    combined oral contraceptive pill for 274
    and infertility 261–2
    and ovarian hyperstimulation syndrome 264
    and ovulation induction 261–2
    and primary amenorrhoea 212
polycythaemia 229, 230
polyhydramnios 25, 46, 388, 400
    and cord prolapse 143–4
    and preterm labour 100
polyps 296, 298
Pomeroy procedure 154
post-term pregnancy, induction of labour 125–6
postmenopausal bleeding 293–4, 295–6, 412

hysteroscopic investigations 293, 294, 296,
    297–8
postpartum complications 157–66
postpartum haemorrhage 126, 134, 139, 140,
    162
    management 159–60
    under-running 159
postpartum psychiatric disorders 165–6
pre-eclampsia 29–32, 34–8, 100
    see also eclampsia
    abnormal changes in 390, 402
    and intrauterine growth restriction 76
    and maternal diabetes 48
    severity of 35–6, 37, 38
precocious puberty 187–8, 393, 403
    aetiology 187–8, 392, 403
pregnancy
    see also delivery; ectopic pregnancy; labour;
        miscarriage; termination of pregnancy;
        twin pregnancy
    abdominal pain during 386, 417
    abnormal presentation 78, 89–94, 386, 398
    adolescent 19–20, 188, 189, 386, 398
    anaesthetic disorders in 105–12
    choriocarcinoma following 351–2
    dating 21–2
    dietary supplements in 385, 398
    use of diethystilboestrol in 390, 401
    drug abuse in 81–8, 390, 401
    early complications 213–24
    and endometriosis 237
    epidemiology 81–8
    in ethnic minorities 386
    following hydatiform mole 356
    hypertensive disorders in 27–38, 48, 112
    infections in 43–4, 51–62, 100, 387, 390, 399,
        401
    isoimmunization 63–72
    medical disorders in 39–50
    multiple 100, 131–2, 262
    and ovarian hyperstimulation syndrome 264,
        265
    post-term 125–6
    postpartum complications 157–66
    prenatal diagnosis and congenital
        malformations 13–26
    preterm labour 95–104
    preterm rupture of fetal membranes 95–104
    social obstetrics 81–8
    vaginal bleeding in 386, 414, 417, 435, 442
premenstrual syndrome
    diagnosis 396, 405
    management 201–2, 273–4
prenatal diagnosis 13–26, 62

pressure deformities 80
preterm babies, and hypothermia 171–2
preterm delivery
  see also preterm labour
  breech 91
  in diabetic mothers 48
  and external cephalic version 91–2
  due to fetal blood sampling 68
  and intrauterine growth restriction 75, 76
  and maternal hypertension 29
preterm labour 95–104
  see also preterm delivery
  aetiology 99
  at-risk groups 99–100
  and domestic violence 88
  incidence 97, 99
  prevention of 99–100
  recurrent 97–8, 100
  risk factors for 98, 99–100
  unpredictable nature of 100
preterm rupture of fetal membranes 95–104,
    417, 442
  and antibiotic usage 100
  and cord prolapse 143, 144
  and herpes simplex infection 58
  inpatient v. outpatient care 103
  in a primigravida 101–3
  due to unstable lie at term 93
primigravida 417, 442
  anhydramnios in 79–80
  fibroids in 227–8
  hepatitis B infection in 55–6
  hypertensive disorders in 29–30, 31–2, 33–4,
    37–8
  induced ruptured uterus in 141–2
  intrauterine growth restriction in 75–6, 77–8
  labour in 133–4
  preterm rupture of fetal membranes in 101–3
  Rhesus (D) antibodies in 67–9
  smoking in 85–6
prioritization 414, 417, 435, 442
proctosigmoidoscopy 253
products of conception, retained 162, 163, 217
proforma 419, 421, 445
progesterone challenge test 276
progestogens 198, 264, 292
  cyclical 194, 200, 212
  for endometrial carcinoma 336
  for endometrial hyperplasia 334
  for endometriosis 282
  locally administered 334
  for premenstrual syndrome 202
  subdermal implants 216
  systemic 334

prolactinoma, pituitary 210
prolapse
  see also genital prolapse
  cord 93, 94, 143–4
  hand 93
prostaglandin synthase inhibitors 194
prostaglandins
  and induction of labour 130, 132, 141–2, 150,
    156, 160, 162, 443
  intramyometrial 160, 162
  and uterine rupture 141–2
protein S deficiency 361–2
proteinuria 29–30, 37–8
protocols 420, 421
Prozac 202
pseudo-diverticulum 138
psychiatric disorders, postpartum 165–6
psychiatric nurse 165, 166
psychiatrist 140, 166
psychologist 252
psychotherapist 252
psychotherapy 202, 328
puberty 189
  precocious 187–8, 392, 393, 403
pulmonary embolism 164, 362
pulmonary hypoplasia 80, 101
pulmonary oedema 32
pulmonary physician 44
purberche 211
pyrexia
  in labour 133–4
  low-grade 283–4
  post-operative 417, 442
  puerperial 163–4
  swinging 164
pyrexia of unknown origin (PUO) 163
pyridoxine 202

quality of care 415, 436
quinagolines 210

radial tachelectomy 322
radiographer 16, 19, 417
radiologist 160, 162
radiotherapist 324, 428
radiotherapy 188, 254, 296
  for cervical malignancy 322, 324, 327–8
  complications of 327, 328, 427
  for endometrial carcinoma 332, 336, 338, 427
  for endometrial hyperplasia 334
  for ovarian malignancy 348
rectal examinations 324
rectocele 305, 307, 308
5-α reductase deficiency 392, 403

Reichter's hernia 359
renal agenesis 80
renal function test 324
respiratory distress syndrome (RDS)
   maternal 36
   neonatal 76, 122, 156, 169–70
reticulocytosis 173
Rhesus (D) isoimmunization 67–9
   and neonatal jaundice 173, 174
   prophylaxis 65–6, 71–2
Rhesus-negative blood 66, 68, 71
rifampicin 44
ringer-lactate solution 110
risk management team 379–80
ritrodine 130
Royal College of Obstetricians and Gynaecologists
   (RCOG) 72, 137, 228, 230, 409, 420, 421, 436,
   441, 445
rupture of fetal membranes 94
   see also preterm rupture of fetal membranes
   artificial 132
   prolonged 133–4
   spontaneous 79–80

sacrocolpopexy 308
sacrospinous fixation 308
salpingectomy 224
salpingoophorectomy
   bilateral
      for chronic pelvic pain 282
      for endometrial carcinoma 296, 332, 336,
      337
      for endometrial hyperplasia 334, 412
      for endometriosis 411, 424
      for ovarian cyst 242
      for ovarian malignancy 348, 364
      for ovarian mucinous cystadenoma 244
      perioperative management of a protein S
      deficient patient 361–2
   left 233
   for ovarian cyst 242, 246
salpingoscopy 260
salpingotomy 224
SANDS 118
sarcoma botyroides 190
screening
   see also biochemical screening; specific
      techniques
   for cervical cancer 315–16, 319, 343–4
   for Chlamydia trachomatis 221–2, 288
   for diabetes mellitus in pregnancy 45–6
   for HIV 53–4
   for ovarian malignancy 343–4
   prenatal 15–16

second trimester
   cervical incompetence testing 98
   congenital malformations and maternal
      diabetes mellitus 46
   in hypertensive mothers 34
   ultrasound scanning in 22
sedation, accidental neonatal 176
selective serotonin re-uptake inhibitors (SSRIs)
   202
semen analysis 271–2, 418, 447
Senior House Officer (SHO) 414, 435, 442
sensitization, against Rhesus disease 66, 67, 71
Sentinel Audit 152
septicaemia 399
   neonatal 173, 176
   in septic incomplete miscarriage 217, 218
SERMS 292
sex assignment 181–2
sex selection 375
sex-linked inheritance 385, 398
sexual abuse 185–6, 189
sexually transmitted diseases (STDs) 55–6, 57–8
   see also specific diseases
   and chronic vaginal discharge 286
   counselling regarding 222
   protection from 216
   and tubo-ovarian abscess 283, 284
   and vulval swelling 250
shaving 206
short essay questions 5–7, 9, 11–380, 383
shoulder dystocia 391, 402, 415, 437
   manoeuvres for 127–8, 437
sickle cell anaemia, in pregnancy 386, 391, 399,
   402
smoking, in pregnancy 85–6, 388, 400
social obstetrics 81–8
social worker
   and domestic violence 88
   and intellectually subnormal mothers 140
   and postpartum psychiatric disorders 165
   and sexual abuse 186
   and smoking mothers 86
   and unexpected diagnosis of Down's syndrome
      at birth 184
sodium citrate 107, 108
sodium valproate 41–2
soft markers, for chromosomal abnormalities 16,
   22, 120, 387, 399
sonoembryology 22
sonography, saline 293
speculum 80
sphincters, artificial 312
spinal block 112
spinal paralysis 110

spironolactone 206
sputum 44, 164
squamocolumnar junction 316
stabilization induction 94
Stamey operation 302
stents, ureteric 366
sterilization 153–4, 156, 396, 406
    by diathermy 271
    by rings 271
    laparoscopic 154, 271
    open 271
    as perimenopausal contraception 277, 278
    reversal 271–2
        macroscopic 272
        microscopic 272
    following termination of pregnancy 215,
        216
steroids
    to prevent preterm labour 98
    to promote fetal lung development 102
stillbirth *see* intrauterine/intrapartum stillbirth
stomach, displacement 107
streptococcus, beta-haemolytic 98, 102
structural abnormalities 443
    see also congenital cardiac abnormalities
    associated with anhydramnios 80
    associated with diaphragmatic hernia 25, 26
    associated with maternal epilepsy 42
    co-existence with congenital cardiac
        abnormalities 20
    exomphalus 17–18
    identification in the first trimester 16
    ultrasound scanning for 22
subdermal implants 154
suction machines 108
sudden infant death syndrome (cot death) 85, 86,
    386, 398
suicide, postpartum 165, 166
superovulation 236–7, 258, 394, 404
    and ovarian hyperstimulation syndrome 264,
        265
support groups
    for alcohol abuse 84
    for coping with stillbirths 118
    for smoking mothers 86
sutures 160, 162, 368
swabs
    endocervical 163, 198, 282, 286
    rectal 286
    urethral 286
    vaginal 102, 163, 190, 198, 282, 286
sympathomimetics 132
symphysiotomy 128, 138, 437
symphysitis 138

syntocinon 32, 94, 132, 134, 159, 218
    and uterine rupture 130, 150
syntometrine 50, 218

tachyphylaxis 292
talipes equinovarus, bilateral 417, 444
tamoxifen 295
temperature, pulse and respiratory (TPR) rate
        recordings 102
tenascin 98, 100
tension free vaginal tapes (TVT) 302, 304, 310
teratogenic substances 390, 401
    alcohol 84
    dexamethasone 98
    Vitamin A 385, 398
terminal care 324
termination of pregnancy 16, 102, 213–24, 443
    Abortion Act (UK) 397, 406
    and amniocentesis 24
    and anhydramnios 80
    due to autosomal recessive conditions 120
    and *Chlamydia trachomatis* screening 221–2
    and chorionic villus sampling 23
    contraception recommendations following
        215–16
    ectopic 223–4
    due to exomphalus detection 17, 18
    and fetal chickenpox infection 60
    late 219
    medical 219–20
    surgical 219–20
testicular feminizing syndrome 212
testicular regression syndrome 392, 403
tetany 169
tetracycline 222
tetracycline derivatives 284, 286
thelarche 211
thermal ablation 196
thermo-neutral environment 171–2
third trimester, beta-sympathomimetic drugs in
        390, 402
threadworms 186, 190, 286
thrombocytopenia 30, 36
    maternal autoimmune 389, 401
thrombophilia 361–2
thromboprophylaxis 36, 38
thrombosis, neonatal 170
tocolytic agents 98, 102
tolterodine detruisitis 304
torsion, ovarian 241, 242, 245–6
trachelorrhaphy, radical 324
Trachomatis vaginalis 286
training, gynaecological 373
tranexamic acid 193–4, 235–6

transfusions *see* blood transfusions
transient tachypnoea of the newborn (TTN) 122, 156
transphenoidal microsurgical excision 210
transverse cervical (Mackenrodt) ligament, shortening 306
trauma
  cervical 162, 219
  neonatal due to shoulder dystocia 128
  surgical bladder injury 367–8
  surgical ureteric injury 365–6
  surgical visceral injury 391, 402
  vaginal 162
  vulval 162, 249, 250
trisequens 201
trisomy 21 21–2
  see also Down's syndrome
tubal ligation 142
tube feeding 176
tuberculosis
  pelvic 200
  in pregnancy 43–4, 390, 401
  and puerperial pyrexia 164
tubo-ovarian abscess 283–4
tumours *see* ovarian tumours
Turner syndrome 212
twin pregnancy 413, 429
  delivery 144, 413, 417, 429, 442
  intrauterine fetal death 388, 400

ultrasound scanning 163, 212, 234
  for cyclical secondary dysmenorrhoea 198
  and endometrial biopsy 293, 294, 297, 298
  for endometrial cancer 208, 336
  for endometrial hyperplasia 333–4
  for follicular tracking 264, 265
  of the liver and gallbladder 174
  for ovarian cyst 242, 245
  for ovarian malignancy 344, 346
  for pelvic abscess 164
  for postmenopausal bleeding 293, 294, 297–8
  during pregnancy 16, 97, 98, 386, 387, 399
    abnormal 417, 443–4
    for anhydramnios 79–80
    for autosomal recessive conditions 120
    booking 80
    for congenital cardiac abnormalities 19
    for dating pregnancy 22
    for the detection of fetal diaphragmatic hernia 25
    for diabetic mothers 48
    for ectopic pregnancy 223–4
    in epileptic mothers 42
    for exomphalus detection 17–18
    for fetal chickenpox infection 60
    in the first trimester 15, 16, 22, 42
    in hypertensive mothers 30, 34, 36, 38
    for intrauterine growth restriction 30, 36, 38, 42, 75, 76
    for preterm rupture of fetal membranes 102
    in response to maternal Rhesus (D) antibodies 68
    in the second trimester 22
    serial 68, 98, 100, 102
    to test for cervical incompetence 97, 98
    for trisomy 21 diagnosis 21–2
    for unstable lie 94
  for primary amenorrhoea 212
  of the renal system 253, 324
  transabdominal 298
  transvaginal 16, 97, 98, 298
  for urinary tract obstruction 230
  for vaginal bleeding in children 190
  for vaginal discharge in children 186
umbilical artery, Doppler velocimetry of 30, 36, 38, 75, 76, 102
umbilical cord, compression 103
umbilical vein, fetal blood sampling from 68
under-running 159
unstable lie, at term 93–4
urea and electrolytes (U&Es) 30, 32, 38, 243
  for congenital adrenal hyperplasia 181
  for endometrial carcinoma 336
  for fibroids 230
urea levels 36
ureter
  catheterization 366
  injury during surgery 365–6
  obstruction 242, 243
  reimplantation 366
ureteric stent 366
urethra sphincter incompetence 397, 406
  see also urinary incontinence, urodynamic (genuine) stress
urethra-vesical junction 311–12
urethral tissue, assessment 310
urgency 309–10
uric acid levels 30, 32, 36, 38
urinalysis 30, 36, 76
  for endometrial carcinoma 336
  midstream specimen of urine 163, 302, 304, 307–8, 310, 327–8
  for neonatal jaundice 174
  for puerperial pyrexia 163
urinary dip-stick tests 30, 36
urinary incontinence 299–312
  assessment 303, 308, 309

detrusor instability 304, 308, 309, 310
low compliance bladder 304, 311–12
recurrent 303–4, 309
urge urinary 309–10
urgency 309–10
urodynamic (genuine) stress 301–4, 308–10,
    397, 406, 411, 414, 425–6, 433
urinary peritonitis 366
urinary retention 109–10
acute 414, 435
urinary tract infections (UTIs) 327, 367
associated with fibroids 229, 230
and preterm labour 98, 100
and puerperal pyrexia 163
recurrent 48
and urinary incontinence 301–2, 303, 304,
    308, 310
urinary tract obstruction 229, 230, 234, 242, 243
urine, diversion of 312
urine microscopy 230
urine welling 365
uroflometry 32, 308, 309, 310, 414
Urograffin 260
urogynaecologist 304, 310
urologist 312, 366
uterine artery embolization
for fibroid treatment 228, 230, 232, 431, 432
for postpartum haemorrhage 160, 162
uterine bleeding, abnormal 333–4
uterine cavity, packing of 162
uterine contractions 159–60, 162
uterine fibroids see fibroids
uterine lesions, benign 225–37
uterine malignancy 329–338
endometrial carcinoma 331–2, 333, 335–6,
    337–8
endometrial hyperplasia 333–4
uterine rupture
in a grande multipara 131, 132
and induction of labour 129–30, 141–2, 150
linear 142
minimization of the risk of 129–30
following previous Caesarean section 129–30,
    149, 155–6
signs of 130, 141
silent 156
treatment options following delivery 142
uterosacral ligaments, excision 236
uterosacral nerve division, laser destruction of
    196
uterus
see also hysterectomy
absent 251
bicornate 219

blood clots in 163
examination under anaesthesia 162
hypotonia of 162

vaccinations
hepatitis B 56
tuberculosis 44
vagina
absent 251
colpocleisis of 308
creation of new 251–2
trauma 162
vaginal bleeding
see also menorrhagia; menstrual disorders
breakthrough 396, 406
in children 189–90
irregular 273, 274, 334
    due to intrauterine contraceptive devices 278
    postmenopausal 293–4, 295–6, 297–8
postpartum 161–2
during pregnancy 386, 414, 417, 435, 442
vaginal carcinoma 253–4
vaginal cuffs 324, 337
vaginal delivery see delivery
vaginal dilators 252
vaginal discharge
associated with Bartholin's abscess 250
in children 185–6, 395, 405
chronic 279–88
vaginal disorders 48, 247–54
vaginal examinations
for anhydramnios 80
consent issues 139, 140
for genital prolapse 302, 307
for herpes simplex type II infection 58
for vigo intacta women 211
vaginal repair 363–4
vaginal stenosis 328
vaginal swabs 102, 163, 190, 198, 282, 286
vaginectomy 253
vaginitis, atrophic 296
VAIN 253
Valsava manoeuvre 50
varicella-zoster immunoglobulin (VZIG) 60
varicella-zoster virus (VZV) infection 60
vasectomy 154
VBAC 130
venflon, large-bore 161
venous thrombo-embolism (VTE) 126, 164, 361
see also deep vein thrombosis
and the combined oral contraceptive pill 193,
    278
in maternal grade III cardiac disease 50
and pain relief in labour 111, 112

venous thrombo-embolism (VTE) – *contd*
   and surgical treatment of menorrhagia 196
ventouse delivery 144
Verre needle 368
vibra aspirators 293–4, 296
vigo intacta 211
vincristine 348
viral load 61–2
visceral injury, and gynaecological surgery 391, 402
vitamin A 385, 398
vitamin B6 202
vitamin C 385, 398
vomiting
   in the hypertensive mother 37
   under general anaesthesia 107–8, 111, 112
von Recklingausen disease, in pregnancy 391, 402
vulval disorders 247–54
   haematoma 249, 250
   recurrent 48
   trauma 162, 249, 250

ward of court orders 140
warfarin 362
weight loss, ovulation induction by 262
white cell count (WCC) 102, 173, 245
wood screw manoeuvre 437
World Health Organization (WHO) 151, 344, 351,
   352, 377
wound infections 164

X-linked inheritance 385, 398
X-rays
   abdominal 186
   chest 43, 164, 253, 336, 346, 347
   cranial 210

Y-linked inheritance 398

Zantac 107–8
Zavanelli's replacement of the head manoeuvre
   128, 437